FOX AND CAMERON'S
Food Science, Nutrition & Health
7th edition

Michael E. J. Lean

MA, MB, BChir, MD, FRCP
Professor of Human Nutrition at the University of Glasgow
Consultant Physician at Glasgow Royal Infirmary
Visiting Research Fellow at the Centre for Human Nutrition,
University of Colorado Health Sciences Center, USA

Hodder Arnold

A MEMBER OF THE HODDER HEADLINE GROUP

First published in Great Britain in 2006 by
Hodder Education, a member of the Hodder Headline Group,
338 Euston Road, London NW1 3BH

http://www.hoddereducation.com

Distributed in the United States of America by
Oxford University Press Inc.,
198 Madison Avenue, New York, NY10016
Oxford is a registered trademark of Oxford University Press

Whilst the advice and information in this book are believed to be true and
accurate at the date of going to press, neither the author[s] nor the publisher
can accept any legal responsibility or liability for any errors or omissions that
may be made. In particular, (but without limiting the generality of the
preceding disclaimer) every effort has been made to check drug dosages;
however it is still possible that errors have been missed. Furthermore, dosage
schedules are constantly being revised and new side-effects recognized. For
these reasons the reader is strongly urged to consult the drug companies'
printed instructions before administering any of the drugs recommended in
this book.

British Library Cataloguing in Publication Data
A catalogue record for this book is available from the British Library

Library of Congress Cataloging-in-Publication Data
A catalog record for this book is available from the Library of Congress

ISBN-10   0 340 80948 5
ISBN-13   978 0 340 80948 8

1 2 3 4 5 6 7 8 9 10

Commissioning Editor: Georgina Bentliff and Jo Koster
Project Editor: Heather Smith and Clare Patterson
Production Controller: Jane Lawrence and Lindsay Smith
Cover Design: Amina Dudhia
Index: Indexing Specialists (UK) Ltd

Typeset in 9.5/12 Berling Roman by Charon Tec Ltd, Chennai, India
www.charontec.com
Printed and bound in India.

What do you think about this book? Or any other Hodder Arnold
title? Please visit our website at www.hoddereducation.com

Contents

Preface to the 7th edition

Fox and Cameron has rightly become the leading textbook in the field of Food Sciences and Nutrition, for use both in colleges and in schools, as well as a reference source for the food and catering companies. The style created by Fox and Cameron was both accessible and authoritative, and not without humour in places.

For this revised 7th edition, a great debt is still owed to B. A. Fox and A. G. Cameron (Brian Fox sadly died in 2002). I have tried to retain their human touch and the balance between presenting up-to-date scientific issues in the context of foods we all know and love (or loathe, in some cases).

I have been helped enormously by the hard work of Dr Wendy Wreiden, Centre for Public Health Nutrition Research, University of Dundee, UK, and we have both relied on help from our secretaries and academic colleagues in the process of revision.

Some of the book is left unchanged from the latest editions. This is in part a testimony to the huge amount of material marshalled by Fox and Cameron. However, all the chapters have been brought up-to-date to incorporate new evidence, new technologies and new emphasis. Reflecting the change in editorship and the changing demands of the food industry to meet the needs of consumers, this new edition includes a great deal more on the impact of foods on health – both through nutrition and through food-borne infections. Referencing is much reduced in this 7th edition. Rather than referring back to older publications, students and their teachers should be accessing the latest scientific regulatory and policy documents on the internet. The impact on the food industry of new, consumer-centred agencies such as the Food Standards Agency and the Joint Health Claims Initiative, are felt throughout this new edition, and students will need to monitor their websites for new information.

The times are certainly changing for the food industry. With continued globalization, and 90 per cent of all food regulations in UK now being derived from Europe, students and workers in the food industry need to keep on their toes. This book is designed to help.

Professor Mike E J Lean
2006

Acknowledgements

'The Water Song' appears on p. 168.
Words and Music by Robin Williamson
© 1968 (renewed) Warner-Tamerlane Publishing Corporation
Administered by Warner/Chappell Music Ltd, London W6 8BS
Reproduced by permission

Preface to the 6th edition

It is universally accepted that an adequate and well-balanced diet is essential for the enjoyment of good health but the scientific principles on which this belief is based are by no means widely understood. This book, which bridges the gap between science and practice in nutrition, is an attempt to make good this deficiency. It is largely concerned with what food *is*, how much of it we should eat and what happens to it – and to us – when we eat it. It provides a comprehensive and up-to-date survey of the body of knowledge which has come to be known as food science, and examines the nutritional significance of this knowledge. This is a more difficult task than might at first be supposed because of the many scientific disciplines involved, the complex nature of many apparently simple foodstuffs and the intricate biochemical reactions that occur when food is digested, absorbed and converted into the stuff of which we are made.

We have sought to make the book as self-contained as possible but a study of food science and nutrition, even at the fairly elementary level at which this book is pitched, is of necessity far-ranging and inevitably involves an assumption of some previous knowledge of basic science. Nevertheless, we hope that the text will be intelligible to all those who might wish to read it, and with this in mind, we have kept the use of structural formulae to a minimum. Unfortunately, it has not been possible to avoid using the combinations of initial letters which serve as abbreviations for frequently used groups of words with particular meanings; these have, in effect, become recognized as part of the specialized vocabulary of food science. To assist the reader in finding a way through this veritable thicket of alphabetic abbreviations a Glossary has been provided which we hope will prove helpful.

We have been encouraged by the consistent popularity of the book over a long period to conclude that it is fulfilling a need and meeting the objectives we set ourselves when it was first written. Consequently, we have not thought it necessary to make radical changes in preparing this sixth edition and it retains the basic structure of previous editions. The first three chapters describe in outline the nature and functions of food, and the changes it undergoes in the body when it is eaten, together with a preliminary exploration of the relationship between dietary factors and good health. A new chapter follows in which the relatively new terms known as dietary reference values, which are used to express dietary requirements, are introduced. These have taken the place of the terms used previously, such as recommended daily amount, and they are employed consistently throughout the remainder of the book. The main body of the text is given over to an account of the nature of nutrients and the foods which contain them and to a description of what happens to food when it is grown, stored, processed, preserved, cooked and eaten. A chapter dealing with the relationship between diet and health discusses the way in which dietary habits can be modified to promote good health and combat disease.

Subsequent chapters look at the related topics of food spoilage and preservation, food poisoning and food hygiene. The final chapter, which is concerned with the important topic of food contaminants and additives, seeks to present a balanced and comprehensive account of what has become a controversial subject. Although there may be risks involved in using some additives, considerable benefits may also be obtained and an attempt is made to balance these two aspects of the use of additives in food.

We have not attempted to provide references to the original sources of the information given in this book; such references would have greatly increased the length and cost of the book and would, perhaps, have been used by relatively few readers. A short reading list is given at the end of many chapters which will assist readers requiring more detailed information. Details of a number of books on food science and nutrition which are of more general interest are given in a General Reading List at the end of the book.

Great care has been taken to ensure that the information contained in this book is as accurate and up-to-date as possible but it is almost inevitable that errors and ambiguities will occur in a book which attempts to summarize a large and expanding field of knowledge. We should be grateful if any such inaccuracies, for which we alone are responsible, can be brought to our notice.

We trust that the book will continue to be of interest and value to all who are concerned with food science and nutrition. It is principally intended for students of Food Science and Technology, Catering and Nutrition and for A-level and BTEC students in schools and colleges. We know that it has also been found to be of interest by many members of the general public who are concerned about the relationship between dietary habits and good health, and who wisely take an interest in 'healthy eating'. We hope that all who read the book will enjoy doing so and that the information it contains will assist them in the pursuit of good health and the avoidance of those life-threatening diseases which are now known to have a nutritional component.

Brian A Fox
Allan G Cameron
1994

Acronyms/terms used

AFD	accelerated freeze-drying		MRL	maximum residue level
ADI	acceptable daily intake		MAP	modified-atmosphere packaging
ACP	acid calcium phosphate		MAS	modified-atmosphere storage
ASP	acid sodium pyrophosphate		MSG	monosodium glutamate
ADP	adenosine diphosphate		MUFA	monounsaturated fatty acid
AMP	adenosine monophosphate		NHDC	neohesperidine dihydrochalcone
ATP	adenosine triphosphate		NPU	net protein utilization
ADH	antidiuretic hormone		PSD	Pesticides Safety Directorate
BV	biological value		PKU	phenylketonuria
BSE	bovine spongiform encephalopathy		PUFA	polyunsaturated fatty acid
COMA	Committee on Medical Aspects of Food Policy		POMC	pro-opio-melanocortin
			PEM	protein-energy malnutrition
CAS	controlled-atmosphere storage		PLP	pyridoxal-5-phosphate
CHD	coronary heart disease		RDA	recommended daily amount
DEFRA	Department for Environment, Food and Rural Affairs		RDI	recommended daily intakes
			RNI	reference nutrient intake
DRV	dietary reference value		SI	safe intake
DHA	docosahexanoic acid		SRSV	small round structured virus
ECG	electrocardiogram		SIADH	syndrome of inappropriate antidiuretic hormone
EFAs	essential fatty acids			
EAR	estimated average requirement		TVP	textured vegetable protein
GMOs	genetically modified organisms		TDT	thermal death time
GDL	Glucono-delta-lactone		TDF	total dietary fiber
HDL	high-density lipoprotein		UHT	ultra-high temperature
HTST	high-temperature short-time		VLCDs	very low calorie diets
JHCI	Joint Health Claims Initiative		VLDL	very low density lipoproteins
LDL	low-density lipoprotein cholesterol		WHO	World Health Organization
LRNI	lower reference nutrient intake			

Food and its functions

The basic function of food is to keep us alive and healthy, to grow and to reproduce. In this book we shall consider how food does this, although we shall also need to think about many other related matters. Indeed, we cannot answer such a fundamental 'How' question without first finding out the answer to some simpler 'What' questions, such as what is food, what happens to it when it is stored, processed, preserved, cooked, eaten and digested. The answers to such questions can only be found out by experiment, and many different sciences play a part in helping to provide the answers. In recent years the study of food has been accepted as a distinct discipline of its own and given the name food science.

Food science exists partly to pursue academic knowledge (the insatiable curiosity of mankind finds in food a universal theme of shared interest). As Samuel Johnson phrased it, 'I look upon it that he who does not mind his belly will hardly mind anything else' (Boswell, *The Life of Samuel Johnson*, Vol. 3, Ch. 9). Its interest lies also in the fact that our knowledge of the subject is growing, leading to an unfolding of new perspectives about what is significant, while new techniques are being developed leading to new methods in food processing and of analysing nutrients, additives and possible contaminants in food. Food science also promotes the fulfilment of a basic human need for a diet that will sustain life and health. To be effective, food science must be applied, in the manufacture and preparation of food and this is the province of *food technology*.

Determining the dietary needs of individuals, or of populations is the realm of *nutritional science*.

The problems involved in determining what foods in what combinations best meet the dietary needs of different countries, or individuals, of the compositional merits of various new foods, of how to store and preserve food with minimum nutritional loss are the provinces of food science. However, in order to use this information it must be applied – food must be grown, stored, processed, preserved and transported on a large scale – and this is the province of *agriculture and food technology*.

It becomes clear that promoting health through diet requires input from human nutritional science, food science and food technology.

In the following pages we shall study the relation between food science, nutrition and health, but first it is important to understand just what we mean by the term food.

FOOD AND FOODS

The definition of what is, and what is not, a food is surprisingly taxing, not least because of the need to provide control and regulation over the things, which, for different purposes, people swallow.

Not everything people eat is food. Children, pregnant women and sometimes others sometimes eat non-food materials such as coal. This behaviour is known as 'pica'. Few people would class coal as food, on the grounds that it is not absorbed and does not contribute in any way to biochemical or physiological function in the body. But where does that leave chewing gum? Chewing gum is produced by 'food companies' with the intention that it should be taken by mouth, recognizing that it will occasionally be swallowed. Although inert, and non-absorbable, chewing gum deserves (and receives) the same regulation as other less ambiguous foods.

According to the Food and Agriculture Organization, 'Food means any substance, whether processed, semi-processed or raw, which is intended for human consumption, and includes drink, chewing gum and any substance which has been used in the manufacture, preparation or treatment of 'food' but does not include cosmetics or tobacco or substances used only as drugs' (ftp://ftp.fao.org/codex/manual/Manual12ce.pdf, p. 41).

It is important to recognize that a food is almost always a complex substance, rather than a pure compound of single, uniform composition. Food is characterized by more than just its chemical composition. There are exceptions of course. Table sugar is indisputably 'a food', although it is a pure industrial preparation of $(CH_2O)_6$. However, for most foods there is a characteristic physical form, containing a variety of nutrients with a range of properties. Some grow that way, others are created by food technology and manufacturers. Some are consumed as grown or produced, others form ingredients of still more complex foods, dishes or meals. In the twenty-first century, we probably have to extend our concept of what constitutes a food, at least as perceived by consumers, to include its packaging and the imagery and descriptive or promotional text included, just as we would include the skin of a banana, or the outer leaves of an onion, as part of 'the food'. We make judgements about food quality from all these components, and packaging, natural or man-made, can influence food composition even if it is not consumed.

Foods contain nutrients – components that contribute to, and in some cases uniquely provide for, biochemical and physiological functions in the body. Foods may also include non-absorbed components which may influence bowel health and function. Some phenolic compounds, such as tannins and classes of non-starch polysaccharides (e.g. cellulose) probably fall into this category. Food may also include contaminants from unusual soil types, or from industrial pollution. Heavy metals, radioactive isotopes, and microbial contamination all have potential negative health effects.

A final and even more tricky consideration is that foods contain a variety of compounds which can be absorbed and which have important biological effects. A good example is caffeine. It is present in several common foods (tea, coffee, chocolate). It is also sold, and prescribed, as a drug. In doses similar to the amount in a cup of coffee it stimulates brain, heart and lung function, with several beneficial (and some potentially harmful) consequences. So, it is perfectly possible for foods to have potent 'pharmacological' actions. Caffeine, depending on how it is packaged, may be subject to either food law or drug law. Fish oils are also currently marketed as drugs while obviously being available as part of fish. The distinction between a 'food product' and a 'drug/medicinal product' is a fine one with scope for interpretation. The European Union (EU) has proposed a definition for a medicinal product as 'Any substance or combination of substances presented for treating or preventing disease in human beings. Any substance or combination of substances which may be administered to human beings with a view to making a medical diagnosis or to restoring, correcting or modifying physiological functions in human beings is likewise considered a medicinal product' (European Parliament, 2001).

For some new products, it can be a close decision whether to market it through food outlets as a 'food product' with permitted health claims to be made, or whether to have it registered and sold on prescription or over the counter in pharmacies as a drug, which permits medical claims. The technology required is identical, although greater controls over content variability may be required for a drug. The main difference lies in the differences between what constitutes a medical claim (drug) and a health claim (food product). Again, there is a grey area for interpretation, and the ultimate practical distinction between a food or a drug lies in the enormous amount of highly expensive research required by drug licensing authorities. For a drug, advertising is restricted, and the market much more limited, but vastly greater prices can be charged and drug patents ensure no direct competition for several years. There is currently great interest in protecting consumers against food companies which make health claims, or even medical claims for their products, often based on no direct evidence at all. The counterargument runs that since antiquity certain foods have been attributed with magical qualities in folklore, and to strip these beliefs from food marketing is to deny a rich and evolving food culture. The leading agency in the UK and Europe is the Joint Health Claims Initiative, a partnership between the food industry, consumer organization and enforcement authorities, which was established to develop a Code of Practice for health claims on foods. The legal and regulatory issues on foods are too complex to be addressed in detail in this book, but a clear and helpful introduction can be found at http://www.jhci.co.uk.

TYPES OF NUTRIENT

The two basic functions of nutrients are to provide materials for growth and repair of tissues – that is, to provide and maintain the basic structure of our bodies – and to supply the body with the energy required to perform external activities as well as carrying on its own internal activities. The fact that the body is able to sustain life is dependent upon its ability to maintain its own internal processes. This means that although we may eat all sorts of different foods and our bodies may engage in all sorts of external activities, and even suffer injury or illness, the internal processes of the body should absorb and neutralize the effects of these events and carry on with a constant rhythm. This is only possible because the components of our bodies are engaged in a ceaseless process of breakdown and renewal (a theme to which we will return).

If the body's internal processes are to be maintained constant despite its ceaseless and varying activity, and in the face of external pressures, there needs to be systems in place to regulate very precisely all the processes needed for life. Thus, nutrients have a third function, namely that of controlling body processes, a function that will be considered in the next chapter.

Although habits and patterns of eating may vary from person to person, and diets may be selected from hundreds of different foods, everyone needs the same types of nutrients and in roughly the same proportions. The relation between nutrients, their

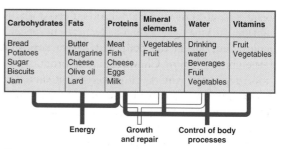

Figure 1.1 *The nutrients: diagram showing their functions and representative foods in which they are found*

functions in the body and important foods that supply them is shown in Fig. 1.1.

Nutrients are often grouped according to their chemical composition. For example, although different oils and fats, such as olive oil and palm oil, do not have identical compositions, they are chemically similar and mostly use the same biochemical pathways for digestion, absorption, transport and metabolism. In the same way, different proteins (and carbohydrates) are constructed and metabolized according to the same general chemical patterns. The three 'macronutrients' (fat, carbohydrate and protein) are therefore conveniently grouped together. Vitamins are not classified according to chemical type; at the time of their discovery in food their chemical nature, which in most cases is complex, was unknown. They were grouped together because it was known that small quantities of them were essential to health and they do not fall into the macronutrient classes. At first they were identified in terms of their effect on growth and health and distinguished by letters as vitamins A, B, C and so on. Their chemical composition is now known, and it has become apparent that they are not chemically related to each other. They all have different functions but it is still convenient to consider them together.

FOOD AS A SOURCE OF ENERGY

Energy is required for sustaining all forms of life on Earth. The prime source of the earth's energy is the sun, without which there could be no life on this planet. The sun continually radiates energy, a tiny fraction of which is intercepted by the Earth and stored in various ways; plants and coal, for example, act as energy storehouses. Living plants convert the sun's energy into chemical energy and some plants of past ages have been converted, over many millions of years, into coal.

Plants, by the process of *photosynthesis*, convert carbon dioxide and water into carbohydrate. Photosynthesis, which is discussed in detail in Chapter 8 (p. 88), can only take place in daylight because solar energy is needed for the process. A complex series of chemical changes occurs which can be represented by the following equation:

$$x CO_2 + y H_2O \xrightarrow{\text{daylight}} C_{12}(H_2O)_y + x O_2$$
$$\text{Carbohydrate}$$

The formation of carbohydrate is, therefore, the method used by plants to trap and store a part of the sun's energy. Sugar-beet, which synthesizes carbohydrate in the form of the sugar sucrose, may be taken as an example:

$$12 CO_2 + 11 H_2O \xrightarrow{\text{daylight}} C_{12}(H_2O)_{11} + 12 O_2$$
$$\text{Sucrose}$$

When sucrose is formed from carbon dioxide and water, energy is absorbed and stored as chemical bonds within the sucrose molecule. It can be stored indefinitely in this form.

Animals, unlike plants, cannot store the sun's energy directly and so must gain it second-hand by using plants as food. Carnivorous animals and man take this process a stage further and also use other animals as food. In this way, chemical compounds which have been photosynthesized and stored in plants are eaten by man and animals and the stored energy made available. For example, the energy that is stored within the sucrose molecule when it is synthesized by sugar-beet is liberated when sucrose reverts to carbon dioxide and water. This breakdown of sucrose into simpler units is brought about in the body by digestion and oxidation, but the overall reaction is simply the reverse of that represented above, namely:

$$C_{12}(H_2O)_{11} + 12 O_2 \rightarrow 12 CO_2 + 11 H_2O$$
$$\text{Sucrose}$$

When sucrose is converted into carbon dioxide and water in this way, the energy stored during synthesis is made available for use by the body, by converting it into short-term storage as ATP, a high-energy phosphate compound, which can release this energy for individual steps in biochemical metabolism. Sucrose may be converted into carbon dioxide and water by burning it in air. The chemical reaction is the same as that represented by the equation above, with exactly the same quantity of heat being liberated as when the oxidation occurs in the body. The difference in the two reactions concerns the speed at which they occur and their efficiency. Oxidation in the body takes place much more slowly than combustion in air as it takes place in a series of steps, thus ensuring a slow, controlled and gradual release of energy to body tissues. The efficiency of combustion within the body is less than that in air because only about two-thirds of the energy of the sucrose becomes available as biological energy, with one-third being 'lost' as heat which helps to maintain body temperature.

Both fat and proteins also contribute in similar oxidations (see Chapter 8).

$$(-CH_2-)_{2n} + (O_2)_{3n} \rightarrow 3n CO_2 + n H_2O$$
$$\text{Fat}$$

The oxidation of proteins depends on which amino acids are included. The nitrogen is removed and thus most are oxidized like carbohydrate while some are oxidized like fat.

The body is sometimes likened to a slow-combustion stove and macronutrients are described as fuel. It is clear that oxidation in the body is a most important process for it enables the energy stored in carbohydrates, fats and proteins to be liberated and made available for use by the body in a closely regulated way.

The energy value of food

Energy is usually measured in units called *calories*. A calorie is the amount of heat required to raise the temperature of 1 g of water by 1°C. As this is rather a small unit, energy derived from food may be expressed in units which are 1000-times larger and known as *kilocalories* (kcal). A kilocalorie is the amount of heat required to raise the temperature of 1 kg of water by 1°C. The common abbreviations for kilocalorie is kcal but Calorie, or Cal (with a capital C) is also used to indicate kilocalories in foods.

Another internationally recognized unit of energy is the *joule* (J), but like the calorie this is an inconveniently small unit with which to express the energy value of food so that the *kilojoule* (kJ), which is 1000-times larger than the joule, is usually used. Sometimes an even larger unit, the *megajoule* (MJ), is used. A megajoule is 1000-times larger than a kilojoule.

The relationship between these units may be expressed as follows:

$$1\,\text{kcal} = 4.19 \times 10^3\,\text{J} = 4.19\,\text{kJ} = 4.19 \times 10^{-3}\,\text{MJ}$$

An average adult usually needs about 1800–2500 kcal/day, which is about 8–10 MJ/day.

In the remainder of this chapter both types of unit are given to illustrate their relation to each other. Elsewhere, however, kilojoules (and megajoules) are used.

In order to compare the energy of different foods it is simplest to determine the amount of energy produced, calculated as heat, when 1 g of the substance is completely oxidized by igniting it in a small chamber filled with oxygen under pressure. The result obtained represents the heat of combustion of food which is usually expressed as kcal or kJ/g. If the calorie value of sucrose is expressed in this way, it is found to be 3.95 kcal/g. This means that when 1 g sucrose is completely oxidized the heat produced is sufficient to raise the temperature of 1000 g of water by 3.95°C. The average values of the heats of combustion of the energy-providing nutrients are shown in Table 1.1.

In order to express the energy value of nutrients in terms of the energy actually made available to the body it is necessary to calculate the available energy values. Such values are always lower than heats of combustion because of losses within the body. A small loss results from incomplete absorption from the intestine; such loss is suffered by carbohydrate, fat and protein, and with protein there is an additional loss because protein, unlike carbohydrate and fat, is incompletely oxidized in the body. In addition a correction may need to be made for non-starch polysaccharides (NSP, see p. 96), previously called dietary fibre. The magnitude of these energy losses may be appreciated from Table 1.1. There is some variation and uncertainty about nutrient availability; the ones quoted may be taken as being sufficiently reliable for most purposes, but in special conditions these may be different. With malabsorptive diarrhoea availability is obviously low, and varies between nutrients. There may, for example, be selective fat malabsorption (steatorrhoea) with liver or pancreatic disease. Mild malabsorption may cause no symptoms.

Although the available energy values given in Table 1.1 are approximate values which can be used to calculate the energy value of any given diet, the available energy value of any food can be found using the average figures, provided that its composition in terms of carbohydrates, fats and proteins is known. The energy value of summer milk, for example, can be calculated from its analysis, as shown in Table 1.2. By similar calculations the available energy value of other foods may be estimated; some average values are given in Table 1.3. This table shows that foods, such as butter and margarine, which contain a high proportion of fat have the highest energy values. Foods rich in carbohydrates, containing a high proportion of sugar (jam) or starch (bread and potatoes), are less concentrated sources of energy. Despite this, such foods supply a considerable proportion of the energy in an average British diet. Indeed, cereal foods contribute no less than one-third of our total energy intake, which is a greater proportion than that supplied by any other class of foodstuff. In many other countries, starchy foods, often in the form of rice, supply an even greater proportion of the total energy content of the diet. As a general rule, the proportion of fat has increased in 'advanced' Western market economies.

Table 1.1 Average energy value of nutrients (per gram)

Nutrient	Heat of combustion		Available energy value	
	(kcal)	(kJ)	(kcal)	(kJ)
Carbohydrate	4.1	17	3.75	16
Fat	9.4	39	9.00	37
Protein	5.7	24	4.00	17

Table 1.2 The energy value of summer milk

Nutrient	Amount in 100 g milk			Energy/100 g milk	
	(g)	(kcal/g)	(kJ/g)	(kcal)	(kJ)
Carbohydrate	4.1	3.75	16	15.4	65.6
Fat	4.0	9.00	37	36.0	148.0
Protein	3.4	4.00	17	13.6	57.8
Total energy provided by 100 g of summer milk				65.0	271.4

Reference: Food Standards Agency (2002). *McCance and Widdowson's The Composition of Foods*, 6th summary edition. Cambridge: Royal Society of Chemistry.
Crown copyright material is reproduced with the permission of the Controller of HMSO and the Queen's Printer for Scotland.

Table 1.3 Typical energy values of some foods with nutrients as percentage of energy

Food	Per 100 g		As percentage of energy		
	(kcal)	(kJ)	Fat	Carbohydrate	Protein
Apples	47	199	2.0	94.0	3.5
Tomatoes	17	73	16.0	68.0	16.5
Lettuce	14	59	32.0	45.0	23.0
Cabbage (boiled)	16	67	22.5	51.5	25.0
Dates	270	1151	0.7	94.5	4.8
Bread (white)	219	931	6.5	79.0	14.5
Potatoes (old)	74	306	1.3	88.5	10.0
Pasta (boiled)	159	677	8.5	75.0	16.5
Rice (white)	138	587	8.5	84.0	7.5
Beef (stewing)	203	852	42.5	0	57.5
Haddock (steamed)	89	378	6.0	0	94.0
Chicken (roasted)	177	742	38.0	0	62.0
Eggs (boiled)	147	612	66.0	Tr	34.0
Milk (summer)	65	270	55.4	23.6	21.0
Cheese (cheddar)	416	1725	75.5	0.1	24.4
Yogurt (plain)	79	333	34.2	37.0	28.8
Jam (fruit)	261	1114	0	99.1	0.9
Sugar	394	1680	0	99.9	Tr
Chocolate	520	2177	53.1	41.0	5.9
Butter	744	3059	99.4	0.3	0.3
Margarine (polyunsaturated)	746	3067	99.9	0.1	Tr
Fat spread (60%) (polyunsaturated)	553	2274	99.0	0.9	0.1
Sunflower oil	899	3696	100.0	0.0	Tr

Tr, trace.
Reference: Food Standards Agency (2002). *McCance and Widdowson's The Composition of Foods*, 6th summary edition. Cambridge: Royal Society of Chemistry.
Crown copyright material is reproduced with the permission of the Controller of HMSO and the Queen's Printer for Scotland.

THE USE OF ENERGY BY THE BODY

As we have already noted, energy is produced in the body from food by a series of precisely controlled steps. Each step results in the release of a small amount of energy which is used in the promotion of bodily functions and may finally produce heat. Without attempting at this stage any chemical explanation of the nature of the steps in the oxidation process, it is possible to gain a simple picture of how energy is used by the body.

Energy is required in the body for *basal metabolism*, which includes all the normal processes of cell respiration, maintenance and repair in the resting status, for *thermogenesis* or heat production, for growth and for physical activity. A proportion of food energy is also used for *diet-induced thermogenesis* to digest and process (store) the nutrients after each meal. This amount is more for protein and carbohydrate than for fat.

Basal metabolism

The term metabolism refers to the sum of all the chemical reactions going on in the body, and the energy needed to sustain the body at complete rest is known as the energy of basal metabolism or the basal metabolic rate (BMR).

The body requires a constant supply of energy to maintain its internal processes even when resting. Even during sleep, when the body is apparently at rest, energy is needed to ensure that essential internal processes continue. For example, energy must be supplied to maintain the powerful pumping action of the heart, the continual expansion and contraction of the lungs and the temperature of the blood. It is needed to maintain the ceaseless chemical activity of the millions of body cells and the tone of muscles. Living muscle must constantly be ready to contract in response to stimuli transmitted to it by nerves. Such a degree of readiness can only be achieved if energy is continually supplied to keep the muscles in a state of mild tension. Muscle tension decreases during sleep but does not become zero, so that a certain amount of energy, which ultimately appears as heat, is necessary to maintain it. The BMR is mainly determined by body weight and composition, which vary with both age (older people tend to have less muscle and more body fat, so relatively lower BMR) and sex (women tend to have higher proportion of body fat, so relatively lower BMR).

Table 1.4 gives average BMR values for men and women of different ages and body weights. It will be noted that the BMR of men is greater per kilogram of body weight than that of women of the same weight. This is because, for a given body weight, women's bodies contain more fat than those of men and fat contributes little to BMR.

Basal metabolic rate also varies with age. As age increases, BMR (per unit weight) falls; this decrease is rather greater for men than for women. Climate also affects BMR, its value being increased by 5–10 per cent in very cold and very hot climates. We are most comfortable, and BMR is lowest, between 20 and 28°C with light clothing. The thyroid gland regulates cellular metabolism throughout the body.

Table 1.4 Basal metabolic rate (BMR) values

| Age (years) | Males | | Females | |
	Weight (kg)	BMR (MJ/day)	Weight (kg)	BMR (MJ/day)
10–17	30	5.0	30	4.6
	65	7.6	60	6.3
18–29	60	6.7	45	4.8
	80	7.9	70	6.4
30–59	65	6.8	50	5.2
	85	7.7	70	5.9

Reference: Department of Health (1991). *Dietary Reference Values for food Energy and Nutrients for the United Kingdom. Report on Health and Social Subjects No. 41.* London: HMSO.
Crown copyright material is reproduced with the permission of the Controller of HMSO and the Queen's Printer for Scotland.

Excess thyroid activity increases BMR. If thyroid function is defective, BMR declines. Many other hormones affect metabolic rate including insulin and adrenaline.

Growth

During the 9 months of pregnancy it is calculated that some 70 000 kcal (293 MJ) (DOH 1991, p. 30) of energy are required to produce the baby, increase the size of the placenta and reproductive organs, allow for the energy (increased BMR) needed for the newly formed baby tissues and create additional stores of fat in the mother which will be used during lactation. Once the baby has been born, lactation requires around 600 kcal (2.5 MJ) per day (Garrow *et al.* 2000).

Newly born infants grow at a remarkable rate and in the first 3 months of life 23 per cent of food energy is required for growth. This figure falls to 6 per cent by the time the infant is 1 year old and to 2 per cent by the fifth year. In general terms it has been estimated that the formation of 1 g of new tissue requires 20 kJ of food energy.

Physical activity

Energy is needed to enable the body to perform external work. Physical activity requires a supply of energy additional to that needed to maintain muscle tone and other internal processes. The simplest physical act, such as standing up, involves the use of many muscles, and the greater the degree of physical activity in daily life the greater is the energy requirement of the muscles. It is useful, therefore, to relate the degree of physical activity to the energy that must be supplied by the diet.

The problem of equating physical activity with energy requirement is complicated by the fact that the body is unable to convert energy that is supplied by food completely into mechanical work. The efficiency of conversion by the body, considered as a machine, is of the order of 15–20 per cent. If the higher value is taken it means that 100 units of energy supplied by food enable the body to perform physical work, for example, running, equivalent to 20 units. The other 80 units appear as heat and account for the fact that heat is lost from the body surface at an increased rate when physical work is done. However, this total energy cost and thus dietary need is 100 units.

Overweight and obese people need more energy for movement, in proportion to their extra weight.

ENERGY REQUIREMENTS

The energy requirement of an individual is the same as energy expenditure, unless there is some growth or weight loss. The *estimated average requirement* for energy by a group of people may be defined using the concept of physical activity level (PAL). This is the ratio of overall daily energy expenditure to BMR. Daily energy expenditure may be calculated by adding together energy expenditure on an hour-by-hour basis at work, in non-work activities and while sleeping.

The values of PAL in different activities are shown in Table 1.5. Different occupations can be grouped

Table 1.5 Calculated physical activity level (PAL) of adults

| Non-occupational activity | Occupational activity | | | | | |
| | Light | | Moderate | | Moderate/heavy | |
	Male	Female	Male	Female	Male	Female
Non-active	1.4	1.4	1.6	1.5	1.7	1.5
Moderately active	1.5	1.5	1.7	1.6	1.8	1.6
Very active	1.6	1.6	1.8	1.7	1.9	1.7

Reference: Department of Health (1991). *Dietary Reference Values for Food Energy and Nutrients for the United Kingdom. Report on Health and Social Subjects No. 41.* London: HMSO. Crown copyright material is reproduced with the permission of the Controller of HMSO and the Queen's Printer for Scotland.

to indicate approximate PAL figures for estimated average 24 hour energy expenditure is as follows:

1 *Light.* Includes professional and technical workers, administrative and managerial, sales representatives, clerical workers,
2 *Moderate.* Includes sales workers, domestic helpers, transport workers, light construction workers, e.g. joiners,
3 *Moderate/heavy.* Includes labourers, agricultural and fishing and forestry workers, heavy construction workers, e.g. bricklayers.

In general terms, most population groups in the UK may be assumed to have light occupations and non-active, non-work activities and, consequently, have a PAL value of 1.4.

The EAR values shown in Table 1.6 are obtained by multiplying the appropriate PAL value by BMR, values of which are shown in Table 1.4.

For people over 60 years of age a standard PAL value of 1.5 is used. The EAR values for men and women aged over 60 years decrease with increasing age, although precise information for the energy requirements of the elderly is lacking. It is estimated that for men and women aged over 75 years the EAR values are 8.8 and 7.6 MJ/day respectively.

For young children and babies EAR values are calculated by interpolating from values calculated from data for older children.

Table 1.6 Estimated average requirements (EAR) for energy (MJ/day)

Weight (kg)	Physical activity level (PAL)				
	1.4	1.5	1.6	1.8	2.0
Males 10–18 years					
30	7.0	7.5	8.0	9.0	9.9
45	8.5	9.1	9.7	11.0	12.2
60	10.1	10.8	11.5	12.9	14.4
Males 19–29 years					
60	9.3	10.0	10.7	12.0	13.4
70	10.2	11.0	11.7	13.2	14.6
80	11.1	11.9	12.7	14.3	15.9
Males 30–59 years					
65	9.5	10.2	10.8	12.2	13.5
75	10.2	10.9	11.6	13.1	14.5
85	10.8	11.6	12.4	13.9	15.5
Females 10–18 years					
30	6.4	6.9	7.3	8.2	9.2
45	7.6	8.1	8.7	9.8	10.8
60	8.8	9.4	10.0	11.3	12.5
Females 18–29 years					
45	6.8	7.2	7.7	8.7	9.7
60	8.1	8.7	9.2	10.4	11.5
70	8.9	9.6	10.2	11.5	12.8
Females 30–59 years					
50	7.3	7.9	8.4	9.4	10.5
60	7.8	8.4	8.9	10.0	11.2
70	8.3	8.9	9.5	10.7	11.8

Reference: Department of Health (1991). *Dietary Reference Values for food Energy and Nutrients for the United Kingdom. Report on Health and Social Subjects No. 41.* London: HMSO. Crown copyright material is reproduced with the permission of the Controller of HMSO and the Queen's Printer for Scotland.

Key points

Definitions
● Nutritional science
  – What people eat and absorb
  – What people are
  – How these effect what people (can) do
● Food science: what is in food
● Food technology: optimises quality and/or profitability of foods

---

Chapter summary

Foods provide a variety of nutrients in a matrix form. All foods and most nutrients contribute to the energy supply, as part of a chain which harnesses energy (calories) from the sun and presents it as a form which can contribute to metabolism, growth and physical activity. Amongst the macronutrients which supply energy, the richest source is fat (9 kcal/g) followed by protein (4) and carbohydrate (3.75).

FURTHER READING

DEPARTMENT OF HEALTH (1991). *Dietary Reference Values for Food Energy and Nutrients for the United Kingdom. Report on Health and Social Subjects No. 41*. London: HMSO.

EUROPEAN PARLIAMENT (2001). Directive 2001/83/EC of the European Parliament on the Community code relating to medicinal products for human use. *Official Journal* L311 28.11 2001, p. 71.

FOOD STANDARDS AGENCY (2002). *McCance and Widdowson's The Composition of Foods*, 6th summary edition. Cambridge: Royal Society of Chemistry. ftp://ftp.fao.org/codex/manual/Manual12ce.pdf

GARROW JS, JAMES WPT, RALPH A (2000). *Human Nutrition and Dietetics*, 10th edn. London: Churchill Livingstone.

Enzymes and digestion

The human body is composed of some hundred-thousand million cells, each of which is a functional unit, enclosed within its cell membrane. These cells are grouped together in the body to form tissues with specialized functions. Thus, some cells comprise connective tissue and bind together the various organs of the body, others are concerned with muscular and nervous tissue, while others form the skeletal framework of bone that contributes strength and rigidity to the body. Most organs contain several functional cell types.

Individual cells are so tiny that their internal structure can only be observed when magnified many hundreds or thousands of times with the help of an electron microscope. Within the cell there are a number of different types of very much smaller 'subcellular organelles'. These have specialized functions, and their size, structure and number vary widely according to demands, or to regulation by local nutrient supply, and instructions delivered by nerves or hormones to the cell.

The complex activities needed to sustain life in the human body take place within the body's cells. The activity of a cell is often likened to that of a chemical factory in which a great variety of raw materials are processed and converted into finished products. In a single cell many different raw materials are required, though they are largely composed of only four elements: carbon, hydrogen, oxygen and nitrogen. The processing stage, which is concerned with the conversion of these simple raw materials into the more complex substances required to carry out

the many functions of the cell, involves thousands of different reactions. Each of these reactions comprises many steps which must be carried out in a definite sequence with the result that the chemical operations of a cell are much more complicated, and need much greater integration, than those of a chemical factory. They must also be capable of adaptation to enormous variations in conditions and fluctuating nutrient supply.

In order to sustain life, the cell's activities must be controlled and organized into a self-regulating and self-renewing pattern. But how can such control be achieved, and how is it that although almost all human cells are built according to the same basic pattern, they are able to perform a multitude of different functions? The answer to these questions is to be found in the existence of a group of crucially important protein substances called enzymes.

Enzymes control all the chemical changes (that is, the metabolism), which occur in living cells. They regulate the building up (anabolic) reactions that result in the formation of complex substances such as proteins from single building units. They also regulate the breaking-down (catabolic) reactions that result in release of energy. Enzymes can activate or catalyse chemical reactions or inhibit them. Enzymes often increase the cycling or turnover of substances in cells (i.e. stimulate both synthesis and breakdown of compounds). This allows processes to be more rapidly regulated (in terms of direction and speed of reaction) by other factors. Anabolic and catabolic processes involve very many steps, and each step is controlled by its own enzyme. This control must be carefully regulated so that the life of the cell continues smoothly at all times, with the whole metabolic process being kept carefully balanced.

ENZYMES

How different cells perform different functions can be explained in terms of the enzymes that are present. Some 1000 different enzymes have been recognized in the body, but in any one cell only a selection are present. Even so, most cells contain about 200 different enzymes, each of which is responsible for controlling a particular step. The complement of enzymes present in a cell automatically selects and controls those reactions which are to proceed. Since enzymes are proteins, their presence in cells in turn depends on the DNA of the cell, including the DNA sequence which for the synthesis of each enzyme and for its own storage and metabolism.

The chemical nature of enzymes

One of the most widely known sources of enzymes is yeast, which is one of the simplest possible types of living organism. This is how the name enzyme arose, for it means literally 'in yeast'. The fermentation of sugar in grape juice by yeast and the leavening effect of yeast in making bread have been used for many centuries. These are actions of enzymes.

A long time elapsed between the discovery of the first known enzyme in yeast and the isolation of an enzyme in the pure state. For many years it was believed that enzymes were living organisms. This idea was only shown to be false at the end of the last century when the German chemist Buchner extracted a cell-free liquid from yeast cells that had a similar enzyme activity to the original living cells. So, although enzymes are made by living cells, they themselves are not living.

All enzymes are proteins, the structure of which is described in Chapter 10. The properties of proteins – their ability to change their shape, their sensitivity to changes of conditions of temperature and acidity, their capacity to oppose changes of acidity that would upset the smooth working of the cell – make them peculiarly suited to control cell metabolism.

A feature of all enzymes is that their tertiary structure includes a site that 'recognizes' and can bind temporarily to immobilize its substrate.

Classification of enzymes

The substance upon which an enzyme acts is called the *substrate*, and enzymes are usually named after this substance. Thus, the enzyme that acts on (breaks down) urea is called urease and that which acts on maltose is called maltase. It is a general rule that enzymes are named after the substrate upon which they act and given the suffix *-ase* (from Latin). In common with most general rules, however, there are notable exceptions, mainly those enzymes which were named before the rule gained general acceptance. Some of these, such as pepsin and trypsin, will be encountered later.

Enzymes may be classified in a number of ways, but one of the most useful is to group them according to the type of reaction which they control. The five main groups of enzyme are shown in Table 2.1. Of these, the first two are the most important in connection with what follows. Hydrolases control the hydrolysis of the substrate, that is its reaction with water and, as we shall see later in the chapter, this type of enzyme is of paramount importance in digestion. Oxidases control the oxidation of the substrate, and this usually takes the form of removal of hydrogen as indicated in the equation shown in Table 2.1. There is often more than one enzyme which carries out a particular function – very similar 'iso-enzymes' may be produced in different tissues – each with its own gene and separate

Table 2.1 Classification of enzymes

Name	Reaction catalysed	General equation
Hydrolases	Hydrolysis	$AB + H_2O \rightarrow AOH + BH$
Oxidases	Oxidation	$ABH_2 \rightarrow AB + 2H$
Isomerases	Intramolecular rearrangement	$ABC \rightarrow ACB$
Transferases	Transfer of a group	$AB + C \rightarrow A + BC$
Synthetases	Addition of one molecule to another	$A + B \rightarrow AB$

system for regulation. A very common feature of enzyme function is that activation of an enzyme, or the expression of the gene, are often inhibited by the product of the reaction catalysed. This prevents wastage of energy on unnecessary metabolism, and prevents accumulation.

Catalytic action of enzymes

Enzymes are organic catalysts; they operate by speeding up a chemical process while remaining unchanged at the end of the reaction. In many respects their action is similar to that of the more familiar inorganic catalysts such as are often used in manufacturing processes. In the manufacture of margarine, vegetable oils are converted into solid fats by chemical reaction with hydrogen. In the absence of a catalyst the conversion of the oils into fats is very slow indeed, but the addition of small quantities of finely divided nickel produces a remarkable increase in the rate of the reaction; moreover, the nickel catalyst may be used time after time, as it is not used up in the process.

It is remarkable that only one part of nickel is needed to catalyse the conversion of several-thousand parts of oil into fat, but this achievement appears quite insignificant when compared with the startling catalytic power of enzymes. One of the enzymes concerned with the breakdown of starch during digestion is amylase, produced by the pancreas. Only one part of amylase is needed to effect the conversion of four million parts of starch into the sugar maltose. Where the efficiency of man-made catalysts is measured in thousands, that of nature's catalysts is measured in millions.

How do enzymes work? We can best approach this by considering first how an ordinary non-catalytic reaction proceeds. Suppose a reaction involves the conversion of reacting substances represented by A into products represented by B. The reaction will not start until A has received a 'push' in the form of energy, often supplied in the form of heat. The reason for this can be appreciated from Fig. 2.1.

Before A can react to form B it must surmount the energy hump shown by moving along path (i), and this requires an amount of energy DG* (uncatalysed). When A has absorbed energy DG* (uncatalysed), known as the *activation energy*, it is in an activated state and can decompose to form B.

This process can be likened to that of transferring a ball from one side of a hill to the other. If Fig. 2.1 represents a hill, the problem is that of transferring a ball from X to Y. If the only path lies over the summit of the hill, then it is necessary to push the ball up the hill – that is, to work on it by supplying energy – until it reaches the top. Once there, it will run down the other side to Y of its own accord. The ball may now be at a lower level than it was at its starting point, as is the case in Fig. 2.1. This means that an amount of energy DG* has been released, though this could not have been achieved without first pushing the ball to the top of the hill, which involved supplying it with energy DG* (uncatalysed).

In the cells of the human body, activation energy cannot be supplied in normal ways, such as heat, because this would damage the cells. The function

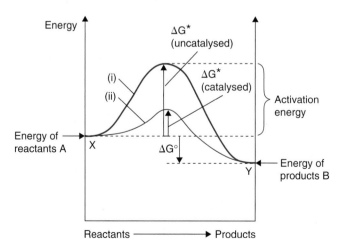

Figure 2.1 *Reaction paths: (i) non-catalytic path; (ii) catalytic path*

of enzymes is to enable the reaction to proceed at a much lower activation energy than would otherwise be possible. In terms of Fig. 2.1, we must replace the reaction path (i) over the summit of the hill by one at a lower level such as (ii) involving a lower activation energy DG* (catalysed).

Enzymes catalyse reactions by replacing a single-step of a high-energy mechanism with a two- or multi-stage process, each step of which involves a low activation energy. If the enzyme catalyst is represented as E and the substrate as A we have:

$$A + E \rightleftharpoons AE$$
$$AE \rightleftharpoons B + E$$

Overall reaction: $A \rightleftharpoons B$

Within each cell is its *nucleus*, which mainly contains genetic material (chromosomes) and this is surrounded by a watery fluid called *cytoplasm*, which contain water-soluble enzymes. The cytoplasm contains a network of membrane-like material, the *endoplasmic reticulum*, which is studded with small dark bodies known as *ribosomes*. The cytoplasm also contains a number of bodies, among which are the egg-shaped *mitochondria* and the smaller *lysosomes*. These bodies contain enzymes which are lipid-soluble within their membranes. Ribosomes are responsible for translating the DNA code in chromosomes by assembling amino acids in the correct order to make proteins and enzymes. Mitochondria house the enzymes for oxidation (combustion) of nutrients to generate chemical energy (as ATP). Lysosomes include the enzymes which release enzymes to attack foreign material and infecting organisms.

Enzymically catalysed reactions proceed by way of a temporary enzyme–substrate complex represented by AE. If both stages require little energy the reaction path is as represented by Fig. 2.1 (ii) and the reaction will be a rapid and near spontaneous one with the enzyme E being regenerated. Thus, we have a simple picture of how enzymes act as catalysts.

It should be noted that although enzymes speed up reactions, and direct substrates towards one specific reaction when others are possible, they cannot turn impossible reactions into possible ones. Neither can they affect the equilibrium position of a reversible reaction; this means that the *amount* of product in a reaction is the same whether an enzyme is involved or not. The presence of the enzyme merely reduces the time taken to reach the equilibrium position. In the absence of the enzyme the reaction may be so slow that, for all practical purposes, it does not proceed at all. In a cell, thousands of different reactions are possible but the function of the enzymes present is to speed up particular ones, so that some reactions proceed rapidly while others proceed at a relatively insignificant rate. In this way, cell metabolism is controlled and directed so that different cells are able to fulfil different functions.

Selectivity of enzymes

Enzymes are usually highly selective in which reaction they catalyse. Frequently one enzyme will catalyse only one cell reaction. It is this characteristic which allows them to preserve order in living cells. Thus, although many other reactions may occur in a cell, the rate at which they proceed is insignificant compared with that of the catalysed reaction.

The selective power of enzymes is sometimes compared with the action of a key in a lock: the enzyme is the lock and only certain molecules can act as the key which exactly fits it. If a reaction between two molecules is catalysed by an enzyme the lock can be imagined as having grooves into which the two molecules fit side by side; this leads to a brief union between the enzyme and the two molecules which are acting as keys, as is shown in stage 2 of Fig. 2.2. The key molecules are thus brought together and converted into an active state which enables them to react with each other. After reaction new molecules are formed, but as shown in stage 3 of the diagram, the enzyme remains unchanged and can catalyse further reaction.

In order to achieve a good fit between lock and key molecules, an enzyme frequently needs the help of another substance to be effective. Three main types of enzyme promotor have been distinguished, namely *coenzymes*, *cofactors* (or activators) and *prosthetic groups* (see p. 149). Coenzymes are smaller than enzyme molecules and are not proteins. They are not permanently bound to the enzyme but may become attached to it during enzyme reaction (Fig. 2.2, stage 1) only to be released later (once stage 3, Fig. 2.2, has been completed). Coenzymes are closely related to vitamins or are the vitamins themselves. One of the functions of the B group of vitamins seems to be to provide the body with suitable

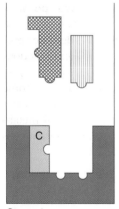

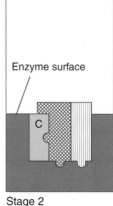

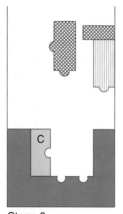

Stage 1
Lock and key molecules
before union.
C is the coenzyme or
prosthetic group

Stage 2
Union and activation of
lock and key molecules

Stage 3
New molecules formed
leaving enzyme surface
unchanged

Figure 2.2 *The lock and key
theory of enzyme reaction*

starting materials from which to make the coenzymes that it needs. The exact function of coenzymes is still only partly understood, but they certainly play an active and vital part in many reactions involving oxidizing enzymes. This is shown by the fact that if a coenzyme needed by an enzyme is absent, the enzyme can exert no catalytic effect. This can be used to measure the status of essential nutrients. For example, thiamine (vitamin B_1) is a coenzyme for the enzyme transketolase. Transketolase activity in blood is a simple laboratory measure of thiamine status.

In some cases it is found that metallic ions, such as magnesium, or non-metallic ions, such as chloride, are required to increase the activity of enzymes. Such substances are known as cofactors (or activators). Prosthetic groups are non-protein groups which are permanently bound to the enzyme.

Sometimes several molecules, which are similar to each other, can approximately fit the grooves of the same lock. In such cases the enzyme does not distinguish between them and acts as a catalyst to them all. In most cases, however, enzymes show great powers of discrimination as the following examples show. The three enzymes, maltase, lactase and sucrase, are present in the small intestine, and during digestion these enzymes catalyse the hydrolysis of the sugars maltose, lactose and sucrose respectively. These three enzymes have considerable specificity, and in the case of lactase, complete specificity, since it will catalyse the hydrolysis of lactose and of no

other substance (not even a similar sugar). Maltase and sucrase, however, catalyse the hydrolysis not only of maltose and sucrose but also that of certain other similar sugars.

A further example of enzymes which show a remarkable selectivity are those which catalyse the hydrolysis of proteins. The three enzymes, pepsin, trypsin and chymotrypsin, each select certain links of protein molecules and catalyse hydrolysis only at these links (see p. 148).

Sensitivity of enzymes

Enzymes are very sensitive to effects of temperature and the environment. All enzyme activity is destroyed on boiling because, being proteins, enzymes are denatured (see p. 141) by high temperatures. At low temperatures enzyme activity is greatly slowed down but as the enzymes are not denatured and, because enzyme reactions have a low activation energy, enzymes may retain some catalytic activity even at subzero temperatures. In general, plant enzymes work best at about 25°C and those in warm-blooded animals at about 37–40°C. An increase in temperature usually increases the rate of a chemical reaction, but in the case of an enzyme reaction it may also lead to inactivation of the enzyme.

Figure 2.3 shows the effect of temperature on the rate of catalysis. At 37°C, the initial rate of reaction is

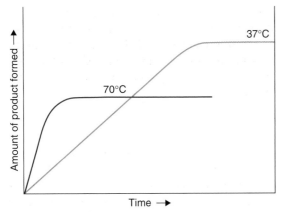

Figure 2.3 *The effect of temperature on the rate of catalysis by an enzyme*

rapid, but after a time the reaction rate slows down and stops, no further product being formed. This may have one of several causes. For example, the reaction may be complete, all the substrate having reacted, or it may be that the products of reaction have made the environment unfavourable for enzyme activity and the enzyme has been deactivated. If the temperature is raised to 70°C, the initial rate of reaction is increased. This is because the greater energy input increases the energy of substrate and enzyme molecules, and these molecules gain the activation energy needed for reaction to take place more rapidly. Although the initial rate of formation of products is rapid, it soon stops because the enzyme is rapidly inactivated at the higher temperature. The net result is that less product is formed at the higher temperature than at the lower. Enzymes catalyse reaction efficiently in man, the temperature being high enough to give rapid formation of products but low enough to avoid inactivation of the enzyme.

Enzyme activity is also dependent upon the acidity or alkalinity (the pH) of the medium in which the enzyme acts. Most enzymes operate most efficiently in an environment that is nearly neutral, and if the medium becomes strongly acid or alkaline the enzyme becomes completely inactivated. Some enzymes, however, can only operate in an acid or alkaline solution. For example, the enzyme pepsin is present in gastric juice and during digestion it catalyses the initial hydrolysis of proteins. It can only act in strongly acid conditions such as are produced by the hydrochloric acid in the stomach. Conversely, the enzyme trypsin which is present in pancreatic juice requires a slightly alkaline medium before it can catalyse protein hydrolysis. When food passes from the stomach into the small intestine the hydrochloric acid is completely neutralized and the medium becomes alkaline. Under these conditions pepsin becomes inactivated and trypsin carries on the digestion of proteins.

CELL METABOLISM

All activities that occur in cells are controlled by enzymes. However, these enzymes are not evenly distributed throughout the cell but are dispersed among the different parts of the cell so that each part has a distinct role in maintaining the life of the cell.

The nucleus of a cell contains all the genes (coded in DNA), which can produce any of the enzymes found in cells. The nucleus also contains a small number of enzymes that, together, specifically control cell (nuclear) growth and division. The surrounding cytoplasm contains water-soluble enzymes that control a variety of anabolic and catabolic processes. The mitochondria are important because they are the powerhouses of the cell and contain a number of oxidases responsible for the manufacture of high-energy materials used for energy production. The important job of protein synthesis in the cell is controlled by enzymes found in the endoplasmic reticulum. Some of the enzymes found only in mitochondria are synthesized from RNA inside mitochondria, rather than from DNA in the nucleus. Mitochondria reproduce in a parallel but separate way to the rest of the cell. Finally, one of the most interesting bodies in the cell is the lysosome, also sometimes called the 'suicide bag'. Lysosomes contain a sufficient variety of hydrolases capable of destroying nearly all the components of the cell. Normally these 'suicide' enzymes are safely contained within the impermeable membrane that encloses the lysosome, but if the cell becomes injured or dies, the enzymes are released and the cell destroys itself and also any infecting agent.

Each cell, and each component of a cell, is surrounded by a membrane. The membrane allows only those raw materials needed by the cell to pass through it, all other substances being prevented from entering. This selection mechanism ensures that only those substances required for a particular job are available, and it also ensures that only those enzymes required to control this function are allowed through the membrane. Most cell membranes are 'semipermeable', that is, they allow water, and sometimes small molecules dissolved in water, to pass freely but larger molecules can only pass through if there are specific transport mechanisms.

In later chapters we shall develop the theme of what happens to nutrients in metabolism in rather more detail, but enough has been said in this introductory survey to show that all the activities and functions of the body which constitute life are entirely dependent upon enzymes.

DIGESTION

'You are what you eat.'

(An error! – Anon)

It is indeed a very odd thing – an extraordinary and remarkable thing – that no matter what we eat, the structure of the body, both flesh and blood, changes very little. There is no obvious similarity between the nature of the food we eat and the nature of our bodies. Yet within a few hours of being eaten, food is transformed into flesh and blood. This transformation is so complete that it cannot be accomplished before food has undergone a drastic breaking-down process known as *digestion*.

Digestion is both physical and chemical: the physical process involves the breakdown of large food particles into smaller ones while the chemical process involves the breakdown of larger molecules into smaller ones. Foodstuffs are mainly complicated, insoluble substances that must be converted into simpler, soluble, more active ones before they can be used by the body. Not all nutrients need digesting, however, as there are some such as water and simple sugars (e.g. glucose) that do not need to be broken down and many vitamins and mineral salts which must not be broken down if they are to be useful. Whether or not nutrients need to be broken down by digestion they cannot be utilized by the body until they have passed into the bloodstream, a process which is known as absorption. The availability of a nutrient, or

food component, is the proportion that is actually absorbed after passing through the two (incomplete) processes of digestion and absorption. Once in the bloodstream, nutrients are distributed to all the cells of the body where they sustain the complex processes of metabolism. So you are *not* what you eat – although what you are reflects what you eat.

The role of enzymes in digestion

The chemical processes involved in digestion are brought about by enzymes. The chemical breakdown of food molecules into absorbable components, which in the absence of enzymes would be very slow indeed, is thereby speeded up so that digestion is completed in a matter of hours. Thus, in the space of some 3–4 hours a remarkable change in the nature of the food has occurred. Substances such as starch, which may contain as many as 150 000 atoms in a single molecule, have been converted into molecules containing only 24 atoms (simple sugars such as glucose). The breakdown of protein molecules is almost equally spectacular, as an average protein molecule is split up into about 500 amino acid molecules during digestion. These two examples perhaps make clearer the magnitude of the chemical task performed by the enzymes of the digestive system.

Each stage of digestion involves hydrolysis and is catalysed by a hydrolysing enzyme or hydrolase. The hydrolysis can be represented:

$$AB + H_2O = AOH + BH.$$

The equation shows how water is involved in splitting up a molecule AB into two smaller molecules AOH and BH. In some instances (e.g. sucrose), a single step involving the breakdown of a molecule into two parts is sufficient to produce a smaller soluble molecule that can be absorbed. In other instances (e.g. proteins), a very large number of hydrolytic steps is required before breakdown is complete.

The digestive process involves a fairly small number of different enzymes which catalyse the chemical breakdown of proteins, carbohydrates and fats. The names of the hydrolases that catalyse the hydrolysis of these different nutrients are shown in Table 2.2. Unfortunately, different authorities use different names for these enzymes. There is an

Table 2.2 Hydrolases involved in digestion

Name	Substrate	Product
Amylases	Starch	Maltose
Maltases	Maltose	Glucose
Lipases	Fats	Fatty acids and glycerol
Peptidases	Proteins	Amino acids

internationally agreed which can be used to classify and identify all enzymes, but the older descriptive terms are still the most widely used. The names given, however, are descriptive of the main changes brought about by hydrolases in digestion. Peptidases can be conveniently subdivided into exopeptidases, which split off amino acids from the ends of protein molecules, and endopeptidases, which attack and split the inside of protein molecules.

We have already noted the high selectivity of some enzymes such as peptidases. Amylases and enzymes which break down sugars show a similar high degree of selectivity. It is therefore evident that a whole series of such enzymes is required to achieve the stepwise breakdown of proteins and carbohydrates. In contrast, lipases are relatively unselective, so that only a few lipases are required to break down fats.

Stages of digestion

The digestive system can be regarded as functioning in a series of tube-like organs which pass through the body from the mouth at one end to the anus at the other, together with associated organs such as pancreas, liver and gall bladder, which produce and release enzymes. The lumen of the gut is thus outside the body. Chewing is important for grading and mixing and also stimulates the flow of salivary juices into the mouth. Saliva contains the first enzymes met by food. For example, if one chews bread it begins to taste sweet. This is because amylase in saliva has catalysed the breakdown of starch in bread into glucose. Food enters the system at the mouth, passes down the oesophagus into the stomach and then through the small intestine and large intestine, being gradually digested and absorbed in the process. Any that remains leaves the body at the other end of the system. In the following text, the stages of digestion are described in a very simple way to provide an

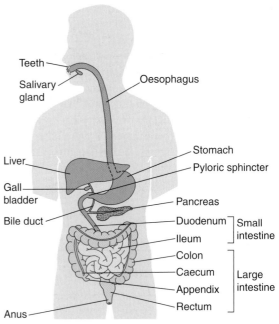

Figure 2.4 *The digestive system*

overall picture of the process. The chemical details will be filled in later after a discussion of the chemical nature of the nutrients concerned. The main parts of the digestive system are illustrated in Fig. 2.4 and the digestive process is summarized in Fig. 2.5.

Digestion in the mouth

When food is chewed, the size of the individual pieces is reduced and saliva is secreted by the salivary glands. The secretion of saliva takes place in response to various sorts of stimuli; the sight of a well-cooked meal, an appetizing smell or even the thought of a good meal may cause the salivary glands to produce saliva. This fluid becomes well mixed with food during mastication, lubricating it and so making it easier to swallow. Saliva is a dilute aqueous solution having a solid content of only about 1 per cent. Its main constituent is a slimy substance called *mucin* which assists lubrication. It also contains the enzyme *salivary amylase*, and various inorganic salts, the most abundant being sodium chloride which furnishes chloride ions that activate the enzyme. The initial hydrolysis of cooked starchy food is catalysed by salivary amylase in the mouth, and this catalytic action is continued as the food moves down the oesophagus and into the stomach. The enzyme soon becomes inactivated in the

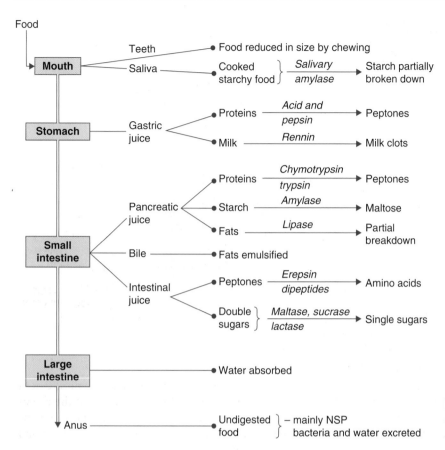

Figure 2.5 *Summary of the digestive process. NSP, non-starch polysaccharide*

stomach, however, because it cannot tolerate a strongly acid environment. In quantitative terms, salivary amylase contributes little to digestion, but does help to make certain starchy foods more palatable by releasing glucose, which sweetens it.

Food is carried down the oesophagus by gentle muscular action called peristalsis. The muscles contract, producing a peristaltic wave and this moves down the oesophagus, carrying the food with it.

Digestion in the stomach

The stomach may be regarded as a reservoir in which food is prepared for the main stage of digestion in the small intestine. This does not mean that no digestion takes place there, however, as cells in the lining of the stomach produce a fluid called gastric juice. The two essential constituents of this dilute aqueous solution are its enzymes and its acid content. The main enzyme is pepsin, secreted as the

inactive pepsinogen and becoming activated when it comes into contact with the hydrochloric acid that forms the acid constituent of the gastric juice.

Some 20 minutes after starting to eat a meal, vigorous muscular movements begin in the lower region of the stomach. Muscular contraction produces an inward pressure and this moves down the stomach wall as a peristaltic wave, so moving food through the stomach and causing it to become intimately mixed with the gastric juice. In this way, the acidity of the semi-fluid food mixture called chyme increases, until the endopeptidase pepsin is able to catalyse the conversion of part of the protein into slightly simpler molecules called peptones. The other major enzyme in the gastric juice is rennin, which also acts in an acid medium and brings about the coagulation or clotting of milk. The acidity of the gastric juice also causes some bacteria, which enter with the food, to be killed.

A copious flow of gastric juice is necessary during a meal and its production is stimulated both by psychological and chemical means. The former is the more important and is governed by involuntary nervous action which may be brought about by the appearance, smell and taste of food. The mere thought of food may be sufficient to stimulate gastric secretion; conversely, the flow of gastric juice may be inhibited by factors such as excitement, depression, anxiety and fear. Certain foodstuffs act as chemical stimulants to secretion. Meat extractives, for example, which are dissolved out of meat when it is put in boiling water, are particularly potent in this respect. Soups and meat dishes in which the extractives have been preserved are therefore valuable aids to digestion in the stomach.

Peristaltic action moves the chyme into the lower region of the stomach which is separated from the upper region of the small intestine, called the duodenum, by the pyloric valve. The valve opens at intervals, so allowing small portions of chyme to leave the stomach. This process continues for about 6 hours after eating a meal until no chyme remains in the stomach.

Digestion in the small intestine

The main stage of digestion occurs during the passage of chyme through the long small intestine. As soon as food enters the duodenum, digestive juices pour forth. There are three sources: the liver secretes bile which is then stored by the gall bladder, and the pancreas secretes pancreatic juice. These two secretions enter the small intestine through a single duct situated a short way down the duodenum; the third secretion is produced in the lining of the small intestine and is called the intestinal juice. They are all produced at the same time and, as they are alkaline, they neutralize the acidity of the chyme. Under these conditions the enzymes of the three secretions are able to exert their catalytic influence.

The pancreatic juice contains enzymes which enable it to help in the digestion of the three main types of nutrient. The endopeptidases trypsin and chymotrypsin, among others, carry on the degradation of proteins begun by pepsin in the stomach; they complete the breakdown of proteins into peptones. Pancreatic amylase is another enzyme present in the pancreatic juice; its capacity for catalysing the hydrolysis of large amounts of starch and converting it into maltose has already been mentioned. Finally,

pancreatic lipase brings about the partial hydrolysis of some fat molecules, converting them into simpler substances which can be absorbed.

The bile has no important enzyme action, but contains bile salts that convert fats in food (liquefied by the warmth of the stomach) into a fine emulsion of tiny oil droplets which may then be acted upon by the lipase of the pancreatic juice. If the liver is damaged, a lack of bile allows dietary fats to remain in a separated, liquid, form which escapes lipolysis. Fat malabsorption then occurs with loose greasy stools (steatorrhoea) and weight loss. With steatorrhoea there is a loss from the gut of fat soluble vitamins (A, D, E and K) and other compounds.

The intestinal juice contains a number of enzymes, three of which have already been mentioned, namely maltase, lactase and sucrase, which break down the double sugars maltose, lactose and sucrose respectively into simple sugars that can be absorbed. In addition to these, a group of exopeptidases, called erepsin, continue the breakdown of proteins begun by the endopeptidases pepsin, trypsin and chymotrypsin. The exopeptidases attack the ends of the chain-like peptone molecules until they are broken down into small units called dipeptides containing only two amino acids. Finally, another group of enzymes called dipeptidases break down the dipeptides into free amino acids which can be absorbed.

Apart from these chemical changes, muscular activity continues, so causing the various substances to move slowly down the small intestine.

Absorption in the small intestine

The digestive process is almost complete after the food material has been in the small intestine for some 4 hours in humans (much quicker in small animals). The most complicated of all nutrients, the proteins, have been converted by stages into amino acids; all carbohydrates, except non-starch polysaccharides (NSPs), have been broken down into simple soluble sugars, while fats have been emulsified and partly split into simpler component parts called fatty acids and glycerol. However, before digested nutrients can be used by the body they must pass through the walls of the digestive tube into the blood, a process known as absorption.

The walls of the long small intestine are folded into finger-like projections called villi (like the pile of velvet) which contain both blood capillaries and a lymph vessel and which have a very large surface area. Non-fatty nutrients, such as the products of protein and carbohydrate digestion, namely amino acids and simple sugars, are absorbed directly through the villi into the blood. Products of fat digestion, namely fatty acids and glycerol, pass through the villi into the lymph vessel where they are resynthesized into fat molecules. However, in the process of being reformed the fatty acids are rearranged so that the resulting fat molecules are more suitable for use by the body.

The large intestine

About 7–9 hours after a meal has been eaten any food that has not been digested and absorbed in the small intestine passes through the ileocaecal valve into a wider and shorter tube called the large intestine. No new enzymes are produced by the body during this stage but the large intestine is a rich source of bacteria. These may attack undigested substances such as NSPs with their own enzymes and partly break them down into 'volatile fatty acids' (e.g. acetate, butyrate and propionate). In addition, vitamin K and certain vitamins of the B group are synthesized (i.e. built up by the bacteria). The small molecules so formed, many which are able to be absorbed, pass through the walls of the large intestine into the blood and they can be particular sources of nutrients for the cells of the colon wall itself. The colonic bacteria also have some capacity to 'rescue' some nitrogenous compounds (ammonia) in the bowel, excreted from amino acid metabolism in the body, and resynthesize useful amino acids. This is a good example of biological synergism, as mammals cannot convert the nitrogen in ammonia back into amino acids.

The main function of the large intestine is to remove water from the fluid mass; this process continues as the fluid passes along, so that by the time it reaches the end of the tube it is in a semi-solid form known as faeces. In a day, between 100 and 200 g of moist faeces may be produced containing undigested food material, residues from digestive juices, large numbers of both living and dead bacteria, and water. After having been in the large intestine for (on average) about 20 hours these materials are passed out of the body.

Transport in the body

Food, after digestion and absorption, provides nutrients that are the raw materials of body metabolism. But this process is not complete without an efficient transport system capable of carrying nutrients to the cells that require them. We have already seen that nutrients, during absorption, pass into the blood and it is the constant circulation of blood through the body system that enables these nutrients to be transported to where they are needed. Blood, which is four-fifths water, contains many substances, such as nutrients and hormones, in solution. Other substances, such as the red blood corpuscles which transport oxygen, are present as cells in the blood and are carried round with it in suspension.

Most digested nutrients, being water-soluble, are easily transported dissolved in blood but the transport of fat is more complicated. Fat is transported in an emulsified form as minute droplets of lipoprotein. Lipoproteins are composed of clusters of fat molecules which have been coated with protein and phospholipids (mainly lecithin) and so converted into an easily transportable emulsion. Lipoprotein chylomicrons are formed in the gut mucosa after absorption of fatty acids, and they are initially transported via the lymphatic system to the thoracic duct, where they enter into the blood.

The heart pumps blood through the arteries and into successively smaller tubes, the smallest of which are capillaries. In the capillaries, nutrients and oxygen from the blood diffuse into the surrounding cells, while waste products from the cells diffuse into the blood. Blood carrying the waste material passes into a network of veins, with carbon dioxide being removed by the lungs while soluble substances are removed by the kidneys. There is also free diffusion of water between the blood and tissue fluid, which enables the fluid bathing the cells to be continually renewed.

Key points

- Enzymes are proteins coded by DNA
  - Any cell contains about 200 enzymes from several thousand in the body
  - The pattern of enzymes in a cell determine the type and function of the cell
- Enzymes are very specific, and very minor (genetic) defects block their functions, leading to disease

Chapter summary

Enzymes in the gastro-intestinal tract modify foods eaten to release nutrients in a form which can be absorbed and digested. Along the gut, different classes of enzymes are made, and released into the gut to mix with food. Enzymes which humans cannot make are also provided by normal bacteria in the colon, to metabolize dietary fibre and ammonia.

FURTHER READING

BANNON G, FU TJ, KIMBER I, HINTON DM (2003). Protein digestibility and relevance to allergenicity. *Environ Health Perspect*, 111(8): 1122–1124.

ENGLYST KN, ENGLYST HN (2005). Carbohydrate bioavailability. *Br J Nutr*, 94: 1–11.

LAYER P, KELLER J (1999). Pancreatic enzymes: secretion and luminal nutrient digestion in health and disease. *J Clin Gastroenterol*, 28(1): 3–10.

SIBLEY E (2004). Genetic variation and lactose intolerance: detection methods and clinical implications. *Am J Pharmacogenom*, 4(4): 239–245.

Food, eating, health and disease

Today, especially in post-industrial countries, most people are able to choose what they eat and how much they eat. It was not always so, however. Since earliest times humans have had a strong instinct for survival, which included a driving force to seek out edible plants and animals. Habitual patterns of consumption were determined by availability. It varied enormously with the seasons, and included periods of semi-starvation. People originally had to be nomadic (hunters) but later learned how to save food, and to plan for the future, which allowed settling into a farming (agrarian) lifestyle. Most agrarian humans stabilized their food supply by breeding animals and by cultivating those crops that proved to be useful sources of food, obviating the need for nomadism, and permitting social development.

Even in the UK as recently as 100 years ago the diet of ordinary people was very restricted and most people simply lived on the food that was available to them. Food choice amounted to selecting food that could be afforded. Some people in these circumstances were very concerned with whether food was 'good' or 'bad' for health, but for many the dominant issue was whether they could find enough food to stave off hunger. Ill health was dominated by malnutrition, which encourages infection.

It was not until the nineteenth century that the origin of infectious diseases was discovered. The appreciation that they were caused by bacteria was a landmark in our understanding of the nature of disease, demonstrating that the presence of something harmful in the environment, whether the air we breathe, the water we drink or more generally the insanitary nature of our living conditions.

The knowledge that infectious diseases were caused by harmful bacteria in the environment allowed preventive measures to be developed to exclude them. For example, contamination of water supplies was a common source of infection, including cholera and typhoid, but installation of sealed sewage systems prevented the problem and the treatment of water by sterilizing it before use caused the destruction of harmful bacteria. Today, in Britain, all water for domestic consumption is carefully treated before use so that it is not injurious to health; a subject treated in more detail in Chapter 12.

DEFICIENCY DISEASES

From the time of Pasteur onwards the part played by harmful bacteria in causing infectious diseases was appreciated. However, the opposite possibility – namely that disease could also be caused by the absence of something – was more difficult to comprehend. With the nutritional knowledge of the nineteenth century the concept is not new: 'Man shall not live by bread alone' probably had its origins in observation and magical qualities had been ascribed to rare or seasonal foods throughout history.

Scurvy is a very ancient disease particularly associated with long sea voyages. At the end of the sixteenth century Admiral Hawkins noted that from his own experience he knew of 10 000 seamen who had died of scurvy. In the 1750s Captain Cook, during a long naval expedition to Australia, added citrus fruits and fresh vegetables to his sailors' diet with the result that scurvy was either prevented or cured. At about the same time (1753) the naval surgeon James Lind published his *Treatise of the Scurvy* in which he produced the first experimental evidence linking diet and disease. He demonstrated, by means of the first controlled clinical trial ever carried out, that adding oranges and lemons to the sailors' diet cured scurvy.

However, Lind himself did not fully accept that this was the only cause of scurvy, and believed that prayer, exercise and salt could all effect a cure. It was not until 1912, in a paper published by Gowland Hopkins, that the nature of vitamins and their vital role in maintaining health was established.

It was only after the discovery of vitamin C that the true features of scurvy (the deficiency disease we now recognize) could be identified. Previously, many other symptoms and signs were attributed to 'scurvy', considered by many to be predominantly a state of moral turpitude. Scurvy was defined, by officers above decks, as a disease of the men below decks.

The discovery of vitamins and the consequent understanding of, and ability to cure, deficiency diseases has been hailed as the greatest advance in nutritional science in the twentieth century. The knowledge that the absence of vitamins from the diet could cause diseases such as scurvy and rickets brought about a fundamental change in attitudes to food. It also focused attention on diet and established it as a major factor in causing disease as well as in maintaining health. The whole science of biochemistry emerged from the discovery of vitamins.

CONCEPT OF A BALANCED DIET

As discussed in Chapter 1, our bodies will only attain and maintain a healthy condition if they receive a supply of food that provides adequate amounts of all the nutrients, and an appropriate amount of energy. Such a diet is known as a balanced diet. A healthy diet will also be one that does not contain anything harmful.

The concept of a balanced diet has arisen mainly in the lay literature. The nutrient needs can, in principle, be defined precisely at a specific time, and under specific conditions. However, conditions (e.g. temperature, exercise, health, stage of growth and reproduction) change over hours, days and over the life cycle. Nutrient needs change with them. In principle, the nutrients provided in food should match these needs, and the 'goodness of fit' is determined by the balance of nutrients from different foods. If the matching or balance is imperfect, then either the body has to adapt by restricting its function, or it has to adapt by developing a system of storage of critical nutrients, to be able to store them when they are in ample supply for use later.

A further constraint is that we only eat intermittently, but metabolism and function must continue. This introduces another potential mismatch between supply and demand, and 'goodness of fit' (of the diet for the needs of the consumer) is improved first by a prolonged period of digestion and absorption, so the nutrients in food do not all arrive at the same moment, and second by having a capacity for short-term (between-meal) storage. For some nutrients (e.g. triglycerides), blood concentrations vary substantially after eating, but for others (e.g. sodium and glucose) blood concentrations cannot fluctuate without causing damage, so there is need for a sensitive, enzyme-based detection and feedback control system.

Until the 1960s protein was considered to occupy a key place in a healthy diet. Great emphasis was given to the need for sufficient protein and to its quality. Animal protein in particular was considered to be especially desirable on account of its high *biological value*, i.e. its goodness of fit, or closeness of matching our needs in terms of specific amino acids. Much less emphasis is now placed on the need to eat plenty of high-quality protein. This is partly because the body's need for protein is less than was previously considered necessary and partly because if the diet contains enough 'energy foods', i.e. carbohydrate and fat, it will almost certainly also contain enough protein. In other words, if the carbohydrate and fat in the diet are right, the protein will look after itself on most western diets.

This does not necessarily apply, however, to restricted diets in the developing world, or to the situation in infancy, pregnancy or recovery from injury, when there may be increased need for specific amino acids. Fat is the most compact source of energy in the diet. The quality and quantity of fat in a healthy diet is the subject of much research and debate which is considered in more detail in Chapter 6. In general, however, there is agreement that the quantity of fat in the diet of affluent countries needs to be reduced and that the quality needs to be adjusted in favour of vegetable and fish oils and fats (or more accurately in favour of polyunsaturated oils and fats) at the expense of animal (or saturated) fats.

One result of promoting the balanced diet concept, which nutritionists were doing until the late 1970s, was that food was thought to be as good as the nutrients that it contained and nutrients were only considered to be those which are essential. That part of food which did not contain nutrients was written off as 'roughage'. Roughage is the indigestible part of food; chemically, it consists mainly of cellulose while physically it consists of the cell walls of plants. Refined foods are those that have been processed so as to remove part or all of the cell walls of the natural foods from which they are derived. Sugar, for example, is a completely refined food. It contains no trace of the cell walls of the sugar-cane or sugar-beet from which it is derived; it is 'pure' sucrose. White flour is a refined food in the sense that a considerable proportion of the cell walls of the wheat from which it is made has been removed. Nevertheless, it is not completely refined, it still contains some 'roughage'. This terminology is unhelpful for human nutrition. Plant cell wall is now recognized to provide non-starch polysaccharide (NSP or dietary fibre). It contains several classes of carbohydrates which escape digestion in the small intestine and which provides the vital source of energy for bacteria in the large bowel. They metabolize most NSP, and as a consequence release nutrients ('volatile fatty acids' – acetate, butyrate and propionate) which are absorbed from the colon. The contribution of NSP to human metabolism (as distinct from starch) is first as a source of non-glucose energy (2–3 kcal/g), second a specific source of locally available nutrients for the colon, third as a modifier of lipid synthesis in the liver (an action of volatile fatty acids) and fourth as the energy source which allows colonic bacteria to perform a variety of important function.

We now acknowledge that food is more than the essential nutrients it contains and that NSP is a necessary part of a healthy diet. At present, there is an emphasis on the need for having plenty of unrefined carbohydrate in the diet while reducing the amount of refined carbohydrate. This can be achieved by eating whole foods rather than processed foods. Apart from protein, fat and carbohydrate (including NSP), the diet must also supply adequate amounts of vitamins and mineral elements. As already noted, examples of vitamin deficiency are now rare in western countries. As for mineral elements, the consensus is not that such diets are deficient in minerals but that one mineral salt, namely sodium chloride, should be restricted as a diet high in salt may predispose to hypertension (high blood pressure). The overall 'balance' of a healthful diet has largely been defined in terms of dietary reference values (DRVs) based on safe intakes to prevent deficiency (Chapter 5). The newer concept of 'optimal diet' is not yet defined in quantities for all nutrients, but is based on the avoidance of chronic diseases. The possible impact on health of other non-essential nutrients, such as caffeine or flavonoids are under research.

DIET AND DISEASES OF AFFLUENCE

The rise in the incidence of 'diseases of affluence' such as obesity, type 2 diabetes, coronary heart disease (CHD) and cancer in the western world has become a major preoccupation of both medical and nutritional science. It is known that these diseases, unlike infectious and deficiency diseases, do not have a single origin, but that a number of different factors are involved – i.e. they are multifactorial in origin. The factors implicated include age, sex, weight, lifestyle (including, for example, exercise and stress), smoking, blood pressure and diet.

Coronary heart disease (CHD) has been more intensively studied than other diseases of affluence, not least because it is a major direct cause of death and disability in developed countries. *Epidemiology*, the study of disease patterns, reveals that CHD is more prevalent in some countries – the developed ones – than in others, and that the disease occurs more in men than in women, mainly in old age but increasingly in middle age. From these observations common diet and lifestyle factors are looked for that might correlate with the distribution of the disease, in order to identify *risk factors*, that appear to have some causal or predisposing connection with the disease.

The main risk factors for cardiovascular disease have been identified as smoking, diabetes and impaired glucose tolerance, raised blood pressure and high blood LDL cholesterol. These last three are closely dependent on being overweight or obese and on being physically inactive. In an ongoing, long-term study of CHD carried out in Framingham, USA (www.nhlbi.nih.gov/about/framingham/index.html), the nature of these risk factors was investigated. Taking men in the 30–62 year age-group, it was found that smoking more than 20 cigarettes a day almost doubled the risk of CHD, that high blood pressure more than doubled the risk and that high blood cholesterol increased the risk by a factor of 2.5. The presence of diabetes compounds the effect of other risk factors.

These risk factors are additive, the risk of CHD increases with each risk factor, as illustrated in Fig. 3.1 which relates to men aged 45 years. Where all three major risk factors are present, the risk of CHD is nearly four times greater than the average. This study also showed that people who live stressful lives – those who are aggressive, competitive and harassed – are more likely to be at risk from CHD than those who lead less stressful lives.

Another major American study, the Boston Nurses Study (Manson *et al.* 1990) showed how all these major risk factors are enormously exaggerated by being overweight or obese. Obese women with high cholesterol, diabetes, hypertension or smoking have a risk of a heart attack up to 12 times that of ideal-weight individuals [body mass index (BMI) 20–21] without the risk factor (Fig. 3.2).

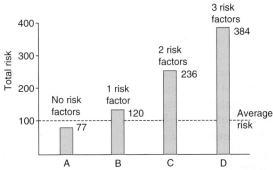

Figure 3.1 *How the number of risk factors increases the risk of coronary heart disease (CHD). A: Men who do not smoke and have normal blood pressure and blood cholesterol. B: Men who smoke and have normal blood pressure and blood cholesterol. C: Men who smoke, have normal blood pressure but very high blood cholesterol. D: Men who smoke, have very high blood pressure and very high blood cholesterol*

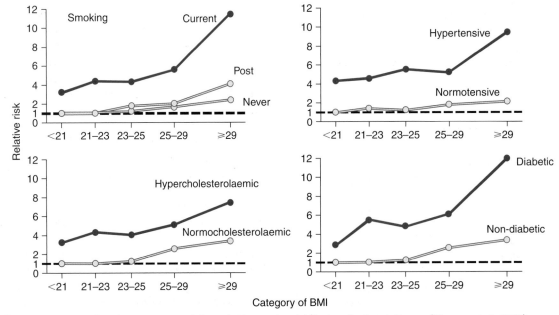

Figure 3.2 *Interactions between overweight and other major risk factors for heart disease (Manson* et al. *1990). Reproduced by kind permission, © Massachusetts Medical Society.*

While classical correlation studies have identified a number of risk factors for CHD, the results fail to explain why the incidence of CHD varies so much from place to place. More recent studies have highlighted the possible importance of *antioxidants* in the body. These studies have shown that there is an inverse relationship between dietary plasma antioxidant levels (e.g. vitamins C, E and β carotene) and CHD, that is antioxidants may exert a protective effect against CHD (see p. 74 for newer theories of CHD).

Correlation studies provide valuable evidence, but cannot prove that a risk factor is a cause. The importance of a risk factor needs to be evaluated in practical ways. There is a hierarchy of evidence from different study designs in epidemiology (Fig. 3.3), but proof can only be concluded with certainty from intervention studies. In these studies, groups of people change their habits in a particular way, showing how changing a particular habit or factor can affect the incidence of the disease.

Many different aspects of diet appear to play a role, including excessive intake of food in general (leading to obesity), excessive intake of particular nutrients (including fat, especially saturated fat) and insufficient intake of polyunsaturated fat and fibre. These nutrient relationships with CHD are derived from information collected about people's food intakes or food purchases. Assumptions have to be made about the composition of foods in order to reach conclusions about nutrients. In many ways, it is often more accurate and more practically helpful to present associations with consumption of foods or food groups. In this way it is possible to show relationships between CHD and high intakes of meat products, or low consumption of fruit and vegetables.

A number of recent reports have been published in the UK and Europe, and by many other nations, which provide a basis for formulating goals for diet, nutrition and health in general, and for producing nutritional and dietary guidelines that could help reduce the incidence of CHD and other diseases of affluence in particular. These reports are considered in more detail in Chapter 17.

CONCEPTS OF HEALTH AND FOOD QUALITY

Health has been defined as 'the attainment and maintenance of the highest state of mental and bodily vigour of which any individual is capable'. The World Health Organization has defined 'health' as a state of complete physical, mental and social well-being and not merely the absence of disease or infirmity. Food contributes to all these components but a complete understanding of health and nutrition leads us to reject the view that food is nothing more than the nutrients.

Nutrients are important, but so is the crunchy texture of an apple, a raw carrot or a nut, the chewiness and aroma of freshly baked wholemeal bread, the satisfying feeling that comes from eating a bowl of muesli and dried fruit, the mouth-watering appearance and smell of fresh strawberries. Food should be fun as well as functional if it is to optimize well-being.

It is unhelpful only to see our bodies as slow combustion machines and food as fuel, just as it is unhelpful to see food as a sort of medicine that can reduce the possibility of disease. Food is for enjoying as well as for doing us 'good'. Health comes not merely from eating the 'right foods' but from our attitudes, approach to life and our lifestyle. Stress and anxiety may contribute as much, or more, to poor health as a poor nutrient balance. Thus, the social and cultural aspects of foods and meals, taste, texture, aroma and even the political conditions of food production can all contribute to well-being, alteration of stress and overall food quality.

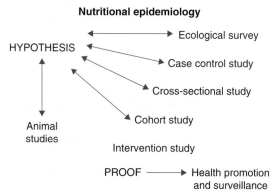

Figure 3.3 *Hierarchy of research methods to establish links between diet and disease*

REGULATION OF APPETITE AND EATING

Conventionally, animals either graze continuously for most of the day, or eat in episodic bouts or meals. Herbivores need such an enormous bulk of green leaves to obtain their energy needs, that grazing is necessary, even with an extra specially adapted stomach (the rumen) which can digest cellulose. When the food supply contains larger amounts of starch, protein or fat, where energy is more concentrated, intermittent meals become possible. This consideration is most apparent with larger animals, whose metabolic rate is lower, in relation to body weight, than smaller animals. A lion will eat only every few days, whereas a cat eats every day.

Humans show some latent grazing tendencies, although we are well-adapted to eating episodic high-energy meals.

Conventionally, we eat, and then feel pleasantly satisfied, or satiated, for a period of a few hours when we do not eat. Then, an appetite develops, which leads us to stop whatever we are doing and seek food. This cycle of eating–satiation–appetite–eating is driven by signals in the hypothalamus, and a great deal is known about the peptides and other hormones involved, and the effect of nutrients or these systems.

If we do not eat when we have an appetite, then hunger develops. Hunger is characterized by physical symptoms in the abdomen and a sense of anxiety. Initially, we are stimulated by hunger preparing us to exert ourselves – or even fight – for food. Subsequently, prolonged food deprivation and starvation results in inactivity and conservation of remaining energy. These phases all have obvious value for survival in a threatening environment where food supplies are intermittent, and evolution has provided us with sophisticated counterbalanced systems to regulate our responses to eating and to food deprivation. Recent scientific interest has focused on the role of adipose tissue (fat) itself. Adipose tissue was usually considered a dull tissue where fat is stored if we eat more than is needed until the next meal, and then released for later energy supply. It has recently come to light that adipose tissue is also a very active endocrine organ, releasing a large number of hormones with different actions (Table 3.1) all regulated by changes in body

Table 3.1 Hormones secreted by adipose tissue

Hormones
Adiponectin
Resistin
Angiotensin
Plasminogen activator inhibitor-1 (PAI-1)
Tumour necrosis factor (TNF)-α
Interleukin (IL)-6
Leptin
Androgens and oestrogens (converted by adipose tissue aromatase)

fat stores. The most celebrated of these hormones is leptin, released when adipose cell fat content is high, but not if it is low. Animal studies show that low, or falling, levels of leptin provide a signal for appetite (or perhaps hunger) and eating, and animals seek food less when leptin levels are low. This system works through another peptide, neuropeptide Y, and is counterbalanced by yet another brain peptide, POMC (pro-opio-melanocortin) which promotes eating. There are many other factors but animals without leptin have huge appetites and become very obese.

In humans, rare genetic abnormalities exist which result in absence of leptin or deficiency of its receptor, and obesity results. However, most obese people have lots of leptin, to which they are resistant for some reason, and their high appetite remains.

All the endocrine factors which regulate appetite in animals exist in humans and present possible targets for new drugs designed to control appetite and eating. However, in every case to date, potent drugs have only very modest effects on eating and on body weight. The reason for this is that human eating patterns appear to respond to influences outside appetite. We are all familiar with the feeling of pleasant fullness, or satiety, after a meal, but know that we can still be tempted by an attractive new food or drink. It takes will-power to resist a chocolate after dinner even when we have no appetite.

Several factors are well-described as stimuli to eating. Boredom is one, and inactivity. Food advertising takes advantage of this when advertising snacks or nibbles to bored, inactive people watching television. Comfort-eating is well described, and again the food industry is ready to market products to be eaten between meals, with the suggestion that they may provide comfort. Most are high in sugar and fat, and so high in energy.

The consequence of this is that for humans, and particularly people with weight problems, eating is less governed by the highly regulated systems of hypothalamic appetite control than by non-appetite systems. These systems are still governed by neuro-endocrine factors, but their interactions with mood and other brain functions mean that drugs are likely to have other unwanted actions before affecting eating. The solution to controlling eating habits lies first in recognizing the complexity of the problem, and then in adopting strategies which will modify boredom, inactivity and comfort other than by food. We need to listen to our bodies more carefully and recognize these signals as distinct from appetite.

METABOLISM AND THE ROLE OF DIET IN REGULATION

Metabolism is a very general term to refer to virtually all the functions and biochemical processes in the body which is not doing external work. Even then, the processes involved in doing external work are essentially the same.

Metabolic rate refers to the total energy turnover of the body (usually expressed as kcal/24 h or kJ/24 h) during a particular activity. At rest, metabolic rate is determined by the necessary work of breathing, or the heart pumping, and of organ functions. The brain uses one-quarter or more of all blood supply and calories used at rest.

When food is consumed, the processing of nutrients involves expenditure of energy, so metabolic rate increases. Both carbohydrates and protein increase metabolic rate considerably, so some calories are wasted on heat; fat does not stimulate metabolism as much. Metabolism increases in organs when they are functioning (especially muscles and heart), and is also affected by a variety of signals from nerves and hormones. Metabolic rate is increased by the nervous system, by adrenaline and by thyroid hormones. Metabolic rate falls if tissues become cold, and when there is a deficiency of thyroid hormones.

OBESITY

Causes and effects of obesity

As mentioned above, obesity is considered to be the result of many factors (see Chapter 5). The most important of these are as follows:

1 *Genetic factors:* there is sound evidence to suggest that a disposition to obesity may be inherited but precise genes are not known.
2 *Composition of the diet:* while it is true that both the nature and quality of food eaten are important in controlling obesity, evidence that any simple component of diet is especially significant in promoting or preventing weight gain is weaker. The totality of the evidence indicates that a diet with high energy density (calories per mouthful) is most likely to promote obesity. This is usually because of a high fat content (and percentage of calories). Snacks and sugary drinks consumed between meals also contribute.
3 *Eating behaviour:* eating behaviour varies from person to person according to various physiological and psychological factors. For example, overweight people have a tendency to underestimate their intake of food. The palatability of food also affects eating behaviour. For example, the wide availability of processed foods that are both convenient and highly palatable has been shown to increase the amount of food eaten and therefore energy intake. People eat more if offered a choice.
4 *Energy expenditure:* the epidemic of obesity over the last 20 years appeared to start when people's physical activity levels dropped below a certain threshold, below which energy expenditure is insufficient for appetite regulation, and a paradoxical increase in food consumption develops. People who avoid weight gain tend to walk more than those who become obese. It is also possible that people having deficient diet-induced thermogenesis (see p. 7) or with a relatively low metabolic rate for their weight may be pre-disposed to obesity.

5 *Other factors:* both hormonal and psychological factors contribute to obesity. Older cigarette smokers have lower body weights than non-smokers, and it is established that giving up smoking frequently leads to weight gain. One reason for this is that metabolic rate decreases after giving up smoking. Young smokers, however, tend to be more overweight.

Obesity is a major threat to health, and this health risk increases progressively through the different grades of obesity. For example, the mortality rate of people with BMI of 35 is about twice that for people of the same age with a BMI of 20–25 (Table 3.2). In particular, obesity has an adverse effect on the cardiovascular system, increasing the hazards from all the major risk factors for coronary heart disease.

Obese people are much more likely to suffer from diabetes than slimmer people and this may lead to kidney failure and blindness, as well as heart disease and stroke. Obese women are more likely to be infertile than slim women and if they do become pregnant they risk having toxaemia and difficulty in childbirth. Obese people (especially women) are more likely to develop gall-bladder disease than slim people because they produce excessive amounts of cholesterol which predisposes to the development of gallstones. Obesity increases the risk of osteoarthritis, especially of the knees, hips and spine and of back pain.

There is considerable evidence, much of it obtained by the American Cancer Society, that increasing obesity gives rise to an increased risk in men of cancer of the colon, rectum and prostate and an increased risk in women of cancer of the breast, cervix and uterus.

Table 3.2 Use of body mass index (BMI) to classify body weight[a]

BMI (weight/height^2)		Description of body weight
Below 18.5	*–*	*Underweight*
18.5–25	*Grade 0*	*Normal*
25–30	*Grade I*	*Overweight*
30–40	*Grade II*	*Moderate obesity*
Over 40	*Grade III*	*Severe obesity*

[a]WHO classification

Depression is a more frequent and more intractable problem in obese people. It is often a reflection of poor self-esteem.

ANOREXIA NERVOSA

The term anorexia means a loss of appetite. However, *anorexia nervosa* is a disease that results from fears of the results of satisfying appetite rather than loss of appetite itself. It is a psychiatric illness where the specific cause is often difficult to diagnose. It mainly affects adolescent girls and while some genetic factors may be involved, environmental factors are much more significant, often including complicated relationships with mothers (who may have weight problems).

The disease results in severe loss of weight and may lead to the cessation of menstrual periods. If unchecked, anorexia nervosa may result in death. Treatment is principally by psychotherapy but also involves dietary help. A number of specific nutrient deficiencies can develop, including iron and zinc, which may generate true anorexia (loss of appetite) and impede recovery. The anorexic patient needs to be encouraged to embark on a gradually increasing intake of food and while no special diet is required it should be nutritionally adequate but without an excessive energy content. Recovery may be slow, taking as much as 2–3 years, and there is the possibility that it may be incomplete, in terms of a totally normal perception of body image and totally normal approach to food and eating.

FOOD INTOLERANCE AND ALLERGY

Food intolerance defined as any reproducible adverse reaction to a food may be caused in a number of ways, the principal ones being listed below. Food aversion is distinguished from food intolerance because it has a psychological origin and is often associated with depression or anxiety. Different types of food intolerance are:

1 *Specific substances in food.* Some foods contain substances that either have direct effects or trigger reactions that produce unpleasant symptoms.

Amines present in wine, cheese, yeast extracts and bananas can cause unpleasant effects as can caffeine contained in tea and coffee. For example, strawberries and tomatoes can cause the release of histamine in some people, producing an irritating rash. Adverse reactions of this kind usually only occur after consuming fairly large quantities of the offending food.

2 *Inability to digest certain foods.* Some people suffer from lactose intolerance. Most people digest milk with ease but in some babies and children, and in some adults, especially in Africa, Asia and South America, this ability is lacking. Milk contains the sugar lactose which is digested in the small intestine with the help of the enzyme lactase. Those who suffer from lactose intolerance produce insufficient lactase to digest lactose, with the result that lactose passes into the large intestine where it is converted by bacteria into lactic acid, causing diarrhoea.

3 *Exaggerated physiological responses to nutrients.* For some people introduction of high-fibre foods (e.g. artichokes) can provoke unpleasant gastrointestinal symptoms.

4 *Food allergy and atopy.* Food allergy is a form of food intolerance involving the body's immune system. Normally, the immune system protects the body against substances such as harmful viruses and bacteria but in food allergy it also reacts to certain harmless substances contained in food. The substance producing an allergic reaction is known as an *allergen* and it is either a protein or bound to a protein (e.g. glycoprotein, see p. 140) that is recognized by antibodies.

Studies among children, in particular, have shown that anxiety about food allergy is much more common than true allergy. Parental anxiety often leads to dietary restriction which proves on formal testing to be unnecessary. The consequence is that histamine and other powerful and irritating substances are released into the bloodstream, producing different symptoms depending on whether the antibodies are found in the skin, the digestive tract or the respiratory system. The symptoms most commonly associated with food allergy are urticaria (nettle rash), eczema, asthma, vomiting and diarrhoea. People who develop true food allergy are called 'atopic'. The syndrome of atopy manifests as allergic reactions,

multiple allergies, as well as asthma and hay fever. Rarely, in extreme cases, very acute allergic swelling of mouth, lips, throat and airways known as anaphylactic shock can develop and may be fatal. This has recently been particularly linked with peanuts, even in miniscule 'trace' amounts.

The treatment of food intolerance is easiest where there is an immediate reaction to food consumed. In this instance it is relatively easy to isolate the food causing the trouble and eliminate it from the diet. Sometimes reaction to allergens does not develop for several hours after eating and the cause may be difficult to identify. The most reliable, but time-consuming, test for allergy is the use of an elimination diet. This involves feeding the patient a limited diet containing foods unlikely to contain allergens and then adding foods containing possible allergens one by one until an allergic reaction is produced. To be effective the suspect foods should be added to the diet without the patient's knowledge, so that psychological aversion to particular foods can be avoided.

The foods and food additives most commonly associated with food intolerance and aversion are cows' milk, eggs, fish, shellfish, nuts, wheat and other cereals, flour, yeast, chocolate, pork, bacon, tenderized meat, coffee, tea, preservatives and artificial colours. Some of these may stimulate allergic reactions, others may contain bioactive compounds. The specific factors in foods such as shellfish may be only intermittently present. Most proteins consumed in foods are broken down by digestion in the gut into amino acids, which are absorbed into the bloodstream (Chapter 2). Very small amounts of proteins are absorbed intact, and these are normally removed by a healthy immune system. At certain times (e.g. in early infancy, or during bowel infections), much larger amounts of intact proteins, especially from common foods such as milk and wheat, reach the bloodstream and sensitize the immune system to cause allergic reactions.

COELIAC DISEASE

Coeliac disease is caused by malabsorption of food resulting in loss of weight and deficiency of mineral elements and vitamins. Coeliac patients are sensitive to the protein gliadin which is part of the gluten (see p. 122) contained particularly in wheat and rye, but only in small quantities in other cereals such as barley, rice and oats. The disease normally originates in childhood after cereals containing gluten are first introduced into the diet, but may develop for the first time in adults.

The cause of the disease is unknown, though it may result from the absence of an enzyme (see Chapter 2) required for the digestion of gliadin. Whatever the cause, sensitivity to gliadin leads to irritation, and eventually destruction, of the villi (see p. 21) in the small intestine which are responsible for the absorption of nutrients and their transfer into the bloodstream. As a result, some nutrients are not absorbed but are excreted from the body, usually as fatty diarrhoea.

Children suffering from coeliac disease do not grow properly, may have a characteristic 'pot belly' and may suffer from anaemia and rickets. In the past, the disease could prove fatal but now it can be cured simply by eliminating all foods containing untreated wheat flour, rye and barley. Such a diet involves avoiding not only the obvious sources of gluten, such as bread and pasta, but also manufactured foods to which wheat flour is added, such as

sausages and sauces. Some manufacturers of baby foods produce gluten-free products, this fact being indicated by a symbol on the label. Gluten-free foods, such as biscuits, bread and flour are made from wheat that has had the gluten removed and such products are widely available. Adults who develop coeliac disease normally present with weight loss and sometimes abdominal pain.

Key points

Food supply affects health:

- Acutely (mainly from microbial infection and toxins)
- Chronically over many years (mainly through subtle balances in the nutrients which affect metabolism)
- By underfeeding and nutrient deficiency (though we are well adapted from evolution)
- By overfeeding (to which evolution did not provide adaptive mechanism)
- By intolerance, including allergies, to certain specific nutrients in some foods

---

Chapter summary

The concept of 'balanced' has various meanings in general speech, but for nutritional science it is used in the same way as in economics. An equal balance of intake and output develops over time, but food and nutrient supply varies and so there is a need for short-term and long-term storage. This is possible for some nutrients (e.g. energy, iron, vitamin B12), but not for others (e.g. amino acids, zinc, vitamin C). In periods of nutrient imbalance, reduced 'goodness of fat' of nutrient supply and demand leads to adaptation and some loss of function, or 'capacity to do'.

FURTHER READING

WORLD HEALTH ORGANIZATION (2003). *Diet, Nutrition and the Prevention of Chronic Diseases.* Geneva: WHO.

MINISTRY OF AGRICULTURE, FISHERIES AND FOOD (1994). *Food Allergy and other Unpleasant Reactions to Food.* London: MAFF.

GARROW JS, JAMES WPT, RALPH A (2000). *Human Nutrition and Dietetics,* 10th edn. London: Churchill Livingstone.

MANN J, TRUSWELL S (1998). *Essentials of Human Nutrition*. Oxford: Oxford University Press.

MANSON JE, COLDITZ GA, STAMPFER MJ *et al.* (1990). A prospective study of obesity and risk of coronary heart disease in women. *New England Journal of Medicine* 882–9.

Website for Anaphylaxis Awareness Group and the Coeliac Association: www.anaphylaxis.org.uk; www.coeliac.co.uk

4

Nutrient dietary requirements and reference values

Chapter 1 outlined the list of essential nutrients but guidance is needed over how much of each to consume. In the past, *recommended daily intakes* (RDI) of nutrients were established for the UK. The RDI was defined as 'the amount sufficient or more than sufficient to meet the nutritional needs of practically all healthy people in a population'. However, as this definition might be interpreted as referring to amounts that individuals must consume rather than averages relating to a group of people, it was later replaced by a recommended daily amount (RDA). This is defined as 'the average amount of the nutrient which should be provided per head in a group of people if the needs of practically all members of the group are to be met'.

There remains the difficulty that RDI, and even RDA, could be, and certainly have been, interpreted as recommended intakes for individuals. In order to overcome this difficulty a new approach was adopted by a specialist panel of the Committee on Medical Aspects of Food Policy (COMA) on dietary reference values, which issued an important report in 1991, 'Dietary Reference Values for Food Energy and Nutrients for the United Kingdom' (DoH, 1991). Terms (and numerical values) from this report are used throughout this book, and an explanation of them is given below.

A healthy diet is often defined in terms of the amount of each nutrient that is required by an individual to prevent signs of clinical deficiency. However, many nutrients have multiple functions and so the amount needed to prevent deficiency may not be the same as the amount of nutrient that will promote optimum health. In addition to the basic need to avoid deficiency, additional amounts may be desirable, so that a nutrient can be stored in the body to provide for times of high demand or low intake. The biological requirement for a nutrient may be altered in illness or by deficiency of another nutrient either upwards or downwards. In other words, the minimum requirement may not be the same as the optimum requirement for an individual, or for groups of people with varying health and needs. Estimating the requirement of each nutrient is complicated, and a variety of approaches have been used. For many nutrients it is not possible, or ethical, to conduct experiments to induce deficiency, in order to define the threshold of adequacy or safety. Moreover, animals' needs are often radically different, so only human data can be used. The earliest (and crudest) method is to measure the consumption of a nutrient in groups of people who do not exhibit deficiency and then to add a safety margin (assuming there is no hazard or toxicity from overconsumption) to define the amount which most people should eat. Consumption by individuals with deficiency, or of populations with a high prevalence of deficiency, can be measured as a guide to the lower reference nutrient intake (LRNI), i.e. the lowest safe intake.

Slightly more sophisticated are balance studies, where a defined dose of a nutrient is fed over a prolonged period, and measures of nutrient status are monitored. Declining status (e.g. plasma vitamin C concentrations) would be an indication of inadequate intake. Increasing excretion of the nutrient (usually measured in urine) indicates an intake in excess of need and saturation of storage capacity, whereas falling excretion is an indication of inadequacy. For some nutrients (e.g. iron) it is possible to obtain blood tests which indicate status in terms of storage (serum ferritin) and of transport (serum transferring or iron-binding capacity). For others, such as zinc, there are no reliable measures of status that can be made on blood tests. Indeed, blood tests can be misleading as serum zinc can be increased or decreased by illness. For some nutrients there are direct effects from regulatory mechanism or from other nutrients which can complicate assessment of status. For example, blood calcium concentration is not a good guide to whole body status. First, because serum calcium is usually maintained in a narrow range (whatever the intake or whole-body status) by a complex regulatory mechanism (parathyroid hormone, calcitonin and vitamin D). Changes in blood concentration usually indicate problems in the endocrine regulation; e.g. magnesium deficiency impairs secretion of parathyroid hormone, which manifests as low serum calcium. High serum calcium indicates parathyroid hormone excess more commonly than any dietary excess. Second, calcium is mainly bound to circulating proteins in the blood, so changes in serum albumen affect serum calcium concentration.

Perhaps the most sophisticated approach towards establishing DRVs involves the use of unusual isotopes of minerals which can be measured, on different dietary intake planes, by mass spectroscopy in body tissues. If a nutrient performs a key role in an enzyme system, then measuring that enzyme function on different intake planes can be used to estimate the level of adequate intake.

With all these more complicated methods intended to define DRVs, there is a gain in precision, but it is often not possible to apply the tests to large numbers of people, or to people across the full range of social and physiological circumstances. Thus, there

always remains the need to build in a 'safety factor' into DRVs. This safety factor attempts to provide a margin of excess intake (based on people of average need) to satisfy higher needs of unusual individuals. It thus becomes important to understand the possible adverse consequences of high intake. Some nutrients are directly toxic in excess (e.g. vitamin A and iron). In general, fat-soluble vitamins (A, D, E and K) tend to accumulate in the body if consumed in excess, and have a greater capacity for toxicity than water-soluble vitamins (B and C). Most minerals are potentially toxic and some have well regulated mechanisms to prevent excessive absorption.

A further complexity, in establishing DRVs is that for some nutrients with widely variable dietary provision (e.g. seasonal fluctuations) or variable need, humans have extensive storage capacity and also the capacity to regulate absorption. For example, we usually absorb only a small proportion of dietary iron or calcium. When exposed to very low intakes, however, or during pregnancy when demand increases, there is increased expression of transport proteins in the gut, and the proportion of dietary iron or calcium which is absorbed increases. This kind of adaptation occurs over time, so may be missed in acute experiments.

The emerging concept of 'optimal health' will probably, in time, change the basis on which DRVs have classically been estimated. There is rapidly accumulating evidence that some nutrients, and possibly many more, have long-term influences on health at levels higher than those needed to avoid deficiency. Thus, folate helps avoid coronary heart disease by supporting serum homocysteine, and this occurs at levels well above those needed to prevent folate-deficient anaemia. These influences may be very specific to certain individuals (e.g. the role of folate is preventing neural tube defects) and this will present challenges to public health in the post-genomic arena.

DIETARY REFERENCE VALUES

The term *dietary reference value* (DRV) is an umbrella term. Dietary reference values relate to healthy people and describe the range of desirable consumption levels of a particular nutrient by a group or population. These reference values recognize that individuals within a group have different needs and that intakes will, therefore, vary. Appropriate intakes are described as being distributed about the *estimated average requirement* (EAR), which is an estimate of the average need for food energy or a nutrient. Individual requirements for nutrients are assumed to be distributed according to a normal distribution curve, as shown in Fig. 4.1. The value of EAR indicated in Fig. 4.1 is an average for a group of people: about half of the people in the group will require less than the average, and about half will require more.

Two other important reference points are indicated in Fig. 4.1. The *reference nutrient intake* (RNI) represents a nutrient intake estimated to meet the needs of 97 per cent of a group. It is two standard deviations above the EAR and is equivalent to the previously used RDI. The LRNI is the nutrient intake estimated to meet the needs of only 3 per cent of the group. Intakes below this level are almost certainly inadequate for most members of the group. The LRNI is two standard deviations below EAR.

It is to be hoped that the use of the term *reference* in place of the previously used *recommended* will help avoid the use of DRVs as anything other than estimates. They can still be used to formulate recommendations, but the precise requirement of an individual within the range of the population will not be known.

It is accepted that for a few nutrients, including some vitamins and minerals, there are not enough reliable data upon which to base DRV. In such cases, a safe intake (SI) has been established. A safe intake is defined as the amount that is enough for nearly everyone but not so large as to cause undesirable effects. Although exceeding SI would not necessarily produce undesirable effects (i.e. it is not a toxic level), there is no evidence that it would produce any benefit. In the USA, the term recommendation is still used. These are published regularly and some show minor differences from European DRVs.

USES OF DIETARY REFERENCE VALUES

1 *Individuals.* Great caution needs to be exercised in applying DRVs to the assessment of individual diets. They should only be used as a general guide to the adequacy of an individual's diet. For example, if nutrient intake is above the RNI, it is very unlikely that any individual will be receiving less than they need. Conversely, if nutrient intake is less than the LRNI, it is likely that an individual is receiving less than is needed. It is unusual to know the exact requirement of an individual for any nutrient, except for energy. This uncertainty commonly leads to overdosage. It is very rare for an individual to need much more than the RNI. The DRVs are established for healthy people who are not deficient in any other nutrient. Under these conditions, nutrient requirements may be increased or reduced.

2 *Healthy diets for groups.* The intention here is to prescribe a diet that will maintain the health of the group. In this situation it is wise to adopt diets that provide the RNI. This will mean that almost all the members of the group will receive an intake of nutrients in excess of their requirements. Here the risk that an individual will suffer from nutrient deficiency is very small. The same principles may be applied when considering the provision of food supplies on a national basis. Within any normal population there will be a range of nutrient intakes consumed by people, habitually, from their choices of normal foods. There will also be a range of individual needs that are affected by size, activity, health, the

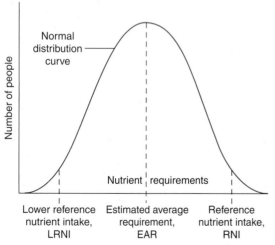

Figure 4.1 *A normal distribution curve of number of people in a population with different nutrient requirements, and the derivation of dietary reference values (DRVs)*

range of other nutrients, variations in the capacity to store a nutrient and by metabolic factors (probably genetic) which influence nutrient metabolism, excretion and function. The DRVs are designed making the assumption that it is very unlikely that an individual with the highest need for a nutrient will be one of those with the lowest intake. In a large population, however, this mismatch will certainly occur.

3 *For labelling of food products.* The EAR values can be used to advantage as a reference point in food labelling. Their use provides a means whereby different products could be compared in terms of their nutrient content, and also a standard form of presentation. Specialist food products, such as baby foods, could use EAR values relevant to a particular age and sex.

The use of EAR on food labels would help consumers appreciate that the values given were nothing more than average values, whereas the use of RDI or RDA values could be misinterpreted to indicate a requirement (or at least an average requirement). With the exception of energy, RDI values are always greater than the requirement. They are set to ensure that the needs of those with very high needs are met, on the understanding that a modest excess of intake would not present a hazard to people with lower needs. This is obviously not the case with energy, where each individual has a very precise need, if weight loss or weight gain are to be avoided.

DRVs are expressed as daily amounts, and it needs to be clearly understood that they apply to groups of *healthy* people; also that the DRVs for any particular nutrient assume that the requirements for energy and all other nutrients are met. Nutrient needs may be very different in others. For many nutrients the requirement varies with age, and in pregnancy and lactation. These are reflected in the DRVs originally published by the UK Department of Health in 1991. They are now kept under review by the Food Standards Agency.

The DRVs for individual nutrients are described in the chapter concerned with that nutrient. Table 4.1 gives some examples of the DRVs for adults aged 19–50 years.

A number of national and international bodies have produced similar sets of recommended nutrient allowances.

In the UK, the food industry has led a novel approach to guiding consumers towards achieving their daily nutrient requirements through food labelling. Guideline daily amounts have been agreed for major nutrients, as a single figure benchmark. The figure is used to describe the amount in a food item or a meal as 'nn% of GDA'. This needs to apply to both male and female consumers of all ages, so the GDAs use the female DRV (EAR) for

Table 4.1 Examples of DRVs for adults aged 19–50 years

	Men aged 19–50	Women aged 19–50
Energy		
EAR, MJ/d [kcal/d]	10.6 [2550]	8.1 [1940]
Macronutrients		
Total fat: % of energy intake	33.0	33.0
Saturated fat: % of energy intake	10.0	10.0
Total carbohydrate: % of energy intake	47.0	47.0
NSP [ENI g/d]	18.0	18.0
Protein [RNI g/d]	55.5	45.0
Folate [RNI µg/d]	200.0	200.0
Vitamin C [RNI mg/d]	40.0	40.0
Calcium [RNI mg/d]	700.0	700.0
Iron [RNI mg/d]	8.7	14.8
Sodium [RNI g/d]	1.6	1.6

Department of Health (1991). *Dietary Reference Values for food energy and nutrients for the United Kingdom. Report of the Panel on Dietary References Values of the Committee on Medical Aspects of Food Policy No 41.* London: HMSO. Crown copyright material is reproduced with the permission of the Controller of HMSO and the Queen's Printer for Scotland.

Table 4.2 Guideline daily amounts

	Men	Women
Calories	2500.0	2000.0
Fat (g/day)	95.0	70.0
Saturates (g/day)	30.0	20.0
Carbohydrates (g/day)	300.0	230.0
Sugars (g/day)	120.0	90.0
Fibre (g/day)[a]	24.0	24.0
Salt (g/day)	6.0	6.0
Sodium (g/day)	2.5	2.5

[a]24 g dietary fibre for food labelling is equivalent to 18 g NSP.

energy (2100 kcal/d) on the guide that overconsumption is usual, and can be permitted for men but not for women, to reduce risk of weight gain. Other GDAs are similarly cautious (Table 4.2). This guidance has been widely adopted and is well accepted. The criteria for computation may need to be reviewed, and possible new developments include guideline meal amounts, to help standardize the size and contents of ready meals, and meals from catering or home-prepared sources.

Key points

- Dietary reference values
  - Define upper and lower amounts to avoid deficiencies and toxicity
  - Do not yet reflect the amount for optimal health
  - Can be used to check and design food supplies for groups or populations
- Should be used with caution for individuals or when attributing disease risk
- Relate to healthy people: different amounts may be needed in diseases

Chapter summary

Dietary reference values include Lower Reference Nutrient Intake, below which most people will become deficient, the Estimated Average Amount for a health population, and the Upper Reference Nutrient Intake which satisfies the needs of nearly all individuals. Both DRVs and Guideline Daily Amounts are used in labels for foods and meals to guide consumers over nutritional adequacy.

FURTHER READING

DEPARTMENT OF HEALTH (1991). *Dietary Reference Values for Food Energy and Nutrients for the United Kingdom. Report on Health and Social Subjects No. 41.* London: HMSO.

FOOD AND AGRICULTURE ORGANISATION, WORLD HEALTH ORGANIZATION (1988). *Requirements of Vitamin A, Iron, Folate and Vitamin B12.* Rome: FAO.

GREGORY J *et al.* (1990). *The Dietary and Nutritional Survey of British Adults.* London: HMSO.

WORLD HEALTH ORGANIZATION (1985). *Energy and Protein Requirements.* Geneva: WHO.
http://www.nal.usda.gov/fnic/etext/000105.html

5

Obesity in the twenty-first century

At several points in this book the food-related issues around obesity are raised. There are many, and the food industry has responded in many ways. Not all are helpful to people with weight problems.

In post-industrial western societies such as the UK, USA and most of Europe, well over half of all people will experience 'a weight problem'. Medically defined obesity – body mass index (BMI) $>30 \, kg/m^2$ or waist $>102 \, cm$ for men, $>88 \, cm$ for women – will be a problem for about one in three as they get older (Table 5.1). Many more will become overweight and almost all adults take some measures to avoid excess weight gain.

The causes of obesity are complicated, but can be reduced to simple terms:

1 A genetic background which predisposes to more weight gain than other people, given the same food supply and physical activity.

2 A reduction in physical activity below the individual threshold necessary for automatic, subconscious balancing of energy in vs. energy out.

3 A food supply characterized by unlimited energy (calorie) availability without the need to work physically for it, with high energy density (calories per mouthful) and with a high proportion of calories (>30 per cent) coming from fat (which does not satisfy appetite as well as carbohydrates or protein).

MEDICAL CONSEQUENCES OF OBESITY

Obesity affects almost every body system (see Table 5.2). The cumulative costs of obesity are colossal, reported at up to 8 per cent of the total spending on health care in the USA.

Table. 5.1 Use of BMI and waist circumference in weight management

		Healthy normal range	Health risks increasing	High risk
			Make personal changes to control weight	*Seek professional help and management*
BMI (kg/m²)		*18.5–25*	*25–30*	*>30*
Waist (cm):	*Men*	*<94*	*94–102*	*>102*
	Women	*<80*	*80–88*	*>88*

Lean MEJ (2003). Management of obesity and overweight. *Medicine* 31, 12–17.

Table 5.2 Medical consequences of overweight and obesity

Medical consequences		
Physical symptoms	**Metabolic**	**Social**
Tiredness	*Hypertension*	*Isolation*
Breathlessness	*NIDDM*	*Agoraphobia*
Varicose veins	*Hepatic steatosis*	*Unemployment*
Back pain	*Hyperlipidaemia*	*Family/marital stress*
Oedema/cellulites	*Hypercoagulation*	*Discrimination*
Sweating/intertrigo	*IHD and stroke*	*Financial*
Stress incontinence		
Anaesthetic/surgical	**Endocrine**	**Psychological**
Sleep apnea	*Hirsutism*	*Low self-esteem*
Chest infections	*Oligomenorrhea/infertility*	*Self-deception*
Wound dehiscence	*Metromenorrhea*	*Cognitive disturbance*
Hernia	*Oestrogen dependent*	*Distorted body image*
Venous thrombosis	*Cancers: breast, uterus, prostate*	*Depression*

PRINCIPLES OF MODERN WEIGHT MANAGEMENT

There is no magic in why some people become obese, and no magic solution will ever be found. No single food or group of foods is responsible, and no new 'diet' will lead to a cure.

There are a variety of behavioural, pharmaceutical and surgical approaches which have been shown scientifically to help people overcome these three problems in controlling their weight. There are literally thousands of products marketed, with a variety of more-or-less implausible claims, which have no evidence for value. It can safely be assumed that they do not work.

For all overweight and obese people (notwithstanding complicated social and psychological backgrounds), there are two components to controlling the problem.

1 *Weight loss.* This is only part of the solution. It can be achieved, with 100 per cent certainty, for 100 per cent of overweight people, by consuming less calories than are used up by metabolism and physical activity. In practice, this means eating fewer calories (not necessarily less volume of food) than at present. All obese people need to eat more calories than thin people in order to stay obese. If they were to eat the same numbers of calories as thin

people, then their weight would all end up much the same (some variation remains because of genetic differences in efficiency, but this is under 20 per cent). To lose weight entails shedding very large numbers of stored calories (7000 kcal/kg of body fat) and to do this means undereating. It is rarely possible for obese people to lose weight purely through physical activity. Recent research and guidelines emphasise that the greatest benefit is losing 5–10 kg. It is not necessary to 'normalise' weight or BMI. This almost will, for example, reduce the incidence of diabetes to less than half what it would be without weight management. All the risk factors contributing to heart disease (e.g. blood pressure, cholesterol, triglyceride, glucose and insulin levels) improve, and so do feelings of depression. This degree of weight loss can be achieved by a variety of interventions including diets, cognitive behavioural therapy, drugs and surgery. All must be considered as appropriate to individual situations.

2 *Weight maintenance.* Achieving energy balance (calories consumed = calories used up) prevents weight gain (or regain) and this is effectively the 'cure' for obesity. Most obese people who are successful in losing weight still find it very difficult to avoid regain – even though the changes from previous (obese) diet and lifestyle are small. Losing a stone (7 kg) reduces metabolic rate by

100–200 kcal/day. To maintain this lower weight, people need either to eat 100–200 kcal/day less – not a big change when the total eaten is 2500–3000 or to increase physical activity to the value of 100–200 kcal/day (e.g. walking 30–40 minutes). These behavioural changes need to be maintained lifelong.

Modern professional weight management is committed to improving health outcomes (physical, mental and social) and so adds two more components.

3 *Identification of people with overweight or obesity.* Two approaches are used. Firstly, in population-directed health promotion, the aim is to alert the public to their rising health risks so that they can take personal action towards preventing further weight gain. BMI >25 kg/m² can be used, but waist circumference >94 cm (37″) for men, or >80 cm (32″) for women are easier to understand and are better guides to health risks. Secondly, screening measurements to identify those who have already reached high levels of risk, in GP surgeries, gyms, worksites etc. BMI >30 kg/m² or waist >102 cm (40″) for men, >88 cm (35″) for women indicate levels which demand professional help to achieve and maintain weight loss of 5–10 per cent.
4 *Prioritization of risk factor management in the overweight and obese.* Because of the interaction between obesity and cardiovascular risk factors, those risk factors (hypertension, high cholesterol and diabetes) need priority treatment in people who are overweight or obese.

DIETS THAT WORK

The dietary keys to achieving, and maintaining, weight loss are the same as those for preventing weight gain in the first place:

1 Foods must be attractive enough to comprise the habitual diet, lifelong.
2 A fat content below 35 per cent, or below 30 per cent for people with proven weight problems generally offers advantages.

Some people find it attractive to follow a 'low-carbohydrate' diet, which has a higher fat and protein content, for a limited time to lose weight, but if

Table 5.3 Energy contents of the macronutrients

	kcal/g
Fat	9
Protein	4
Carbohydrate	3.75
Dietary fibre	2–3

continued into the long-term, 'low-carb' diets tend to increase serum low-density lipoprotein (LDL) cholesterol and also to promote weight regain.

There is some debate as to whether the key element is low fat, or low energy-density of foods which help combat obesity. In practice, these two go together (see Table 5.3).

Other dietary components that contribute to achieving energy balance include a high intake of non-starch polysaccharide (NSP, in foods and not as a supplement) and higher intakes of fruits and vegetables. The last two work probably mainly by displacing other higher energy density, higher-fat foods from the diet.

The nearer to a totally vegetable-based (e.g. vegan) diet, the harder it is to stay overweight or to gain weight. People who eat a large bowl of salad before each main meal tend to be filled up, eat fewer calories in the meal, and find it easier to overcome a weight problem. Drinking a large glass of water before each meal can have the same effect. Both lead to a lower energy-density of the meal.

Almost any diet plan which restricts food choice will help some people to control a weight problem. Cafeteria or buffet-style wide choices encourage greater food, and calorie, consumption.

PORTION SIZE CONTROL

Over the last 20 years, led by a global food market from USA, portion sizes have increased steadily. Research shows that the more food people have in front of them, the more they will eat – especially people with weight problems.

Why people chose larger portions, knowing they have a weight problem, is hard to understand. It may be to do with memories of food shortage, or simply of greed. People are very reluctant to leave or throw away food.

These issues need to be overcome in order to maintain energy balance, by behavioural training and use of smaller plates, etc., and the food industry needs to facilitate this.

FOOD INDISCIPLINE AND BEHAVIOURAL THERAPY

People with weight problems tend to eat in chaotic ways. Some may go to the extreme of bulimia ('eating like a bull' – binging, and often then inducing vomiting). Many eat episodically without following a 'normal' meal routine. The availability of ready-to-eat food at every street corner and petrol station has contributed, and the impact of the ubiquitous bottle of cola or lemonade/soda (10 per cent sugar solution: 400 kcal/L) must not be ignored. Children who drink sugar-free drinks gain less weight.

Again, there needs to be a new balance between the commercial excesses of the 'free market' and the need of a responsible society to safeguard the health of its members. As a first step, it can be suggested that the food industry should find ways of remaining profitable and sustainable while helping the more ignorant and vulnerable to avoid unwanted accumulation of fat.

At an individual level, a number of simple behavioural measures have been found helpful in regulating food choice and eating (see Tables 5.4 and 5.5). They need to be adopted as part of usual, lifelong behaviour.

SLIMMING CLAIMS

There are countless products marketed with claims that their use will cause weight loss (interestingly, few are promoted as ways of avoiding weight gain, which consumers would actually find more valuable). At present, it is not necessary for a food company to do specific research, or produce any evidence, to support these claims. The consequence is that many are fraudulent. Vulnerable, often desperate, obese people spend vast amounts of money in pursuit of completely impossible targets using completely improbable dietary measures. Some of

Table 5.4 Behavioural measures in regulating food choice and eating

Behavioural measures
Eat three meals a day
Eat nothing outside the three meals
Only ever eat sitting down
Never eat with your fingers
Never eat with the television on
Always check the calories on labels
No second helpings – ever
Always choose 'small' items
Prepare breakfast (e.g. porridge) in the evening, so that it is ready for morning
Write a timetable or menu for the day's (or next day's) meals
Make more time for shopping: fruit and vegetables need to be bought twice a week

this may be due to ignorance, but sometimes it is a way of defraying criticism that they have failed to take action in a responsible way. Some obese people feel better about continuing to overeat, and lying about it, if they spend money on a product which promises a cure, even if they know this is fraudulent. New EU regulations (2005) are in preparation which will require there to be evidence for claims on foods.

'ON THE MOVE' FOR OBESITY PREVENTION

At present, the best way forward appears to be to follow the simple, small-change programme of America on the Move (www.americaonthemove.org). The essential elements of America on the Move are:

1 *Increasing steps walked each day by 2000 above current level.* Using a cheap step-counter provides a daily target, and also self-monitoring. People learn ways to increase their steps – by an amount equivalent to walking about 20 minutes, or 1 mile (1.6 km) daily – and then incorporate them into their normal lifestyle. They will also feel better, with less chance of depression. Avoiding physical inactivity, especially TV watching, has been found to be effective for preventing weight gain in children.

Table 5.5 Measures outlined by the Glasgow Weight Management Service

Behavioural measures	
Self-monitoring	This is the foundation of CBT approaches and forms the cornerstone of self-management. Daily records of food intake and activity levels can provide the information required to identify links in the behaviour chain that require to be targeted for change. Also, keeping records of eating and activity behaviours encourages compliance. Regular monitoring of weight is also recommended.
Stimulus control	One of the central elements in behavioural treatment based on the theory that eating is triggered by a number of external and internal cues. These cues for eating are learned as a result of repeated associations between the stimuli and eating food. Individuals are taught how to recognize and avoid triggers that prompt unplanned eating, i.e. habits are developed through repeatedly pairing eating with other activities such as watching TV or mood states like feeling bored. These habits have to be modified for successful weight management in the long term.
Problem-solving	This is the systematic method of identifying and analyzing problems and identifying possible solutions. Individuals are encouraged to consider a range of options to solve problems rather than think there is always a 'perfect solution'.
Contingency management	Involves developing strategies to help with recovery from episodes of overeating or weight regain. Rewarding positive responses reinforces their use in the future.
Relapse prevention	Teach skills to recover from lapses and deal with high risk situations with a 'plan of action'. This promotes maintenance and helps individuals accept the chronicity of managing their weight and the necessity of keeping vigilant in their new habits. Central to this approach is the increase in self-efficacy that develops when individuals learn how to cope with risky situations without giving up on their new habits.
Stress management	Used to minimize the negative impact of stress on positive eating and activity behaviours. This is important if overeating is triggered by a range of emotions (either positive or negative) and food is habitually used to aid emotional regulation.
Disordered feeding	The initial goal is to establish regular eating patterns. Rigid or chaotic eating patterns are discouraged in favour of flexible, balanced choices. This helps to displace episodes of binge-eating that may be triggered in response to feelings of deprivation.
Cognitive restructuring	Cognitive restructuring helps individuals to think in a more balanced manner by teaching them to identify and modify those unhelpful thoughts that undermine weight control, i.e. typically thoughts concerning the impossibility of achieving weight loss; rigid, unrealistic goals; self-critical responses to any episodes of unplanned eating or weight gain. Self-monitoring of feelings/thoughts in relation to eating and activity is used to identify negative thoughts and then individuals are taught how to make more balanced judgements. Cognitive techniques also help patients accept realistic, but less-than-desired, weight losses by considering the impact of body image. Inappropriate feelings of failure after achieving modest but clinically important weight loss can lead to relapse and weight regain so should be targeted for intervention.
Social support	Social support from family members and friends is important for modifying lifestyle behaviours. Helping individuals consider the impact their relationships have on their lifestyle decisions and dealing with barriers is useful in creating a social structure supportive of weight management.

2 *Reducing energy intake by 100 kcal/day.* Amazingly, this small amount is more than enough to prevent the weight gain of almost all people with obesity. America on the Move has produced lists of up to 100 simple ways to cut 100 kcal. As with physical activity, the aim is for people to adopt these small changes as part of their habitual diets, and the food industry has the potential to modify products and their marketing to facilitate these changes.

3 *Working with employers and others towards a less obesogenic environment.* It is in the commercial interest of employers to prevent obesity in their workforce. America on the Move has pioneered ways of persuading employers to present better opportunities for staff to be physically active and to be able to cut 100 kcal/day – using educating approaches and also changes in catering arrangements.

The On the Move programme thus represents a low-cost, consumer-centred approach, which is potentially sustainable. It has shown prevention of weight gain in Families on the Move, and has been applied to schools, in College Students Worksites and Churches on the Move. Research is ongoing, and a Britain on the Move partnership is being developed.

Key points

- Obesity is defined epidemiologically by BMI $>30\,kg/m^2$
- Clinically and for health promotion
  - Waist $>80\,cm$ (women); $>94\,cm$ (men) (Action Level 1 – for personal action)
  - Waist $>88\,cm$ (women); $102\,cm$ (men) (Action Level 2 – needs professional help)

Chapter summary

Obesity is the most costly disease in 22% of adults in UK, 30% in USA are now obese – i.e. above 15%, the WHO critical threshold for intervention in epidemics. There is then a need for political, social and economic intervention for prevention and also clinical intervention for treatment of obesity. There are many misleading claims made for foods, diets and treatments for obesity. High-fat, energy dense, cheap foods and physical inactivity conspire as causes, and must be addressed for effective management. Weight loss 5–10 kg brings major medical benefits, and maintenance to prevent regain needs structured approaches. Only small changes (walk an extra 2000 steps a day, and cut 100 calories) are needed for prevention of weight gain, but environment change is necessary for sustainability.

FURTHER READING

DEPARTMENT OF HEALTH (2004). *Choosing Health: Making Healthier Choices Easier.* London: Department of Health.

DEPARTMENT OF HEALTH (2005). *Choosing a Better Diet: A Food and Health Action Plan.* London: Department of Health.

DEPARTMENT OF HEALTH (2005). *Choosing Activity: A Physical Activity Action Plan.* London: Department of Health.

International Association for the Study of Obesity: www.iotf.org

SWINBURN B, EGGER G (2004). Influence of obesity-producing environments. In Bray G, Bouchard C, (eds). *Handbook of Obesity: Clinical Applications,* 2nd edition. New York: Marcel Dekker.

WORLD HEALTH ORGANIZATION (2004). Global strategy on diet, physical activity and health. Geneva: WHO. [www.who.int/dietphysicalactivity/en/]

6

Fats, oils and lipids

The term *lipid* is a general one that is used to describe a large group of naturally occurring fat-like substances. They form a diverse group of compounds that have little in common except that they are soluble in organic solvents such as chloroform and alcohols but are not soluble in water. Lipids are essential, structural and functional components of all membranes. Indeed, the appearance of lipids was essential to the emergence of life. Lipids in plants, animals and foods also provide a base in which other 'lipid-soluble' compounds can dissolve. They are organic compounds which all contain carbon, hydrogen and a small amount of oxygen. Many lipids are derivatives of fatty acids. Fatty acids are essentially acid groups attached to chains of carbon atoms, with two hydrogen atoms added to each like the inorganic paraffin oils. Oils and fats, waxes and phospholipids are examples of lipids that are fatty acid derivatives. Steroids are also classified as lipids, though they are not direct fatty acid derivatives and they are dissimilar in structure to the rest of the group.

Oils and fats are of major importance in food and nutrition. Chemically they belong to a class of substances known as esters, which result from the reaction of 'fatty' acids with alcohols, which in turn result from the hydrolysis of fatty acids. Fats are esters of the trihydric alcohol glycerol. The three hydroxyl groups of the glycerol molecule can each combine with a fatty acid molecule and the resulting ester is called a triglyceride. The simplest type of triglyceride results when the three acid molecules are all the same. For example, if three molecules of stearic acid react with a molecule of glycerol, the fat formed is glyceryl tristearate tristearin:

$$\begin{array}{ccc} & \text{HOCH}_2 & \text{C}_{17}\text{H}_{35}\text{COOCH}_2 \\ & | & | \\ 3\text{C}_{17}\text{H}_{35}\text{COOH} + \text{HOCH}_2 \rightleftharpoons \text{C}_{17}\text{H}_{35}\text{COOCH} + 3\text{H}_2\text{O} \\ & | & | \\ & \text{HOCH}_2 & \text{C}_{17}\text{H}_{35}\text{COOCH}_2 \end{array}$$

Stearic acid   Glycerol   Tristearin

In terms of chemistry, the words oils and fats are interchangeable; the only distinction between them is that at normal temperatures oils are liquids while fats are solids. However, this distinction is rather vague, as a 'normal' temperature cannot be accurately defined, and some 'oils', such as palm oil, are usually solid at the prevailing temperatures of the British climate. Some oils are volatile, and have a characteristic odour. Oils in biological systems and foods should be distinguished from the inorganic hydrocarbon paraffin oils, the main constituents of petroleum.

Phospholipids are important substances concerned with the transport of lipid in the bloodstream. Lecithin is one of the most significant phospholipids; it is made up of a group of substances that play a major role in the digestion of fats and, as such, it has already been encountered in Chapter 2. Phospholipids are similar to fats in that they have a structure based on glycerol but instead of the three hydroxyl groups being combined with a fatty acid (see below) only two are so combined, the third being combined with phosphate linked to choline. Lecithin is found in some foods, notably egg yolk. It is not an essential part of the diet for healthy individuals as it is manufactured by the body.

Steroids, as already indicated, are very different in structure from other lipids but include the important substances cholesterol, cortisone and sex hormones. Cholesterol is a white fat-like substance which is present in body tissues and is found in a variety of animal foods, notably brain, kidney, liver and egg yolk. Meat and fish contain small amounts and dairy foods contain a little. The body of an adult contains about 140 g cholesterol, found in all parts including the membranes of every cell, especially nerve cells. Cholesterol is also important in the body as the source of raw material from which bile acids and several hormones – including cortico-sterone from the adrenal gland and sex hormones – are made. The fat-soluble vitamins (A, D, E and K) and related compounds are based on cholesterol. The body obtains some cholesterol from the diet (except strict vegetarian diets) but most is made in the body, especially by the liver, although all body cells can make cholesterol.

Waxes are indigestible compounds made from fatty acids combined with any alcohol except glycerol. Animal waxes are often esters of cholesterol. Waxes are of no particular importance in food science and will not be encountered again in this chapter.

OILS AND FATS

Oils and fats are of great importance in food science since they are used in their own right, for example, in cooking, in salad oils and as spreads, and as ingredients in many manufactured and cooked foods. They are important in nutrition as the most compact energy source available (9 kcal/g) and they play an important role in body metabolism. The specific roles of different fatty acids in promoting health and disease, a subject considered in the next chapter is of major public health concern.

Fatty acids

Fatty acids are those organic acids which are found in fats chemically combined with glycerol. Fatty acids are known as carboxylic acids because they contain the carboxyl group –COOH. Over 40 different fatty acids are found combined as part of triglycerides. It should be noted that where fatty acids are referred to as being part of fats this means that they occur chemically linked with glycerol and not as free acids. Natural fats never consist of a single triglyceride but are mixtures of triglycerides with different fatty acids contents. Commonly, more than one type of fatty acid is bound to glycerol in a triglyceride molecule.

Fatty acids consist of a chain of carbon atoms (each with hydrogen atoms attached) with a carboxyl group at the end. The length of the carbon chain varies, but the number of carbon atoms is always an even number between four and 24. The commonest fatty acids contain 16 or 18 carbon atoms (see Table 6.1). For example, stearic acid, $CH_3(CH_2)_{16}COOH$, contains 18 carbon atoms. There are three types of fatty acid which may be classified as follows.

1   *Saturated fatty acids* in which the carbon atoms are linked together by single bonds. Thus, the carbon

Table 6.1 Fatty acids most commonly found as part of triglycerides

Saturated		Monounsaturated		Polyunsaturated	
Butyric	$C_{4:0}$	Palmitoleic	$C_{16:1}$	Linoleic	$C_{18:2}$
Caproic	$C_{6:0}$	Oleic	$C_{18:1}$	Linolenic	$C_{18:3}$
Caprylic	$C_{8:0}$	Erucic	$C_{22:1}$	Arachidonic	$C_{20:4}$
Capric	$C_{10:0}$			Eicosopentanoic	$C_{22:5}$
Lauric	$C_{12:0}$			Docosahexanoic	$C_{22:6}$
Myristic	$C_{14:0}$				
Palmitic	$C_{16:0}$				
Stearic	$C_{18:0}$				

chain consists only of repeated CH_2 groupings: $—CH_2—CH_2—$. An example is stearic acid, whose formula is noted above.

2 *Monounsaturated acids* in which there is one double bond in the carbon chain (see below). Thus, the chain contains two 'unsaturated' carbon atoms each joined to only one hydrogen atom: $—CH= CH—$. For example, the component oleic acid, $CH_3(CH_2)_7CH=CH(CH_2)_7COOH$, is a monounsaturated fatty acid.

3 *Polyunsaturated fatty acids* (PUFAs) in which there are two or more double bonds in the carbon chain: $—CH=CH—CH_2—CH=CH—$. For example, linoleic acid, $CH_3(CH_2)_4CH=CHCH_2$ $CH=CH(CH_2)_7COOH$, contains two double bonds in its carbon chain. There are two main classes of PUFA, n-3 and n-6 (or omega-3 and omega-6 using an alternative terminology) defined by the place of the first double bond.

The nature of single and double bonds

The distinction between saturated and unsaturated fatty acids is that the former contain carbon atoms linked by single bonds, whereas the latter contain at least two carbon atoms linked by double bonds.

A carbon atom contains four electrons in its outer shell, and when it combines with other elements, such as hydrogen, it does so by sharing these electrons in order to gain the stable structure conferred by eight electrons in the outer shell. The combining together of elements by electron sharing is known as covalence; the bond so formed is a covalent bond. A covalent bond consists of a shared pair of electrons where each of the two atoms involved provides one electron for sharing. When carbon atoms link together to form a chain consisting of single bonds each carbon atom can combine with two hydrogen atoms:

$$\begin{array}{cc} H & H \\ | & | \\ —C—C— \\ | & | \\ H & H \end{array} \quad \text{or} \quad —CH_2—CH_2—$$

Each dash between atoms represents a shared pair of electrons, i.e. a single covalent bond. In order to gain a stable octet of electrons each carbon atom forms four covalent bonds with adjacent atoms.

Carbon atoms can also link together so as to form chains containing double bonds. Four electrons are involved in the formation of a double bond – two from each of the carbon atoms concerned – so that fewer electrons are available for forming bonds with hydrogen. Each carbon atom can now only combine with one hydrogen atom in order to gain its stable octet of electrons. A double bond is represented by a double dash:

$$\begin{array}{cc} H & H \\ | & | \\ —C=C— \end{array} \quad \text{or} \quad —CH=CH—$$

the more double bonds that a carbon–hydrogen chain possesses the greater is its degree of unsaturation.

The degree of unsaturation of a fat is important in determining its physical and chemical or nutritional properties. All natural fats found in foods contain a mixture of saturated and unsaturated fatty acids (always combined with glycerol), but the greater the proportion of the latter the lower is the melting point of the fat. Fats which are high in unsaturated fatty acids (e.g. olive oil, sunflower seed oil) are therefore liquid at room temperature (i.e. they are oils) while those rich in saturated fatty acids are solid at room temperature but soft at body temperature (e.g. butter or lard) (see Table 6.2). Thus, animal fats tend to be more saturated, so stay slightly soft at normal body temperature, whereas cold-blooded fish and vegetable fats tend to be more unsaturated, so stay as oils which are slightly firmer at environmental temperature. Cell membranes function best when neither hard nor completely liquid.

The degree of unsaturation of an oil or fat can be measured by its iodine value. When iodine (in practice the more reactive iodine monochloride is used) is added to a triglyceride formed from an unsaturated fatty acid, it reacts with the double bonds in the molecule, and the degree of unsaturation may be calculated from the amount of iodine absorbed:

$$—CH=CH— + I_2 \rightarrow —CHI—CHI—$$

One molecule of iodine is used to saturate each double bond. The result is usually expressed as the iodine value which is the number of grams of iodine needed to saturate $100\,g$ of oil. For example, the iodine value of butter is 26–38, while the iodine value of olive oil is 80–90.

The fatty acids most commonly found as part of edible oils and fats are shown in Table 6.1. Oleic acid is the most commonly occurring fatty acid in nature,

Table 6.2 The per cent combined fatty acid content of oils and fats

| Oil or fat | Saturated | | | Monounsaturated | PUFA | |
	Myristic $C_{14:0}$	Palmitic $C_{16:0}$	Stearic $C_{18:0}$	Oleic $C_{18:1}$	Linoleic $C_{18:2}$	Other PUFAs
Butter	8	22	9	16	1	1
Lard	1	24	14	39	9	1
Margarine	5	23	9	33	12	1
Margarine (polyunsaturated)	1	12	8	22	52	1
Fish oil	6	13	3	18	3	28
Olive oil	0	10	3	72	8	0
Palm oil	1	42	5	37	10	0
Rapeseed oil	0	4	2	58	20	9
Corn oil	0	11	2	29	50	1
Soya bean oil	0	11	4	21	52	7
Sunflower seed oil	0	6	4	20	63	0
Safflower seed oil	0	7	2	11	74	0

PUFA, polyunsaturated fatty acid.
Sources: Ministry of Agriculture, Fisheries and Food (1998) *Fatty Acids – Supplement. McCance & Widdowson's The Composition of Foods.* RSC/MAFF, Cambridge/London.

and in most fats it forms at least 30 per cent of the total fatty acids. Its name refers to its abundance in olive oil. Palmitic acid is also widely distributed and is found in every natural fat, usually accounting for 10–50 per cent of the total fatty acids.

Table 6.1 uses a convenient shorthand method for describing fatty acids. Butyric acid $C_{4:0}$ means that it contains four carbon atoms but no double bonds, while linolenic acid $C_{18:3}$ contains 18 carbon atoms and three double bonds.

Table 6.2 shows the contribution made by fatty acids in combination with glycerol (as triglycerides) to some important oils and fats. The total fatty acid content is taken as 100, the figures for the individual combined acids are average values, as oils from different places vary in composition. Some other fatty acids not shown in the table occur in these oils and fats. In particular, butter contains 13 per cent $C_{4:0}$ to $C_{12:0}$ fatty acids ('medium-chain fatty acids'), rapeseed oil used to contain as much as 33 per cent erucic acid although the amount of erucic acid in foods is now restricted by law due to its adverse effect on digestibility, growth and heart muscle. About 40% of PUFAs in fish oil is arachidonic acid.

It is often stated that animal fats are saturated while vegetable oils are unsaturated. While there is

some considerable truth in this generalization, it must be recognized that all these fats and oils are mixtures of both, as Tables 6.2 and 6.3 demonstrate. This table shows the more important dietary sources of saturated and polyunsaturated fats, those of animal origin being shown in italics. From the above generalization it might be presumed that when the label on a packet of margarine declares that it is made from blended vegetable oils, it would contain a high proportion of PUFA. However, if it is a cheap brand, it may well be made from palm and coconut oils and will therefore contain a high proportion of saturated fatty acids.

Essential fatty acids and n–3 fatty acids

Polyunsaturated fatty acids include the essential fatty acids (EFAs), which, although essential to the body, cannot be made by the body and so must be supplied by food.

There are two essential fatty acids, linoleic acid and alpha-linolenic acid. In addition, there are several other PUFAs (including arachidonic acid and docosahexanoic acid (DHA)) which have important functions in the body. They are not regarded as EFAs

Table 6.3 Sources of saturated and polyunsaturated fats

Sources		
High in saturated fats	Dairy products	Butter, cream, milk, cheese
	Meat	Liver, lamb, beef, pork
	Others	Coconut oil, palm kernel oil, palm oil, hard margarine, lard
High in mono-unsaturated fats	Certain vegetable oils	Olive oil, rapeseed oil and margarines made from them
High in polyunsaturated fats	Vegetable oils	Corn (maize) oil, soya bean oil, safflower seed oil, sunflower seed oil
	Nuts	Most, except coconut and cashew nuts
	Margarines	Many soft varieties especially soya bean and sunflower seed

because they can be made in the body in limited amounts from linoleic and alpha-linolenic acids. However, their synthesis may be limited in infancy, and in illness, at which times they effectively become 'essential', i.e. required in foods to avoid deficiency diseases. These essential fatty acids and their important products are in the n-3 series of PUFAs.

Most vegetable oils and some fish oils are good sources of essential fatty acids. In the UK, the main sources of linoleic acid are vegetables, fruit, nuts, cereal products and fat spreads, while the main sources of alpha-linolenic acid are vegetables, meat and meat products, cereal products and fat spreads.

The amount of EFAs required by the body is small and deficiency in human nutrition is rare. In western countries most adult diets provide 8–10 g/day, which is adequate. The DRVs are derived on the basis of preventing EFA deficiency, and it is recommended that linoleic acid should provide at least 1 per cent of total energy and that alpha-linolenic acid should provide at least 0.2 per cent of total energy. Although there is no evidence that a high dietary intake of PUFAs is associated with any threat to health, it is nevertheless recommended that dietary intake of PUFAs should not exceed 10 per cent of total food energy.

Essential fatty acids have important functions in the body: they form part of the structure of all cell membranes, they help in the regulation of cholesterol metabolism and they provide the raw materials from which the hormones known as prostaglandins are made.

Isolated deficiency of EFA is unusual and almost entirely restricted to infants – mainly those born prematurely. It more commonly occurs in complicated disease situations and in association with other nutrient deficiencies. Most organ systems and functions are affected, but the most obvious outward signs of EFA deficiency are growth failure and skin lesions. These were observed many years ago (1947) in infants fed on diets providing less than 1% of energy as linoleic acid.

The EFAs and their (n-3) derivative DHA are particularly important during fetal life and early infancy because they are needed for normal brain development. If they are not provided in sufficient amounts the body uses n-6 fatty acids instead. This can have serious functional consequences (e.g. for intellectual function and visual pathways). The provision of EFAs in milk (especially to pre-term infants) is critical. Similarly, the synthesis of normal prostaglandins is corrupted by utilization of n-3 fatty acids if the n-6 EFAs are not available, and this can accelerate vascular disease.

Although essential fatty acids are essential for early development, large amounts, as widely sold as 'food supplements', are not of extra benefit. Some research in this field is of dubious reliability.

Cis and trans fatty acids

When two carbon atoms are joined by a double bond, there is no freedom of rotation about the axis of the double bond. Consider oleic acid (Fig. 6.1). In one form the two parts of the hydrocarbon chain are on the same side of the double bond (cis form), while in the other they are on opposite sides of the double bond (trans form).

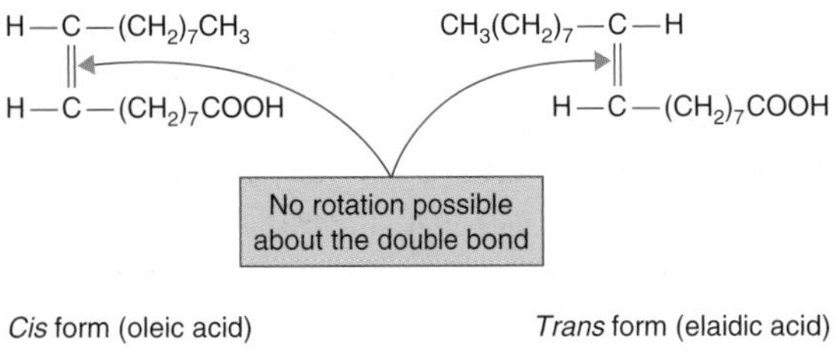

$$H-C-(CH_2)_7CH_3 \qquad\qquad CH_3(CH_2)_7-C-H$$
$$H-C-(CH_2)_7COOH \qquad\qquad H-C-(CH_2)_7COOH$$

No rotation possible
about the double bond

Cis form (oleic acid)   *Trans* form (elaidic acid)

Figure 6.1 *The* cis *and* trans *forms of a fatty acid*

Naturally occurring unsaturated fatty acids mainly have *cis* forms. Enzymes can recognize the difference between *cis* and *trans* forms, acting on the former but not the latter.

The distinction that is drawn between *cis* and *trans* fatty acids may seem like an unnecessary complication, but it will be seen later (p. 70) that it has some relevance when considering the relationship between the types of fat we eat and our health. *Trans*-fatty acids can accumulate and have similar effects to saturated fatty acids.

The physical nature of oils and fats

Having considered the chemical nature of oils and fats, it is now necessary to consider their physical nature.

The physical characteristics of oils and fats are important in many food applications, such as their use in cake and pastry mixes and in mayonnaise and ice-cream. Unlike pure chemical compounds, fats do not melt at a fixed temperature but over a range of temperatures. In this range they are plastic, that is they are soft and can be spread, but they do not flow. In other words, their properties are intermediate between those of a solid and a liquid. This property is important for the fats in cell membranes, and also for food science.

The plasticity of a fat results from it being a mixture of a number of different triglycerides, each triglyceride having its own melting point. If a large proportion of the triglycerides are below their melting point, the mixture will be solid and will consist of a network of minute crystals surrounded by a smaller quantity of liquid triglycerides. The solid network is not rigid, however, and the crystals can slide over one another, giving rise to the plastic character of the fat. If the temperature of the fat is raised an increasing proportion of triglycerides melt, the

solid network gradually breaks down and the plasticity of the mixture increases until it becomes liquid, when all the triglycerides have melted.

The melting point of fats is also affected by the fact that many triglycerides can exist in several crystalline forms; that is, they are polymorphic. Each crystalline form has its own melting point and when oils are cooled different mixtures of these separate crystalline forms, and therefore of different melting point, may be obtained depending upon how the cooling was carried out. The way in which an oil is cooled therefore affects the texture and consistency of the product formed. Such considerations are important in commercial methods of fat manufacture.

Animal fats

The two most important isolated animal fats are lard and butter, the latter being considered in Chapter 7 together with other dairy products. Lard is prepared by melting pig's fat and is virtually 100 per cent fat. As can be appreciated from Table 6.2, lard is relatively low in PUFA. Natural lard is a low-melting fat with good properties as a shortening agent, an acceptable white colour and bland flavour, but it suffers from the disadvantage that it has poor creaming properties and is therefore not a desirable fat for cake making.

The creaming properties of lard, i.e. its ability to incorporate air when beaten, may be improved by interesterification and industrial chemical processes which, as the name implies, involves a rearrangement of the combined fatty acids between the triglyceride ester molecules. This regrouping process results in a more random distribution of fatty acids. To understand why this should be so it is necessary to consider the arrangement of combined fatty acids in the triglycerides of lard. Lard is peculiar among fats in that the saturated fatty acids, mainly palmitic, are found predominantly in the middle position of the triglyceride molecules. It is this factor which causes lard to form large coarse crystals that prevent it from creaming well.

During interesterification the fatty acids change position, thus reducing the proportion of triglyceride molecules with a saturated fatty acid in the centre position. Interesterification is carried out by heating lard at about 100°C in the presence of a catalyst such as sodium ethoxide, $NaOC_2H_5$. This gives a product with greatly improved creaming properties and so more suitable for incorporation in margarine and cooking fats.

Marine oils

Whale and fish oils are characterized by their high content of long-chain polyunsaturated fatty acids containing 20 and 22 carbon atoms and up to six double bonds (see Table 6.2). Fish oils are rich sources of the longer chain fatty acids eicosapentanoic acid (EPA) and DHA which are omega-3 fatty acids. These have been found to have anti-inflammatory effects and may affect immune function. The omega-3 fatty acids in fish have also been shown to help protect against coronary heart disease particularly by reducing serum triglycerides. The best sources are foods naturally rich in omega-3 fatty acids, not 'good supplements'.

Vegetable oils and fats

Vegetables constitute the most important source of edible oils and fats. Most vegetable oils are liquid at 20°C, although there are a few notable exceptions such as palm oil, palm kernel oil and coconut oil which melt above this temperature (Fig. 6.2). The nature of the combined fatty acids in vegetable oils can be appreciated from Table 6.2, which shows the relatively high proportion of monounsaturated and polyunsaturated fatty acids they contain compared with animal fats.

Soya beans are grown extensively in China and the USA and soya bean oil is now the most important edible vegetable oil. The residue left when the oil has been extracted from the bean constitutes a valuable source of protein and as such is discussed on p. 165. Soya bean oil is the major vegetable oil used in margarine manufacture and large quantities are also used in cooking fats.

Vegetable oils are normally extracted from seeds, kernels and nuts, either by mechanical pressure or by solvents. The latter method involves the use of a liquid solvent of low boiling point in which the oil is soluble. After the seed or nut has been ground, it is shaken with the solvent, the oil is extracted and a solid residue remains. When the liquid mixture is heated, the low boiling solvent evaporates, leaving the oil. Groundnut oil, for example, occurs in groundnuts (i.e. peanuts) to the extent of 45–50 per cent by wet weight, most of which may be extracted by means of a screw-press which squeezes out the oil. In some modern methods a two-stage process is used. After an initial extraction with the press, a solvent is used to extract the remaining oil. The residue is not wasted, in fact its high protein content makes it a valuable substance, and it is used as a cattle food.

Another useful source of edible oil is the palm tree, which is not to be confused with the more slender coconut palm. The fruit of the palm tree grows in large bunches, which may contain over 1000 fruit. Each fruit is rather like a plum, having a thin orange to dark red skin covering a fleshy interior in which is embedded a hard shell containing the kernel. Palm oil is extracted from the fleshy part of the fruit and palm kernel oil from the kernel. Both these oils are edible, and palm oil is extensively used in the UK for the manufacture of margarine and cooking fats.

The olive is also valuable as a source of oil, with over a million tonnes of olive oil being produced annually. Olive oil is notable for the large proportion of oleic acid it contains (see Table 6.2) and for its purity. The finest olive oil does not need purification and is used for all manner of purposes in the Mediterranean countries, where olives have been cultivated for thousands of years. It is one of the key elements of the 'Mediterranean diet', which is encouraged worldwide for its protective value against coronary heart disease, partly by supplementing saturated fats in the diet and partly for the high vitamin E content and in oil from nuts and seeds. Unsaturated fatty acids are unstable and easily oxidized when exposed to oxygen free-radicals unless they are protected by antioxidants. The most important lipid-soluble antioxidant in plants is vitamin E, so vegetable oils are the major source of vitamin E, in foods such as cereals and in purified oils. They are also natural sources of the lipid (and antioxidant) carotenoids some of which are used to make vitamin A.

Refining of crude oils

Crude olive oil is exceptional in that it can be used for edible purposes without refining. Most vegetable

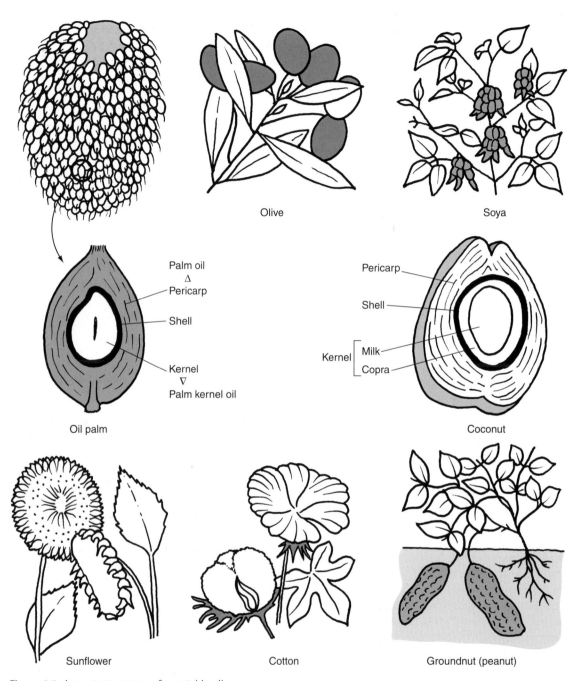

Figure 6.2 *Important sources of vegetable oils*

oils, however, contain a number of impurities such as moisture, free fatty acids, colouring matter, resins, gums and vitamins. These impurities affect flavour (owing to rancidity caused by oxidation of free fatty acids), odour and clarity, and are removed during refining. The refining process is carried out in a number of stages which may be considered in turn.

1 *Degumming.* Crude oils often contain impurities in suspension which in the presence of water form gums. The impurities are removed by adding hot water to the warm oil, which is then transferred to a centrifugal separator. The separator revolves at a high speed and the gum particles, which have a higher density than the oil, are thrown to the bottom of the vessel, leaving an upper layer of clarified oil.

2 *Neutralizing.* Owing to spoilage, all crude oils contain a small proportion of free fatty acids and low-grade oils may contain considerable quantities. The acids are removed by neutralizing the oil with a solution of caustic soda, which converts the fatty acid into an insoluble soap. The soap is then removed by allowing it to settle to the bottom of the neutralizing tanks. If the acid impurity is palmitic acid, for example, insoluble sodium palmitate is formed:

$$C_{15}H_{31}COOH + NaOH \rightarrow C_{15}H_{31}COONa \downarrow + H_2O$$

Palmitic acid   Sodium palmitate

3 *Washing and drying.* In order to remove the last traces of soap from the oil, it is washed with warm water. Two layers form and the lower water layer is run off, leaving the oil layer, which is then vacuum dried. In modern industrial plants these separate stages are being replaced by a continuous automatic process in which the neutralizing stage is carried out very much more quickly in a centrifugal separator. The oil is now clear and free from acid, but it is usually yellowish in colour and still has a distinct odour. It is, therefore, bleached and deodorized (see below).

4 *Bleaching.* The oil is warmed and fuller's earth and activated carbon are added. Both these materials have a large capacity for adsorbing coloured matter. The mixture is stirred and a partial vacuum is maintained. When all the coloured matter has been adsorbed, the oil–earth mixture is passed through filter presses, from which the oil emerges as a clear, colourless liquid.

5 *Deodorizing.* The oil is heated under vacuum in a tall tank and steam is injected so that the liquid mixture is violently agitated. In one method it is sprayed upwards as an umbrella-shaped fountain, so that a large surface area of liquid is continually exposed, and the volatile odoriferous substances and remaining free fatty acids are stripped from the oil.

The oil is now pure and ready for use, or, as is usually the case, ready for blending. It is desirable that the oil should not come into contact with air once it has been refined, as this leads to deterioration due to oxidation, particularly if the natural antioxidant vitamins have not been returned. In some modern extraction plants, therefore, the oil is stored under an inert atmosphere of nitrogen. It is becoming standard practice to add vitamin E to spreadable fats. This not only acts as an antioxidant but also provides a source of vitamin E in the diet. There are no European directives or UK regulations on the addition of vitamin E to oils or spreadable fats. Vitamins A and D have to be added by law. The added vitamin E in oils and spreading fats now form the main dietary source for much of the world. Its high consumption is one factor which may be contributing to falling rates of heart disease.

Hydrogenation of oils

Hydrogenation is the process whereby an oil is converted into a fat (i.e. by which it is hardened). This important process has resulted in a considerable increase in the use of hardened vegetable oils at the expense of animal fats, which were once such a staple feature of the diet.

Hydrogenation is simply the addition of hydrogen to the double bonds of unsaturated fatty acids combined with glycerol in an oil. During hydrogenation one molecule of hydrogen is absorbed by each double bond:

$$-CH{=}CH- + H_2 \rightarrow -CH_2-CH_2-$$

The most commonly occurring unsaturated fatty acids found in combination with glycerol in vegetable oils, namely oleic, linoleic and linolenic acids, contain one, two and three double bonds, respectively. As they all contain 18 carbon atoms, complete hydrogenation converts them all into stearic acid. Stearic acid has a much higher melting point (70°C) than any of the other three, so the hydrogenated oil is harder than the original. The equation below illustrates the conversion of liquid triolein into solid tristearin, which takes place when a molecule of triolein absorbs three molecules of hydrogen.

$$
\begin{array}{ll}
CH_2OCOC_{17}H_{33} & CH_2OCOC_{17}H_{35} \\
| & | \\
CHOCOC_{17}H_{33} + 3H_2 \rightarrow & CHOCOC_{17}H_{35} \\
| & | \\
CH_2OCOC_{17}H_{33} & CH_2OCOC_{17}H_{35} \\
\text{Triolein} & \text{Tristearin}
\end{array}
$$

Hydrogenation only proceeds at a reasonably fast rate in the presence of a catalyst (finely divided nickel being used industrially). The nickel is usually made by reducing finely divided nickel carbonate or nickel formate. The catalyst is added in small quantities to the oil, which is contained in large, closed steel vessels called converters, operating at a temperature of about 170°C and high pressure. The oil is stirred and hydrogen gas is pumped in. The oil is heated to start the reaction, but as the reaction is exothermic, further heating is not necessary. After hydrogenation the oil is cooled and filtered to remove the nickel, which can be reused.

The way in which a catalyst affects a reaction was considered in Chapter 2 and it will be recalled that catalysts reduce the energy required for a reaction to proceed (i.e. the energy of activation: see Fig. 2.1). Nickel, similar to enzymes, catalyses a reaction by providing a surface upon which the reaction can take place, and converts a single-step high-energy mechanism into one involving several low-energy stages.

The first stage of hydrogenation is the adsorption of reactants, in this case hydrogen and oil, onto the nickel surface. Adsorption takes place only at certain preferred parts of the surface known as active centres and results in the adsorbed hydrogen and oil molecules being brought close to each other. Exchange of energy between the nickel and the reacting molecules weakens the internal bonds of the latter and activates them sufficiently to provide them with the necessary energy of activation. Reaction occurs, after which the hydrogenated oil molecules are desorbed (i.e. they leave the nickel surface which is then available to catalyse further reaction). These stages of hydrogenation are illustrated in Fig. 6.3.

Surface catalysts, such as nickel, are easily poisoned by substances which are adsorbed in preference to the hydrogen and oil molecules. Carbon monoxide and sulphur compounds, if present in even minute quantities, poison the catalyst owing to their strong adsorption by the nickel. This means that the hydrogen gas, which is often produced from water gas (a mixture of carbon monoxide and hydrogen), must be most carefully purified before use and that the oil to be used must be carefully refined before hydrogenation.

Hydrogenation is a selective process, with some triglycerides becoming saturated more rapidly than others. The most unsaturated triglycerides are partly hydrogenated before the less unsaturated ones react, so that in terms of the fatty acids combined in the triglycerides, more linolenic acid is converted into linoleic acid in a given time than linoleic to oleic acid. The relative rates of reaction of oleic, linoleic and linolenic acid are in the ratio 1:20:40. This fact enables the hydrogenation to be controlled, and food oils are only partly saturated with hydrogen.

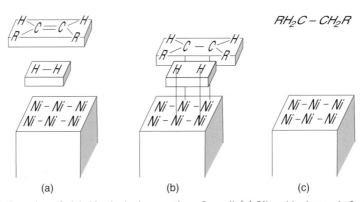

(a)　　　　　(b)　　　　　(c)

Figure 6.3 The catalytic action of nickel in the hydrogenation of an oil. (a) Oil and hydrogen before reaction. (b) Molecules adsorbed and activated on nickel surface. (c) Hydrogenated oil after reaction

Hydrogenation of oils not only converts unsaturated fatty acids into saturated ones, but it also converts naturally occurring *cis* forms of unsaturated fatty acids into their *trans* forms. Such *trans* forms are treated by the body in the same way as saturated fatty acids, so a high consumption of hydrogenation trans-fatty acids, e.g. from pastry, biscuits and other baked foods, contributes to causing coronary heart disease.

Careful control of the hydrogenation process is important. For health reasons it may be desirable to retain a degree of unsaturation in the partly hardened oil. In addition, complete hydrogenation would make fats too hard and lacking in plasticity for use in food preparation. Apart from its hardening effect, hydrogenation is advantageous in that it also bleaches the oil and increases its stability.

Rancidity

Oils and fats are liable to spoilage which results in the production of unpleasant odours and flavours; such spoilage is usually described by the general term rancidity. Different types of oil and fat show varying degrees of resistance to spoilage; thus, most vegetable oils deteriorate only slowly, whereas animal fats deteriorate more rapidly and marine oils, which contain a relatively high proportion of combined highly unsaturated fatty acids deteriorate so rapidly that they are useless for edible purposes unless they have been refined and hydrogenated.

Spoilage may occur in many ways, but two important types of rancidity may be distinguished, namely hydrolytic rancidity and oxidative rancidity.

Hydrolytic rancidity

Hydrolytic rancidity occurs as a result of hydrolysis of triglyceride molecules to glycerol and free fatty acids and it is brought about by the presence of moisture in oils. The rate of hydrolysis in the presence of water alone is negligible, but it is hastened by the presence of enzymes and microorganisms. Oils and fats that have not been subjected to heat treatment may contain lipases which catalyse hydrolysis. They may also contain moulds, yeasts and bacteria present in the natural oil or they may become contaminated with them during processing. Such microorganisms hasten hydrolytic breakdown.

The nature of the unpleasant flavours and odours produced by hydrolysis depends upon the fatty acid composition of the triglycerides. If the triglycerides contain combined fatty acids of low molecular weight containing 4–14 carbon atoms, hydrolysis yields free acids having characteristically unpleasant odours and flavours. For example, hydrolysis of butter yields the rancid-smelling butyric acid, while palm kernel oil yields considerable amounts of lauric and myristic acids. Oils containing combined fatty acids with more than 14 carbon atoms are not liable to hydrolytic rancidity as the free acids are flavourless and odourless.

Oxidative rancidity

Oxidative rancidity is the most common and important type of rancidity and it results in the production of unpleasant rancid or 'tallowy' flavours. It is caused by the reaction of unsaturated oils with oxygen and its occurrence does not depend, therefore, on the presence of impurities or moisture in an oil; oxidation can consequently affect pure and refined oils. The actual mechanism of the oxidation is complex and not completely elucidated, but the main features are known and are as follows.

The oxidation of oils takes place by means of a chain reaction which is a type of reaction that is characterized by extreme speed. A chain reaction takes place in three stages known as initiation, propagation and termination. In the initiation stage, which is slow to occur, a hydrogen atom is removed from an unsaturated triglyceride molecule with the production of a free radical ($R^•$). Free radicals, which are groups containing an 'unpaired' electron, are extremely unstable and immediately react with another molecule to form a more stable substance. This initiation stage only occurs under the influence of catalysts in the form of minute traces of metals, particularly copper, which are always present despite refining, and in the presence of heat and light.

The slow initiation stage is followed by a fast propagation stage in which free radicals from the initiation stage combine with atmospheric oxygen to form an unstable peroxyl free radical which reacts with molecules of unsaturated oil to form another free radical and an unstable hydroperoxide.

It can be seen from the sequence shown below, that for every free radical R$^\bullet$ used up another is generated, with the result that the reaction is self-generating. The site of the reaction in the unsaturated oil is a methylene (–CH$_2$–) group adjacent to a double bond and we can represent such molecules by RH, H being the hydrogen atom of the methylene group adjacent to a double bond.

As the reaction proceeds hydroperoxide is continually formed and, being unstable, it breaks down to form ketones and aldehydes, which are responsible for the off-flavours of rancid fats. The reaction continues either until all the oxygen (or oil) is used or until the free radicals which are responsible for maintaining the reaction are removed. Many fats, particularly vegetable oils, contain natural substances, such as vitamin E, known as antioxidants which help to retard rancidity by reacting with peroxyl free radicals (RO$_2$$^\bullet$) so that they are no longer available for the propagation stage. Synthetic antioxidants such as synthetic vitamin E, are also added to fats to control rancidity (see p. 278).

LIPIDS IN AQUEOUS MEDIA: COLLOIDAL AND EMULSIONS

The physical nature of a solution is familiar enough. An aqueous sugar solution, for example, consists of sugar molecules dispersed through water, the whole system being homogeneous. However, if we consider what happens when we add to water a substance made up of relatively large molecules, such as a starch or a protein, we find that the system formed is not homogeneous but consists of two distinct parts or phases. The large molecules dispersed through water form one phase, known as the disperse phase and the

water forms the other phase, known as the continuous phase, the complete system being described as colloidal.

A colloidal solution is usually called a sol and contains particles, consisting of single large molecules or groups of smaller molecules, that are intermediate in size between small molecules and visible particles. Such systems have properties that are intermediate between those of true solutions and suspensions of visible particles.

All types of colloidal systems are similar to sols, in that they contain two distinct phases and in that the disperse phase contains particles intermediate in size between small molecules and visible particles. The disperse phase may be solid, liquid or gaseous, but in every case the properties of colloidal systems depend upon the very large surface area of the disperse phase. Colloidal systems are found in life – for example, most intracellular fluid is colloidal and lipids can only be transported as colloidal suspensions (emulsion) in the blood or in milk. Colloidal systems are important for the structure and properties of many foods. Part of the early phase of digestion in the small intestine involves the generation of emulsions and other colloidal systems in the gut contents, which permit further digestion and absorption. Bile acids are made in the liver and cycled through the gall bladder into the duodenum where they function to create emulsions from dietary fats. After absorption of the fat, the bile acids are reabsorbed and transported back to the liver. Colloidal systems are ultimately unstable, and the two phases can separate if conditions change, e.g. temperature, pH or by centrifugation.

The types of colloidal systems which are important in food are summarized in Table 6.4, and will be considered in the following pages.

Table 6.4 Types of colloidal systems

Disperse phase	Continuous phase	Name	Examples
Solid	Liquid	Sol	Starch and proteins in water
Liquid	Liquid	Emulsion	Milk, mayonnaise
Gas	Liquid	Foam	Whipped cream, creamed fat, beaten egg white
Gas	Solid	Solid foam	Ice cream, bread
Liquid	Solid	Gel	Jellies, jam, starch paste
		Solid emulsion	Butter, margarine

Emulsions and emulsifying agents

When oil is added to water it forms a separate layer above the water; the oil and water do not dissolve in each other and are said to be immiscible. If oil and water are shaken vigorously the two liquids become dispersed in each other and an emulsion is said to be formed. Such an emulsion is unstable, however, and on standing it reverts to the original two layers. Emulsions are described as being either oil-in-water (o/w) or water-in-oil (w/o) emulsions. An o/w emulsion is one in which small oil droplets form the disperse phase and are dispersed through the water (Fig. 6.4), whereas a w/o emulsion is one in which small water droplets are dispersed through the oil.

Although food emulsions are described as being either o/w or w/o, these terms may be misleading in that the oil and water may contain other substances. Thus, in addition to triglycerides the oil phase may contain other lipids and fat-soluble materials, and the water phase may, for example, be saline, vinegar or milk (which is already a natural emulsion and colloidal system). Table 6.5 gives details of some important food emulsions.

Why is it that once water drops have been dispersed in oil they come together again and form a continuous water layer? The answer is to be found in the fact that the action of dispersing water through oil in the form of drops increases the area of oil and water in contact. In order to do this, work must be done against the force of surface tension which causes a liquid to assume minimum surface area.

The natural tendency is, therefore, for the water drops to coalesce, for by so doing the interfacial area is decreased and a more stable system is produced.

In order for oil and water to form a stable emulsion a third substance called an emulsifying agent or emulsifier must be present. Although the complete mechanism by which emulsifiers facilitate the formation of stable emulsions is complex, variable and incompletely understood, an outline of the main factors can be given.

As the surface tension between oil and water, known as interfacial tension, is great, it is difficult for a stable emulsion to be formed. Emulsifiers lower interfacial tension by becoming adsorbed at the oil–water interface and forming a film one molecule thick round each droplet. The adsorbed film prevents the droplets from coalescing and, in some instances, may form a film which, by virtue of its mechanical strength, imparts stability. For example, protein emulsifiers are notable for the mechanical strength of the adsorption film that they produce. If an emulsifier contains charged groups, the adsorption process gives rise to charged droplets which repel each other. Such droplets will not coalesce and this factor therefore promotes emulsion stability.

Emulsifying agents are substances whose molecules contain both a hydrophilic or 'water-loving' group and a lipophilic (fat-loving) group and is hydrophobic or 'water-hating'. The hydrophilic group is polar (i.e. it carries a tiny electrical charge and is attracted to the water) while the non-polar hydrophobic group, which is frequently a long chain hydrocarbon group, is attracted to the oil. This is because water (H_2O) is readily polarized (H^+ plus OH^-), whereas fats cannot

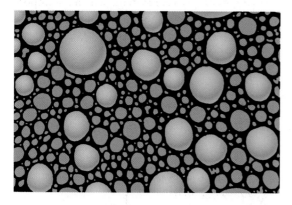

Figure 6.4 *Diagram of an oil-in-water emulsion based on a photomicrograph. The diameter of the oil droplets (light shading) is in the range 10^{-4}–10^{-6} mm*

Table 6.5 Examples of food emulsions

Example	Type	Main emulsifiers present or added
Milk, cream	o/w	Proteins (casein)
Butter	w/o	Proteins (casein)
Mayonnaise, salad cream	o/w	Egg yolk (lecithin), GMS, mustard
Margarine	w/o	Proteins (casein), lecithin, GMS
Ice cream	o/w	Proteins (casein), GMS, plus stabilizers (gelatin, gums, alginates)

o/w, oil in water; w/o, water in oil; GMS, glyceryl monostearate.

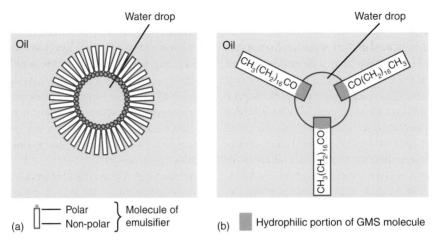

Figure 6.5 *(a) Molecules of emulsifier adsorbed at a water–oil interface forming a complete protective film round a water droplet. (b) The adsorption of glyceryl monostearate (GMS) in a water-in-oil (w/o) emulsion*

be polarized. Thus, in a w/o emulsion the emulsifier is adsorbed in such a way that the polar 'heads' of the emulsifier molecules are in the water and the non-polar 'tails' stick out into the oil, as shown in Fig. 6.5.

The type of emulsion formed by an oil–water system depends upon a number of factors, including the composition of the oil and water phases, the chemical nature of the emulsifying agent and the proportions of oil and water present. If the polar group of an emulsifier is more effectively adsorbed than the non-polar group, adsorption by the water is greater than by the oil. The extent of adsorption at a liquid surface depends upon the surface area of liquid available and increased adsorption of emulsifier by water is favoured by the oil–water interface becoming convex towards the water, thus giving an o/w emulsion.

The relative proportions of oil and water also help to determine whether an o/w or w/o emulsion

is formed. If more oil than water is present the water tends to form droplets and a w/o emulsion is formed. Conversely, if more water than oil is present an o/w emulsion is favoured.

Many substances show some activity as emulsifying agents, and among naturally occurring ones phospholipids, proteins and complex carbohydrates such as gums, pectins and starches are important. Natural food emulsions are often stabilized by proteins and milk, for example, is stabilized by the casein and other proteins present. Artificial emulsifiers are added during the preparation of many emulsions, though in the UK only those on a permitted list (see p. 301) may be used. Of these glyceryl monostearate (GMS) is the most important and will serve as an example.

Glyceryl monostearate is a monoglyceride which is formed when one hydroxyl group of glycerol is esterified with stearic acid as shown in the following equation.

$$
\begin{array}{ccc}
\text{CH}_2\text{OH} & \text{CH}_2\text{OH} & \\
| & | & \\
\text{CHOH} + \text{CH}_3(\text{CH}_2)_{16}\text{COOH} \longrightarrow & \text{CHOH} & + \text{H}_2\text{O} \\
| & | & \\
\text{CH}_2\text{OH} & \text{CH}_2\text{O}\!\!-\!\! \boxed{\text{CO}(\text{CH}_2)_{16}\text{CH}_3} &
\end{array}
$$

Hydrophobic portion
of glyceryl monostearate

One part of the GMS molecule is hydrophilic because it contains hydroxyl groups and the rest of the molecule, as indicated in the formula, is hydrophobic. When GMS is added to a w/o emulsion, the hydrophilic parts of the molecules are adsorbed onto the surface of the water droplets and the lipophilic parts are adsorbed onto the surface of the oil round the drops, as illustrated in Fig. 6.5b.

Commercial GMS is not a single substance and in addition to glyceryl monostearate it contains some diglycerides and triglycerides. It is widely used in food manufacture and is added, for example, to margarine, mayonnaise, salad dressing and ice cream.

The phospholipid lecithin is an important natural emulsifier which favours o/w emulsions and which is present in egg yolk and many crude oils, particularly vegetable oils. Lecithin is extracted from vegetable oils, notably soya bean oil, and added to some manufactured products.

Sometimes stabilizers are added to products in addition to emulsifiers, their function being to maintain an emulsion once it has been formed. Such substances improve the stability of emulsions mainly by increasing their viscosity. As viscosity increases, the freedom of movement of the dispersed droplets of the emulsion is reduced and this lessens the chance of their coming into contact and coalescing. Stabilizers are high molecular weight compounds, usually proteins such as gelatin, or complex carbohydrates, such as pectins, starches, alginates and gums. For example, starch or flour may be added to thicken gravies, sauces and salad cream and several stabilizers, such as gelatin and gums, are added to ice cream.

Uses of emulsifying agents

A number of natural foods are emulsions (milk is the prime example) and are stabilized by natural emulsifiers which are present as constituents of the food. Here we are concerned, however, not with natural foods but with manufactured foods to which emulsifiers are added. Emulsifiers are added to several products containing fat, such as margarine, cooking fats, salad dressings and ice cream.

Mayonnaise and salad cream

Emulsifiers play an important part in making salad cream and mayonnaise, which are o/w emulsions.

The term salad cream means, according to a now-revoked legal definition (1991 No. 1231 The Food (Miscellaneous Revocations) Regulations 1991) 'any smooth, thick stable emulsion of vegetable oil, water, egg or egg yolk and an acidifying agent, with or without the addition of one or more of the following substances, namely vinegar, lemon juice, salt, spices, sugar, milk, milk products, mustard, edible starch, edible gums and other minor ingredients and permitted additives. The minimum proportions of vegetable oil and egg yolk solids that used to be allowed in Britain were 25 and 1.35 per cent, respectively. However, the compositional standards are no longer enforceable.

Mayonnaise is normally thicker than salad cream and contains a higher proportion of both oil and egg yolk (and thus less carbohydrate and water). The finest oil for making salad cream is undoubtedly olive oil; however, because of its higher cost, other vegetable oils are often used. Such oils must be of high purity, light colour and bland flavour and they are therefore refined, bleached and deodorized before use. As they must also be liquid, vegetable oils such as groundnut oil, soya bean oil, cottonseed oil and maize oil are employed. Unfortunately, they cannot capture the flavour of olive oil.

Salad cream should be viscous and have a creamy consistency, which can only be achieved if the o/w emulsion is stable. In order to produce such a product, emulsifying agents must be present, the chief one being lecithin contained in egg yolk. The stability of the emulsion formed is increased by the addition of stabilizers which increase viscosity. Such an increase in viscosity becomes more important the smaller the oil content, and is brought about by the addition of starches and gums such as xanthan gum.

Ice cream

Manufactured ice cream is one of the successes of food technology and is noteworthy in that air is a major ingredient. Without air, ice cream would simply be a frozen milk ice, but with air it becomes a highly complex colloidal system. It consists of a solid foam of minute air cells surrounded by emulsified fat together with a network of minute ice crystals that are surrounded by watery liquid in the form of a sol.

Ice cream is made from fat, non-fat milk solids, sugar, emulsifiers, stabilizers, flavourings and colour.

A typical ice cream contains by weight 12 per cent fat, 11 per cent non-fat milk solids, 15 per cent sugar and about 1 per cent minor ingredients, the rest being water. During processing air is incorporated and accounts for about half the volume of the final product; as ice cream is sold by volume this latter point is not unimportant. A process which allows the sale of air is likely to be profitable. In the UK the description of ice cream is not allowed for any food other than the frozen product containing a minimum of 5 per cent fat and 2.5 per cent milk protein by weight. To be classified as a 'dairy' ice cream, all the fat must be milk fat (The Food Labelling Regulations 1996). 'Non-dairy' ice cream contains suitable vegetable fats, such as hydrogenated coconut oil.

In the manufacture of ice cream the ingredients are mixed together, pasteurized (see p. 80) and homogenized. The latter treatment, together with the added emulsifiers, produces a stable o/w emulsion. The emulsion is cooled to a temperature which partly freezes the mixture; at the same time air is whipped in. A solid film forms on the walls of the freezer and this is continuously scraped off. The temperature is subsequently reduced further and this causes the rest of the water to freeze and the product to harden.

Fat plays an important role in determining the texture of ice cream, and also flavour if milk fat is used. Fat converts the ice cream mix into an o/w emulsion and when air is incorporated into the mixture it aids the formation and stabilization of a foam by forming a stable fat film round the air bubbles. The main components of the aqueous phase of the emulsion are sugar and non-fat solids. The latter are important because they contain proteins which are natural emulsifiers in ice cream. During pasteurization the milk proteins become denatured (see p. 140) and form a solid film of considerable strength around the oil droplets. This prevents the oil droplets from coalescing and thus stabilizes the emulsion.

An important function of synthetic stabilizers added to ice cream is to increase viscosity rather than aid emulsification. Gelatin, gums and alginates are all used and help to promote the firm texture, smooth taste and good keeping qualities associated with modern ice cream. These stabilizers also assist the formation of a weak network of hydrated molecules through the ice cream and this gives a firm-textured product which is slow-melting and resistant to the formation of large ice crystals. The use of gelatin exemplifies this.

Gelatin molecules are relatively large, have a thread-like shape and are hydrophilic. When gelatin is added to the ice cream mix its long, thin molecules are dispersed through the emulsion, and water molecules are attracted and held at the large surface area of gelatin exposed. In this way, the water molecules lose their freedom of movement, and melting, which occurs when the freedom of movement of molecules suddenly increases, is made more difficult. The gelatin molecules, by forming a three-dimensional mesh (or gel) also give added firmness to the structure.

When an ice cream emulsion is frozen, ice crystals are formed. If ice cream is to give a sensation of smoothness when it melts in the mouth, the crystals must be very small. Because gelatin molecules are dispersed through the emulsion and because of their hydrophilic nature, they ensure that the water molecules are also dispersed. In this way, the formation of large ice crystals, which can only occur when large numbers of water molecules come together, is prevented. If ice cream is allowed to melt completely the air is released from the colloidal system, and it cannot be reconstituted by refreezing.

Margarine

Margarine is a manufactured food which was invented by a French scientist, Mège-Mouriés, in 1869. The nineteenth century saw a rapid rise in the population of Europe so that the increasing demand for the two most common fats – butter and lard – soon outstripped their production. Mège-Mouriés's intention was to make a fat that would resemble butter as closely as possible. His recipe was extremely odd; he obtained an oil called *oleo oil* from beef tallow and mixed the warm oil with chopped cow's udder, milk and water and stirred them until a solid mixture called *oleo margarine* was obtained.

Today's margarine is, happily, made by a very different process from that employed by Mèges-Mouriés. His method was based on animal fat which was available as a cheap industrial waste product but as such fat became increasingly scarce it was necessary to find an alternative source for making margarine.

For many years whale blubber was cheap and margarine making contributed to decimating the world's whale population. Although vegetable and fish oils were available, these were liquids and the problem was how to turn them into solid fats resembling butter. The problem was solved by the invention of hydrogenation at the beginning of the twentieth century.

Margarine is now made from a water-in-oil emulsion, the aqueous phase being fat-free milk and the oil phase being a blend of different oils. The two phases are mixed together and, with the aid of suitable emulsifiers, a stable emulsion is formed. The emulsion is processed until it forms a solid product having the desired consistency.

1 *The oil blend.* Several different oils are blended together in preparing the oil phase. The blend may include animal, vegetable and marine oils; the actual oils being selected at any time depending upon cost and availability, as well as the type of product it is desired to make. Today, the major vegetable oils used include those derived from soya, sunflower, palm, rapeseed, safflower, maize, cotton seed, coconut and groundnut. The animal fats may include beef and pig fat trimmed from carcasses. It is important that the oil phase should have a bland taste and a wide plastic range; to achieve the former oils are carefully refined and to achieve the latter some are hydrogenated. It has already been pointed out that in order to have suitable plasticity both liquid and solid triglycerides must be present. In margarine, the desired liquid to solid ratio is obtained by selective hydrogenation of the oils used. After hydrogenation oils are refined again as shown in Fig. 6.6 and pass to the blending tank in which they are heated until they are all liquid.

2 *The aqueous blend.* The skimmed milk is matured after pasteurization by adding a 'starter' in the form of lactic acid bacteria, and the ripening and souring is allowed to continue until the desired flavour is produced. Small amounts of other materials are added to the ripened milk and these have an important influence on the nature of the final product. Artificial flavouring and colouring agents, vitamin A and D and salt are all added.

3 *Emulsification.* The oil and aqueous phases together with emulsifying agents, such as lecithin and GMS, are now mixed together in large cylindrical tanks. These are fitted with two sets of paddles which rotate in opposite directions and mix the fluids until they form a stable emulsion, which has the appearance of a thick cream.

4 *Processing the emulsion.* The emulsion is now passed on to a roller, which slowly revolves and which is cooled internally. When the emulsion comes into contact with the cold surface of the roller it is rapidly cooled and converted into a solid film. The film is scraped off the roller, and after being stored for about a day it is worked until it gains a smooth, even texture. This involves breaking up the structure of the flakes of fat, by passing it through rollers and by kneading it.

In the more modern continuous process, using a machine known as a 'votator', the emulsifying and processing stages follow one another directly and take place in closed machines. This saves time, and prevents the margarine from coming into contact with air.

Finally, the margarine is packed by weighing it into blocks, wrapping and labelling it. The label must state that the product is margarine and give the vitamin content.

The term 'margarine' no longer describes a single product, but a whole range of products that provide a wide variety of different blends of oils and flavours to meet every need and taste. Hard margarines are available as an alternative to butter for table use and also for baking. Soft margarines are available in abundance resulting from the use of different oil blends including those, such as sunflower oil brands, which are designed to be high in PUFAs (and low in cholesterol).

Early varieties of margarine contained oils and fats that had been completely hydrogenated and as a result contained no combined EFAs. Modern methods of manufacture, involving careful selection of vegetable oils rich in PUFAs, including linoleic acid, and selective hydrogenation that allows some oils rich in PUFA to escape hydrogenation, produce margarines containing EFA.

Margarine produced by early methods was significantly inferior to butter in its vitamin content but all table margarine now manufactured contains added vitamin A and D. The vitamin content is controlled by UK law, so that it contains 800–1000 μg

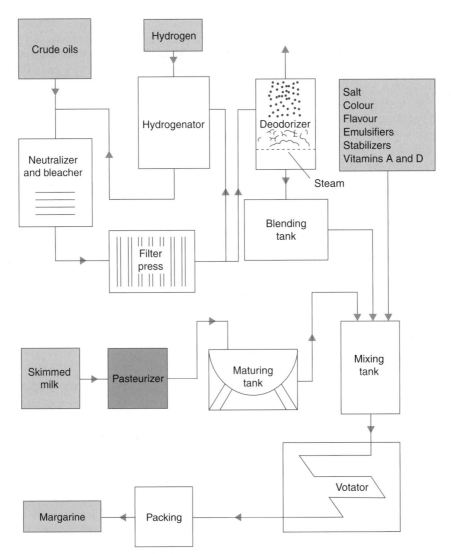

Figure 6.6 *Flow diagram of margarine production*

vitamin A/100 g (as retinol equivalent) and 7–9 μg vitamin D/100 g. This means that the vitamin content of margarine is equal to that of summer butter.

A typical margarine contains 81 per cent fat by weight and has an energy value of about 3000 kJ/100 g. This compares with an average value of 82 per cent fat for butter and an energy value of 3140 kJ/100 g. The water content of margarine is controlled by law and must not exceed 16 per cent.

In terms of nutrition, margarine (or spreading fats) vary considerably, and have different implications for health. In general, the softer the spread the

greater the proportion of polyunsaturated fatty acids (PUFAs) and monounsaturated fatty acids (MUFAs). The firmer the spread, the more saturated fatty acids. Thus, a hard margarine is particularly likely to contribute to increasing blood cholesterol. However, the process of industrial hydrogenation introduces a proportion of *trans*-fatty acids which are chemically and physically similar to PUFA or MUFA, but function more like saturated fatty acids. Some manufacturers have recognized this health hazard and have modified their processes to avoid or minimize *trans*-fatty acids, and this has

Table 6.6 Composition of typical fat spreads per 100 g

	Energy (kJ)	Protein (g)	Fat (g)	Energy from fat (%)	Carbohydrate (g)	Sodium (mg)
Margarine[a]	3042	0.2	81.7	99.4	1.0	880
Fat spread[b]	2556	0.5	68.5	99.2	0.8	800
Reduced-fat spread (41–62% fat)	2339	0.1	62.7	99.2	1.1	600
Low-fat spread (41% or less)	1503	4.9	37.6	92.6	1.8	650

[a]Soft not polyunsaturated.
[b]70% Fat, polyunsaturated.

proved a valuable marketing point as consumer and media understanding of nutrition rises.

It is important to recognize that the composition of a food such as a spread can be expressed in terms of food science (usually %g/100 g or g/serving by weight). To understand the nutritional implication, however it is necessary to use nutritional terms (per cent energy contributed by different components such as fat; Table 6.6). It is worth reflecting that spreads and oils are never consumed alone, so their nutritional impact depends on how they are combined with other foods rather than on their flavour.

Low-fat spreads

Owing to the considerable body of opinion which believes that we should, for health reasons, reduce our intake of fat, a number of low-fat spreads are now available. Low-fat and reduced-fat spreads contain 40–80 per cent fat compared with margarine, which must contain a minimum of 80 per cent fat (see Table 6.6). This difference is created by altering the emulsification conditions, allowing the addition of more water. Adding air can make the spread softer, but does not change its composition by weight. Such products may be based either on butter or margarine. They cannot be called margarine because they do not comply with the legal requirements for that product name.

Cooking fats

Cooking fats, or *shortenings* as they are sometimes called, differ from margarine in that they are pure fat products rather than solidified emulsions. Because they will be melted during cooking there is no need

for emulsification. They are made from an oil blend which may contain animal, vegetable and marine oils. The actual blend will depend on the nature of the product required and on the availability and cost of suitable oils. The oil blend is partly hydrogenated so as to give a product having the required plasticity and after refining and blending, the fat blend is cooled and processed in a 'votator'-type of machine similar to that used in making margarine. After the oil blend has been cooled down it is a near-white solid but, during processing, air is sometimes incorporated and it is transformed into a pure white, thick creamy liquid. While in a liquid condition it may be forced under pressure through a texturizing valve, which ensures that on cooling the product sets into a smooth-textured soft mass.

Superglycerinated fats and their use in cake making

In commercial practice, cooking fats are often required for specific purposes, such as cake making, and these incorporate an emulsifier. Such fats are called superglycerinated or high ratio fats. The emulsifying agent most frequently used is GMS. The efficiency of such a fat is measured in terms of its creaming, emulsifying and shortening powers. The use of high-ratio fats allows the use of a higher ratio of sugar to flour than with ordinary cooking fats.

The creaming power of a fat is measured by its capacity for incorporating air bubbles when it is beaten. This power is dependent upon the plastic properties of the fat which enable it to entrap air bubbles within its structure without loss of mechanical strength, which would certainly occur if it were in a liquid condition. In the first stage of making a rich type of cake, fat is warmed to increase its plasticity and then the softened fat is creamed with sugar by beating the two together until sufficient air becomes trapped in the mixture. This entrapped air assists the action of baking powder in the aeration of the cake during baking and has an important influence on the volume and evenness of texture of the final product.

When creaming of the fat and sugar is complete, eggs are usually beaten into the mixture and mixing is continued until the whole is light and foamy. The result is an emulsion, usually of the o/w type, because egg yolk tends to emulsify fat as an o/w emulsion. The emulsion is stabilized by the lecithin of the egg yolk and the GMS of the superglycerinated fat. The presence of the GMS greatly increases the stability of the emulsion and enables a large amount of water to be emulsified with the fat. As the amount of sugar that can be used depends on how much water there is to dissolve it, the use of high-ratio fats enables cakes of high sugar and moisture content to be produced. Looking at it in another way, a cake having a certain sugar and moisture content can be produced using less of a superglycerinated fat than of a normal cooking fat. This has led to the term 'fat extender' being used to describe such a fat.

After eggs have been beaten into the mixture, flour and baking powder (and milk if it is used) are added. A foam is created, each tiny air bubble being surrounded by an oil film, which, at this stage, is not very strong. When the cake mixture is put into the oven, the air and water vapour trapped within the bubbles expand due to the rise in temperature. If the cake is to rise evenly during baking to give it the desired lightness of texture, the foam must be stable. Rupture of the oil films will produce the familiar 'sad' or 'sinking' effect. The protein of the egg white acts both as a foaming agent and a foam stabilizer. The protein becomes adsorbed onto the interface between the air and the oil film, and, as the temperature rises and the bubble expands, the protein stiffens, or coagulates, so forming a rigid wall around the bubble. This prevents the bubble from bursting and also prevents the production of very big bubbles which would spoil the evenness of the texture. If the ratio of fat to egg is too high, the foam structure is weak and during baking some bubbles break and the cake sinks.

As already indicated, a fat must not only act as a creaming and emulsifying agent but also as a

'shortener'. This function is of primary importance in the production of biscuits and shortbread but is also an important factor in cake making. Fat coats the starch and gluten of the flour with an oily film, so breaking up the structure and preventing the formation of a tough mass. This leads to a cake that has a tender and 'short' crumb, whereas the use of too little fat produces a cake that is tough and of poor keeping quality. The greater the proportion of fat in the mixture, the greater the shortening effect.

If a cooking fat is to be an effective shortening agent it must have good plasticity because this enables it to spread over a large area of flour, coating the surface with a film of oil. Such a fat must be neither too hard, in which case it will have poor spreading power, nor too liquid as with an oil, in which case it tends to form globules rather than a film. In other words, a soft fat is required; this may be achieved by suitable blending of the oils used in manufacture. Blends which contain a high proportion of PUFA have better shortening power than those composed of mainly saturated fats. The presence of monoglycerides, such as the GMS added to superglycerinated fats, and diglycerides, also improves shortening power.

Fat substitutes

In recent years there have been developments in food science to develop replacements for fats and oils in foods. One of these substances is formed by the reaction of sucrose and fatty acid esters from edible fats. The resulting product is known as Olestra. Olestra is not absorbed, and therefore does not provide the kilocalories of fat but has similar properties to fat in food preparation. Olestra thus allows for lower energy consumption when it is used in place of fats for food manufacture, and helps to reduce blood lipids if it replaces saturated fatty acids. It is permitted for use in certain snack foods in the USA but has not been approved for use in the UK (Institute of Food Science and Technology Current Hot Topics http://www.ifst.org.uk/hottop13.htm).

LIPIDS IN THE DIET

Lipids in the diet mainly occur in the form of fats, but also include a number of fat-soluble compounds

Table 6.7 The fat content of selected foods

Food	Fat (%)
Lard	99.0
Margarine	81.0
Butter	82.0
Cream cheese	47.0
Cheddar cheese	34.0
Pork sausage	32.0
Herring	19.0
Beef, rump steak	14.0
Eggs	10.9
Milk	3.8
Bread, white	1.7
Rice	1.0
Haddock	0.6
Potatoes	0

Table 6.8 Cholesterol content of some foods

Food	Cholesterol (mg/100 g)
Egg yolk	1120
Kidney, pig's, stewed	700
Whole egg	391
Liver, pig's, stewed	290
Butter	213
Cheese, Cheddar	97
Chicken, white meat	70
Beef, average	58
Milk whole	14
Vegetable oil	0

like cholesterol. Dietary fat is usually considered in two forms, the 'visible' fats such as butter and margarine and 'invisible' fats which occur in foods such as milk and eggs where the fat is in a highly emulsified form. Some foods, such as meat, contain both forms of fat. The amount of fat in selected foods is shown in Table 6.7.

Fat has four functions in the diet. First, it serves as a source of energy. As fat has a higher energy value (9 kcal/g) than either carbohydrate (3.75 kcal/g) or protein (4 kcal/g), foods containing a high proportion of fat form a compact energy source. They are energy-dense. A man doing heavy work expends about 14 MJ per day. If he obtained all his energy from fat he would need to eat only 378 g of fat. A less fatty diet containing a large amount of carbohydrate would be more bulky. Second, fat makes diets more palatable. It contributes importantly to food structure and texture. Fat provides a base for the enormous range of fat-soluble compounds which provide flavour; lipids more readily cross the cell membranes of taste buds. The amount of fat in diets varies considerably, the higher the standard of living the higher is the proportion of fat in the diet. For example, in the poorest countries fat may only contribute about 10–20 per cent of the total energy in the diet, whereas in the wealthiest industrialized nations, fat may contribute 40 per cent of the total energy of the diet. Moreover, in wealthier countries a greater proportion of the fat in the diet is animal fat. Third, fats provide

the body with essential fatty acids. Fourth, they provide the body with fat-soluble vitamins.

Cholesterol is another lipid that is provided by the diet, although only about 20–25 per cent of body cholesterol comes from food, the rest being made by the body itself. A person of average weight will have rather more than 100 g of cholesterol in their body and the body makes about 700 mg of cholesterol each day. The actual amount varies with the individual and also with the amount received from food. If the amount supplied in the diet is reduced, the body compensates by making more for itself. The body normally has more cholesterol than it needs and some of the excess is made into bile salts which help with the digestion of fat. Cholesterol is transported in the bloodstream in the form of lipoproteins; synthesized in gut and liver. The blood cholesterol concentrations – more specifically the low-density lipoprotein (LDL) cholesterol – is a major determinant of coronary heart disease. Dietary fat – specifically saturated fat – is important in defining blood LDL-cholesterol. Dietary cholesterol is of much less importance for most people. Table 6.8 shows the cholesterol content of some foods.

Dietary reference values for fat

Apart from EFAs, there is no dietary requirement for fat or for specific fatty acids. There is an absolute need for dietary energy, but there is scope for variation in the amount provided by each macronutrient. However, DRVs are considered to be useful because of the possible relationship between fat/fatty acids and coronary heart disease (CHD) and cancer.

Table 6.9 Dietary reference values (DRVs) for fat for adults as a percentage of daily total dietary energy intake (including alcohol)

Type of fatty acid	DRV
Saturated fatty acids (maximum)	10
cis-Monounsaturated fatty acids	12
cis-Polyunsaturated fatty acids	6
Glycerol	3
trans-Fatty acids (maximum)	2
Total fatty acids	30
Equivalent to total fat	33

DRVs are calculated by adding individual reference values, as shown in Table 6.9.

Total fat intake is calculated from the sum of fatty acid intakes plus glycerol, i.e.

Total fat intake = saturated fatty acids
+ cis-monounsaturated fatty
acids + cis-polyunsaturated
fatty acids
+ trans-fatty acids
+ glycerol.

The 1991 Committee on Medical Aspects of Food Policy (COMA) report on dietary reference values recommends that an increase in consumption of any fatty acid should be avoided and hence the DRVs shown in Table 6.9 should not be exceeded. This means that not more than 10 per cent of total dietary energy (including that derived from alcohol) should be derived from saturated fatty acids and not more than 30 per cent from all types of fatty acid. The variations in total energy needs of individuals mean that the absolute intakes of all these fatty acids will vary, to provide a fixed percentage of energy. This can have implications for portion sizes during menu planning, since so many foods are presented in fixed size units.

Lipids in the body

Lipids in the body have three main functions.

1 In the fat depots of the body – the adipose tissue – they provide the chief store and source of energy for the body.
2 In all body tissues lipids form the main part of the structure of cell membranes.

3 Lipids provide the raw materials from which many hormones are made.

When fatty foods are eaten they pass through the digestive system in the manner described in Chapter 2. In the small intestine they are partly hydrolysed by lipase, one fatty acid molecule being split off from a fat molecule at a time, so that the result is a mixture of free fatty acids and monoglycerides and diglycerides. Because the hydrolysis is not complete, little free glycerol is produced. During absorption of fats, fatty acids and glycerol pass through the villi into the lymph vessel where they are resynthesized into fat molecules, being rearranged in the process so that the new fat molecules formed are more suitable for use by the body.

Fat, since it is insoluble in water, cannot be carried round the body dissolved in blood. Instead, it is transported in the form of complex lipoproteins which are made up of two parts: a lipid component of triglyceride, cholesterol and phospholipid together with a protein component. Thus, fat is carried by the blood in emulsified form as tiny droplets of lipoprotein. The lipoprotein complex responsible for transporting lipids from the small intestine is in the form of chylomicrons. It is the chylomicrons that are responsible for the 'milky' appearance of blood plasma that occurs after a meal rich in fat has been eaten.

The lipoproteins may be divided into four types, distinguished from one another by their different densities when they are separated by ultracentrifugation for analysis. They vary from chylomicrons with a high triglyceride content and correspondingly low density to high density lipoproteins with a low triglyceride content. These differences are shown in Table 6.10.

Chylomicrons carry triglyceride to both muscle and adipose tissue where lipoprotein lipases rapidly hydrolyse them. Some of the free fatty acids produced plus the remains of the chylomicrons (minus the triglyceride component), together with glucose from foods, pass to the liver where they are converted to triglycerides and then transported as very low density lipoproteins (VLDL) to muscle and adipose tissue.

Most body fat lies under the skin as adipose tissue. It was once supposed that such fat formed an inert store that was drawn upon when the body required

Table 6.10 Per cent composition of blood plasma lipoproteins

Lipoprotein	Abbreviation	Protein	Triglyceride	Cholesterol	Phospholipid
Chylomicrons	–	2	85	4	9
Very low density	VLDL	10	50	22	18
Low density	LDL	25	10	45	20
High density	HDL	55	4	17	24

energy. However, it is now known that adipose tissue is a source of considerable metabolic and synthetic activity. Triglycerides (as part of both chylomicrons and VLDL) are constantly being broken down and reformed within adipose tissue. Glucose derived from carbohydrate is also converted into fat in adipose tissue, this process being promoted by the hormone insulin. The constant breaking down and reforming of triglycerides involves the inter conversion of fatty acids between triglyceride molecules and the formation of many different triglycerides. Essential fatty acids must be provided by the diet, however, as these cannot be produced by the body's metabolic processes.

When the body requires energy from its reserves triglycerides from adipose tissue can be used, and they are broken down to fatty acids which are carried by the blood to muscles and other tissue. Glycerol is also produced and it is broken down to carbon dioxide and water and energy by a process involving adenosine triphosphate (ATP) and the Krebs cycle (see p. 103).

The production of energy from fatty acids involves, first, an activation step, the energy for which is provided by ATP – an energy-rich molecule – which is considered in more detail in Chapter 8. In this step a molecule of coenzyme A (containing the B vitamin pantothenic acid) is added to the fatty acid. This active form is then acted upon by about four enzymes (which contain B vitamins) in a series of steps, each of which involves the removal of a fragment containing two carbon atoms. Each two-carbon fragment is in the form of acetyl coenzyme A, which is then oxidized in a complex cycle of reactions known as the citric acid cycle (or Krebs cycle). It appears that the final oxidation of both carbohydrate and fat follows the same pathway; also, both nutrients finally yield the same products, namely carbon dioxide, water and release energy which is captured for use in metabolism by

converting ADP to ATP. This process, known as beta-oxidation is a highly controlled pathway of oxygen whose purpose is to release energy, just as burning does in an uncontrolled way.

If energy is not required immediately, molecules of glycerol and fatty acid recombine (using up some energy) and are deposited again as fat. There is, therefore, a dynamic equilibrium between the molecular breakdown and rebuilding processes.

Ketosis

During normal fat metabolism small amounts of acetoacetic acid, CH_3COCH_2COOH, and beta-hydroxy butyric acid, $CH_3CH(OH)CH_2COOH$, are produced by combination of two-carbon fragments. Acetone, CH_3COCH_3, is also produced from breakdown of acetoacetic acid. These three substances are known as ketone bodies and if they accumulate in the blood, ketosis is said to occur. Ketone bodies can be used as an energy source by most tissues, including the brain, in place of glucose.

Ketosis occurs when fat rather than carbohydrate is the prime energy source. This occurs during starvation or on a fat-rich diet in healthy people. Ketones are detectable in urine and can sometimes be faintly detected by their fruity, 'nail varnish remover' aroma on the breath. Provided that ketosis is controlled it is probably beneficial, particularly as it allows ketones to act as an energy source for the brain when carbohydrate energy sources have been exhausted.

A much more serious situation arises with severe insulin deficiency when carbohydrate cannot be metabolised, usually in type 1 (occasionally type 2) diabetes. Severe acido-ketosis may be fatal, partly because of the toxicity of the ketone bodies themselves and partly because the accumulation of acetoacetic acid and beta-hydroxy butyric acids reduces the pH of blood (i.e. increases acidity). If the pH is reduced from its normal value of 7.4 to a value of 7.2 or lower acidosis is said to occur. This condition may result in a coma, which, if untreated, may be fatal.

Lipids and cardiovascular health

In recent years there has been a growing debate as to the quantity and quality of lipids that are desirable to ensure a healthy diet. In wealthy countries, as already noted, fat contributes up to 40 per cent of the energy content of the diet, while in poorer countries it only contributes some 10 per cent. Moreover, in affluent countries a much larger proportion of the fat eaten is derived from animals, so the proportion of saturated fatty acids is commonly 15–20 per cent of energy.

In the western world, during the twentieth century, certain 'diseases of affluence' have appeared, as described in Chapter 3. Among these diseases CHD has become prominent as the most frequent cause of death. The study of this disease has been, and continues to be, intense. It has been established that there is no single cause, while correlation studies (see p. 25) indicate that the four main risk factors are smoking, diabetes/impaired glucose tolerance, raised blood pressure and high blood (LDL) cholesterol. Underpinning these major risk factors are diets and lifestyles which result in weight gain (particularly high-fat diets) and physical inactivity. The major metabolic risk factors (type 2 diabetes/impaired glucose tolerance, hyperlipidaemia and hypertension) tend to cluster in high-risk individuals who commonly show two or three of these risk factors as they gain weight and grow older. People with these multiple risks have metabolic syndrome and commonly show a central fat distribution, with high waist circumference even before they are markedly overweight. Insulin resistance is a primary problem. The expression of this syndrome, mainly accelerated CHD, is stimulated by high fat diets and inactivity. Fat is stored preferentially in the intra-abdominal space – a genetic trait linked directly to the other features of metabolic syndrome. The increased mass of metabolically active intra-abdominal fat floods the liver with excess free fatty acids which aggravate insulin resistance. The factors believed to contribute to CHD are shown in Fig. 6.7.

Of all the factors implicated, diet is the one that has been most studied and is the one of most concern in this book. Although we do not know the causes of CHD, we do know that it is associated with the build-up of fatty material, especially cholesterol, in the blood. Much research therefore is directed towards trying to discover the way in which diet affects blood cholesterol. First, however, it is necessary to explain the nature of CHD.

Coronary heart disease can be regarded as the result of two processes: arteriosclerosis and thrombosis. An early feature is reduced flow of blood to the coronary arteries which supply blood to heart muscle. A healthy coronary artery has the features shown in Fig. 6.8. Blood flows through the artery which is surrounded by the *endothelium*, a smooth lining to the artery which allows blood to pass through it without resistance. This in turn is surrounded by a layer of the protein *elastin*, which has an elastic character, and a thick layer of smooth muscle and connective tissue called the *media*.

With increasing age there is some 'hardening of the arteries', or atherosclerosis, which involves the formation of a swelling between the elastin and endothelium layers and consequent narrowing of the channel through which blood flows. The swelling (or atheroma) involves accumulation, initially inside scavenging macrophage cells, of a mixture of cholesterol and other fatty substances together with complex carbohydrates, blood, calcium and fibrous material. Macrophages later die, leaving their corrosive contents. The thick rough area of the arterial wall containing this material is called plaque.

If the growth of plaque restricts blood flow unduly, symptoms occur and the greater the amount of plaque formed the more severe the symptoms become. Undue restriction of blood flow produces angina in the form of stabbing pains which normally occur during exercise and which subside following rest.

The processes involved in the formation of a thrombus are not fully understood, but it is known that when cells are damaged various 'clotting factors' are released into the blood. This results in the formation of the blood protein thrombin, which initiates the conversion of another protein fibrinogen into strands of fibrin. These strands form a protein network that traps red blood cells and clumps of blood platelets, which together form a blood clot. Atheroma plaques become unstable or brittle and can rupture suddenly, resulting in thrombosis and a block to blood flow. Coronary thrombosis (myocardial infarction)

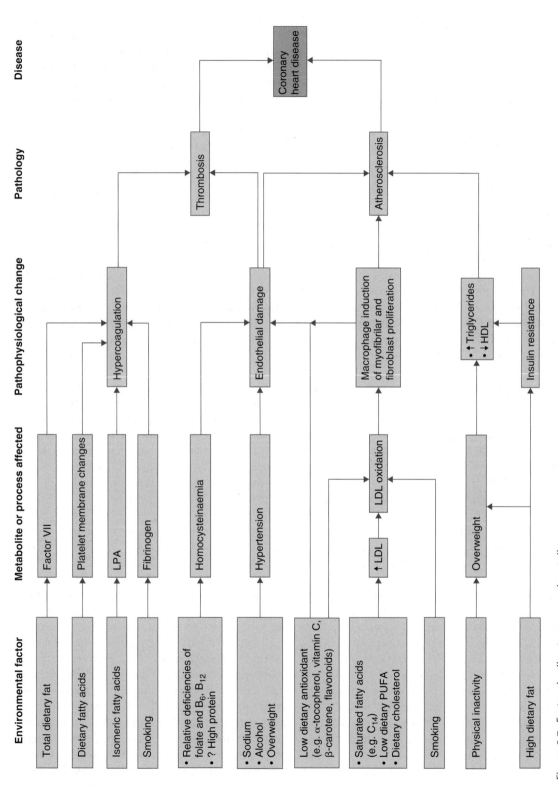

Figure 6.7 *Factors leading to coronary heart disease*

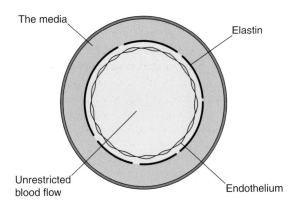

Figure 6.8 Cross-section through a healthy artery

classically presents as severe chest pain, commonly with breathlessness, which does not resolve with rest. The function of the heart as a pump is affected: first the normal rhythm of contractions is often upset and in up to a half of cases ventricular fibrillation develops – very rapid uncoordinated electrical activity which causes death in 2–5 minutes. Heart failure, which may be associated with other less serious rhythm disturbances (such as atrial fibrillation) results in accumulation of fluid in the lungs (left ventricular failure) or in the legs (right ventricular failure). As judged from characteristics electrocardiogram (ECG) changes, up to half of all myocardial infarctions are silent – i.e. they have no symptoms.

The development of arteriosclerosis is very slow, while thrombosis occurs rapidly. If thrombosis occurs where other arteries have been severely narrowed by arteriosclerosis a fatal heart attack is likely.

Cholesterol and dietary factors in CHD

It has been recognized for over 50 years that high serum cholesterol is an important correlate of CHD in epidemiological studies which compare CHD and blood test results in different countries. The association between high total fat intake with serum cholesterol and CHD have also been established for 50 years, from the work of Ancel Keys *et al.* (see Further reading). This was in the context of countries whose high fat intake also included large amounts of saturated fats, from animal-food sources. The links between dietary fat and CHD have

subsequently been refined. The strongest associations are with dietary saturated fatty acids and *trans*-fatty acids which rather specifically elevate LDL cholesterol – the most artherogenic fraction. Monounsaturated and polyunsaturated fatty acids have variably neutral or even protective actions.

The effects of dietary fat are most marked in individuals with the genetic predisposition to metabolic syndrome, about 20–40 per cent of the population who have central fat distribution raised serum triglycerides and low serum HDL-cholesterol. These factors are also closely related to physical inactivity. The causal pathway involves elevated blood levels of 'small dense LDL-cholesterol', which is readily oxidized and fails to be cleared by LDL receptors, thus accumulating at points of stress in arteries.

It needs to be understood, that cholesterol intake from food will, at best, have only a very small effect on total cholesterol in the body. In particular, consumption of low-cholesterol margarines rather than butter will have no appreciable effect on total body cholesterol. Butter and margarines with the highest content of cholesterol contain only about 0.2 per cent cholesterol, so that the amount of cholesterol we receive from such foods is insignificant compared with the cholesterol we receive from other foods (see Table 6.8), and even less significant when compared with the amount of cholesterol made by the body. The effect of saturated acid vs. PUFA in spreads is more important.

Modification of diet as a means of reducing risk of CHD

The hierarchy of evidence linking diet to heart disease appears in Fig. 6.7. Most of the evidence which links diet and CHD is observational. Epidemiology, at its simplest level links data on the incidence of CHD in different countries with data on diet composition. Ecological research of this kind is cheap, using existing databases, but risky since the data were not gathered for this purpose and are always incomplete. Many associations of CHD have emerged, the consistent ones being with high amounts of total fat, high saturated fat and low amounts of fruits and vegetables and low amounts of fish. High salt consumption is also related to CHD more weakly, although it associates more closely with stroke.

Cohort studies, where large groups of people are characterized and followed up to see who develops CHD over the years, generally support these associations. Cohort studies also offer more specific information such as physical activity (which protects against CHD) and on related diseases such as smoking, obesity, hypertension, hyperlipidaemia and type 2 diabetes (all of which increase CHD). The observational, epidemiological evidence is therefore convincing support for short-term experiments that high-fat, high-saturated fat diets lead to increases in LDL cholesterol, and they support the view that this is an important dietary step in accelerating CHD, where other major risk factors are similar. A consistent relation supports the view that fish, fruits and vegetables are also directly protective.

These studies provide enough evidence for many people to propose dietary targets for protection against CHD – on the evidence that other diseases would not be aggravated. Indeed, the same targets for CHD risk reduction are advocated to reduce diet-related cancers.

Critics, particularly from medical backgrounds with a concern for evidence-based drug prescribing, still call for experimental evidence to provide proof that dietary change would indeed have net benefit. A difficulty is that sufficiently large and long-term studies are colossally expensive since CHD develops slowly, modifications to the process take many years to be clear and thousands of subjects covering different ages, genders, ethnic backgrounds, etc., are needed for absolute certainty and safety. There is also a methodological problem that 'control groups' tend to make dietary changes when they enrol in dietary studies, becoming more like the intervention groups.

Quicker results are possible from studies in people who have very high risk of CHD (e.g. in secondary prevention after a heart attack, in diabetic or hyperlipidaemic individuals), but the extent to which the remainder of the population would benefit remains uncertain. Viewing the totality of the available (but always incomplete) evidence, the dietary associations identified in epidemiology still appears to be supported. The evidence is uncomfortable for some parts of the food industry, and over the years there have been frequent attempts to 'muddy the water' with apparently conflicting data or even completely spurious suggestions.

The best evidence from long-term intervention at a population level is probably from the North Karelia Project in Finland. A multisectoral programme sustained over 25 years resulted in substantial reduction in saturated fat and in salt consumption, together with reduced smoking, greater physical activity and a doubling or trebling of fruit and vegetable consumption. There were reductions of 50–70 per cent in the rates of CHD, stroke and also cancers. It was not possible to be certain which dietary element was most valuable, and in a sense that is not a useful question.

The changes were not particularly complicated or expensive, and to make any dietary change involves changing the whole dietary package. The new diet came to be more similar to a Mediterranean diet, which has also been popularized as protective against CHD. A completely different diet also associated with low rates of CHD is the Japanese diet. These diets are dissimilar in several ways but all represent balanced, food-based packages which would probably offer reduced rates of CHD if adopted more widely.

For health promotion directed at the general population, clear, quantifiable targets are needed, with a time scale to achieve them. Sets of targets have been produced in Scotland (Table 6.11), in England and Wales (COMA, Table 6.12) in USA in the NCEP step 1 and step 2 diets and by WHO (2003, Table 6.13).

These sets of dietary targets are always compromises between what might be theoretically optimal and what is practically possible. They are also mostly derived from the same evidence bases, so differences between them mainly reflect changing emphasis. Dietary targets to reduce CHD have changed little over the past 20–30 years and the popular view that the nutritionists are constantly changing their minds is largely a fabrication of the media, fuelled by misinformation from elements in the food industry.

The classical and dietary risk factor for CHD provide only part of the explanations for this disease, so making radical changes will not abolish the disease. It is estimated that 30–50 per cent of CHD is 'diet-related' so this is the maximum prevention possible by dietary change alone. As further information accrues this may be increased, but only slightly. There are numbers of additional contributors for CHD, which follow.

One such trial is the Oslo study, the details of which are summarized in Table 6.14. In this study

Table 6.11 Scottish dietary targets

Targets	
Fruit and vegetables	Average intake to double to more than 400 g per day
Bread	Intake to increase by 45 per cent from present daily intake of 106 g, mainly using wholemeal and brown breads
Breakfast cereals	Average intake to double from the present intake of 17 g per day
Fats	Average intake of total fat to reduce from 40.7 per cent to no more than 35 per cent of food energy
	Average intake of saturated fatty acids to reduce from 16.6 per cent to no more than 11 per cent of food energy
Salt	Average sodium intake to reduce from 163 mmol per day to 100 mmol per day
Sugar	Average intake of NME sugars in adults not to increase
	Average intake of NME sugars in children to reduce by half to less than 10 per cent of total energy
Breastfeeding	The proportion of mothers breastfeeding their babies for the first 6 weeks of life to increase to more than 50 per cent from the present level of around 30 per cent
Total complex carbohydrates	Increase average non-sugar carbohydrates intake by 25 per cent from 124 g per day through increased consumption of fruit and vegetables, bread, breakfast cereals, rice and pasta and through an increase of 25 per cent in potato consumption
Fish	White fish consumption to be maintained at current levels
	Oil-rich fish consumption to double from 44 g per week to 88 g per week

Scottish Office (1996). *Eating for Health: A Diet Action Plan for Scotland.* Edinburgh: HMSO. Crown copyright material is reproduced with the permission of the Controller of HMSO and the Queen's Printer for Scotland.

Table 6.12 National Cholesterol Education Programme and American Heart Association recommendations to reduce blood cholesterol and prevent CHD

NCEP and AHA recommendations	

Step I and Step II diets (NCEP)

Restricted total fat intake	less than 30 per cent of total calories

Step I diet

Saturated fat	less than 10 per cent of total calories
Cholesterol	less than 300 mg/day

It was intended as the starting point for patients who had high cholesterol levels

Step II diet

Saturated fat	less than 7 per cent of total calories
Cholesterol	less than 200 mg/day

Intended for people already at the Step I goals or for patients with a high-risk cholesterol level (240 mg/dL or higher) or who have already had a heart attack

Therapeutic lifestyle changes (TLC) diet (AHA)

As for Step II, plus:

Therapeutic options for LDL-lowering

Plant stanols/sterols	2 g/day
Increased viscous (soluble) fibre	10–25 g/day
Total calories (energy)	Adjust total calorie intake to maintain desirable body weight/prevent weight gain
Physical activity	Include enough moderate exercise to expend at least 200 kcal/day (e.g. brisk walking for 40–60 min)

Third Report of the NCEP Expert Panel on Detection, Evaluation and Treatment of High Blood Cholesterol in Adults (Adult Treatment Panel III). *Circulation*, 106: 3143–3421 (2002). Reproduced by kind permission of Lippincott, Williams & Wilkins. http://www.americanheart.org/presenter.jhtml?identifier=4764

Table 6.13 WHO summary of strength of evidence on lifestyle factors and risk of developing cardiovascular diseases

Evidence	Decreased risk	No relationship	Increased risk
Convincing	Regular physical activity Linoleic acid Fish and fish oils (EHA and DHA) Vegetables and fruits (including berries) Potassium Low to moderate alcohol intake (for coronary heart disease)	Vitamin E supplements	Myristic and palmitic acids Trans fatty acids High sodium intake Overweight High alcohol intake (for stroke)
Probable	α-Linolenic acid Oleic acid NSP Wholegrain cereals Nuts (unsalted) Plant sterols/stanols Folate	Stearic acid	Dietary cholesterol Unfiltered boiled coffee
Possible	Flavonoids Soy products		Fats rich in lauric acid Impaired fetal nutrition Beta-carotene supplements
Insufficient	Calcium Magnesium Vitamin C		Carbohydrates Iron

EPA, eicosapentaenoic acid; DHA, docosahexaenoic acid; NSP, non-starch polysaccharides.
Diet, nutrition and the prevention of chronic diseases (2000). Geneva: World Health Organization (WHO Technical Report Series No. 894).
Reprinted with permission. http://www.who.int/hpr/NPH/docs/who_fao_expert_report.pdf

Table 6.14 Detail of the Oslo study, showing results after 5 years

	Intervention group	Control group
At start of trial:		
Age in years	45	45
Cases of CHD	0	0
Smokers as per cent	70	70
Serum cholesterol as mg/100 mL	328	329
After 5 years:		
Dietary fat as percentage of energy intake	28	40
Saturated fat as percentage of energy intake	8	18
Serum cholesterol as mg/100 mL	263	341
Deaths from CHD per 1000	31	57

CHD, coronary heart disease.

men with high cholesterol levels were chosen. The intervention group reduced both total fat and saturated fat intake and reduced smoking. The results after 5 years showed a convincing reduction in death from CHD compared with the control group.

From the evidence gained from intervention trials it seems fair to conclude that for middle-aged men who are in the high-risk category by virtue of high levels of blood cholesterol or because there is a family history of CHD, there is enough positive evidence to recommend a reduction in the quantity of fat in the diet and a change to a diet involving less saturated fat and more polyunsaturated fat.

The COMA report on dietary reference values (1991) sets a desirable level for total intake of fat equal to 33 per cent of total energy intake. It also sets a desirable intake of saturated fat equivalent to 10 per cent of total energy intake.

Other contributors to CHD

The classical risk factors and the diet/fat theories of CHD fail to explain the full extent of the variance in incidence of the disease. There are now a number of other recognized factors that are gradually assuming a greater importance in predicting risks of CHD.

1 *The free radical theory.* Normally, PUFAs, which are present in high concentrations in cell membranes, are protected by the presence of antioxidants, particularly beta-carotene. The free radical theory proposes that in the absence of antioxidants, free radicals are produced (see p. 55) and these attack the unstable double bonds of PUFA molecules and, in the presence of ions of copper and iron which act as catalysts, oxidize the PUFA to lipid peroxides, which damage surrounding cells.

   It has been established that lipid peroxides are present in arteries that have been damaged by arteriosclerosis, but there is as yet only epidemiological evidence to support the theory that it is the absence of effective antioxidants that leads to the production of lipid peroxides which give rise to arteriosclerosis.

   This free radical theory has an important dietary consequence. It means that whereas in the diet fat theories it is the presence of too much fat in the diet that is suspect, in the newer theory it is the presence or absence of antioxidants that is significant. Evidence from dietary analyses and blood tests have related low levels (or intakes) of vitamin E, beta-carotene and vitamin C to higher rates of CHD. However, interventions with these antioxidants do not reduce CHD and in the case of beta-carotene appear to make matters worse. It seems that the benefit of fruit and vegetables – which contain a variety of other antioxidants such as flavonoids – cannot be replicated by high-dose vitamins or beta-carotene. This was an important lesson for nutrition.

2 *Cardiac arrhythmia.* Most of the risk factors considered in relation to CHD have to do with arteriosclerosis, but recently more attention has been given to risk factors associated with thrombosis.

The electrical activity of the heart normally follows a regular pattern throughout life but sometimes the electrical activity can become irregular and this condition, known as arrhythmia, can cause death. Death from arrhythmia is becoming more common and there is some evidence that the balance of fatty acids in the diet may be one of the risk factors. There is also some evidence that linoleic acid in the diet may protect against arrhythmia.

3 *Environment in early life.* As early as 1977 it was suggested that deprivation in infancy followed by relative affluence in later life could increase the risk of CHD. Later research studies have tended to support this finding. However, these findings are statistical in nature and are being followed up by experimental studies. An overview of this fascinating research indicates that poor fetal growth (shortness and lightness at birth) is a predictor of diabetes, hypertension, high cholesterol, CHD and stroke in adult life. This association has been described as 'fetal programming', but is most marked in countries where becoming overweight is common: adults who remain thin are at less risk. Poor fetal growth could be related to poor nutrition *in utero* (e.g. reduced amino-acid supply) or to stress. There is no good evidence that changing diet in pregnancy would be beneficial but common sense urges against weight loss by pregnant women. The main solution is avoiding adult weight gain and obesity.

Key points

- The water-insoluble nature of fats and oils reflect their chemical structure (triglycerides) and their nutritional roles (calorie-dense and association with fat-soluble lipid nutrients)
- The health impact of fatty acids is determined by chain length and degree of saturation
- Essential fatty acids are needed only in minute amounts and larger amounts as supplements can be hazardous
- Oxidation of fats in foods causes rancidity, and in the bloodstream promotes atheroma and heart disease
- Oxidation is preventable by fat-soluble antioxidants (e.g. Vitamin E)
- Fats and oils can be dispensed and transported in water as emulsions, in foods and in the body

Chapter summary

Dietary fats are important as contributing to (saturated, *trans*- and oxidized fatty acids) or protecting against (fish oils, omega-3) cardiovascular disease. All fats are very calorie-dense (9 kcal/g) and contribute to weight gain and obesity when comprising over 30 per cent of dietary energy. Fats and fat-soluble compounds (lipids) contribute texture and flavour to foods. They can be emulsified using artificial emulsifiers in foods and bile acids in the gut and lymph to be dispensed in water. They need to be protected (especially PUFAs) by endogenous or dietary antioxidants.

FURTHER READING

THE FOOD LABELLING REGULATIONS (1996): www.opsi.gov.uk/si/si1996/Uksi_19961499_en_1.htm

Institute of Food Science and Technology Current Hot Topics: www.ifst.org.uk/hottop.htm

DE LORGERIL M, SALEN P (2001). Mediterranean type of diet for the prevention of coronary heart disease. A global perspective form the Seven Countries Study to the most recent dietary trials. *Int J Vitam Nutr Res*, 71(3): 166–172.

DEPARTMENT OF HEALTH (1991). Dietary reference values for food energy and nutrients for the UK. Report of the Panel on Dietary Reference Values of the Committee on Medical Aspects of Food Policy No. 41. London: HMSO. www.nutrition-matters.co.uk/misc/1991COMAreport.htm

EVERETT DH (ed.) (1988). *Basic Principles of Colloid Science*. London: Royal Society of Chemistry.

VAN DEN HOOGEN PC, SEIDELL JC, MENOTTI A, KROMHOUT D (2000). Blood pressure and long-term coronary heart disease mortality in the Seven Countries Study: implications for clinical practice and public health. *Eur Heart J*, 21(20): 1639–1642.

Milk and dairy products

Dairy products constitute an important group of foods, as Tables 16.1 and 16.2 (p. 237 and 238) show. Like all foods, dairy products contain a mixture of nutrients. Milk is the sole food of young, growing calves, so contains most of the nutrients needed by all animals, including humans in generally similar proportions. However, cows' milk is for calves, not humans, and does contain more sodium (salt) than is safe for humans, and a greater proportion of saturated fatty acids than is safe if large amounts are consumed. It also contains more protein and a different profile of proteins to human milk. Although traditionally dairy products have played an important role in the British diet, their reputation has suffered recently on account of doubts expressed about the quantity and nature of fats in the diet. The animal fats and cholesterol present in dairy products have both been linked with modern 'diseases of affluence'. On the other hand, the high calcium content of milk and dairy products may help prevent osteoporosis – a scourge of the 'civilized' elderly.

MILK

Milk is a food of outstanding interest. It has been drunk by humans since the earliest prehistoric times and still forms the basis of national economies. It was designed by nature, or more correctly evolved naturally, to be a complete food for very young animals. Its extremely high nutritional value is a consequence of this and cows' milk – which is the main focus of this chapter – is not only a complete food for young calves but is also an excellent food for young children and valuable for adults. Milk is an interesting and complex colloidal system, the properties of which are of great practical importance in making butter and cheese and in other ways of processing milk. The complexity of this colloidal system can be judged from the fact that, despite much research, there is still much that is not fully understood.

Milk is an oil-in-water emulsion containing 3.5–4 per cent fat. In addition to milk fat, the fat phase contains fat-soluble vitamins, phospholipids, carotenoids and cholesterol, while the aqueous phase contains proteins, mineral salts, sugar (lactose) and water-soluble vitamins. The composition of different specimens of milk may show some variation with factors such as breed of cow, the nature of its food and the season of year. The figures which are given in Table 7.1 are, therefore, average values which refer to fresh summer milk. Winter milk contains only about two-thirds as much vitamin A as summer milk. The table also shows the percentage contribution made to the nutritional allowances of a man and a child by one pint (568 mL) of fresh milk each day, assuming that proteins contribute to energy. The figures given indicate the importance of milk as a source of calcium

Table 7.1 Composition of fresh summer milk and its contribution to the diet

| Nutrient | Amount in 100 g milk | Per cent contributions to nutrient RNI by 500 mL of milk daily | |
		Man with daily expenditure of 10.6 MJ	Girl 4–6 years with daily expenditure of 6.5 MJ
Energy	271 kJ	13	25
Carbohydrate	4.7 g	4	8
Fat	3.8 g	6	12
Protein	3.4 g	22	34
Water	88 g	–	–
Ascorbic acid	1.5 mg	55	75
Calcium	103 mg	86	69
Iron	0.1 mg	1	2
Niacin	90 mg	4	9
Riboflavin	170 mg	48	95
Thiamin	50 mg	17	33
Vitamin A	56 mg	17	29
Vitamin D	0.1 mg	–	3 (maximum)

RNI, reference nutrient intake.

and riboflavin; they also show why milk is regarded as such a valuable food, for it makes contributions to every class of nutrient. The main nutrients in which fresh milk is deficient are iron, niacin and vitamin D, while milk, as received by the consumer, may also be deficient in ascorbic acid. Milk does not contain dietary fibre in the form of non-starch polysaccharide, but in physiological terms the high level of lactose probably fulfils the role of dietary fibre. Lactose is only partly hydrolysed and absorbed in the intestine, the remainder (a proportion which increases with the total amount fed) passes into the large bowel where it is fermented as a fuel for bacterial metabolism.

Milk fat

The fat of milk is in the form of minute oil droplets, most of which have diameters of 5 μm – so small that a single drop of milk contains several million of them. The fact that milk is so highly emulsified makes it particularly easy to digest: it is digested more easily than any other fat. Milk fresh from the cow contains uniformly distributed oil droplets but when it is allowed to stand, the oil droplets, being lighter than the aqueous phase, tend to rise to the surface and form a layer of cream. As the oil droplets rise

they coalesce and form larger droplets, but the emulsion does not break down.

Milk may be homogenized by heating it to 65°C and forcing it through a small hole under pressure. This breaks up the oil droplets and reduces their diameter to 1–2 μm. This may not sound like a dramatic reduction in size but it increases the number of droplets by a factor of about 500 and results in a tremendous increase in surface area of fat. Such treatment has a considerable effect on the properties of milk; for example, it prevents the cream from separating out and it gives the milk a higher viscosity and richer taste. Homogenized milk coagulates more easily and has greater proneness to off-flavours and rancidity than unhomogenized milk.

Milk, whether homogenized or not, is a stable emulsion and the fat–water interface is stabilized by adsorbed natural emulsifiers present in the milk. The main emulsifier is protein, which is adsorbed around each oil droplet forming a protective monolayer, but other emulsifiers such as phospholipids (e.g. lecithin) and vitamin A also play a part.

The triglycerides of milk fat contain many different combined fatty acids. However, relatively few are present in significant amounts, chief of which are the saturated fatty acids shown in Table 7.2.

Table 7.2 The more important fatty acids in cow's milk

Fatty acids		g fatty acid/100 g total fatty acids
Saturated		61.1
$C_{4:0}$	Butyric	3.2
$C_{12:0}$	Lauric	3.5
$C_{14:0}$	Myristic	11.2
$C_{16:0}$	Palmitic	26.0
$C_{18:0}$	Stearic	11.2
	Others	6.0
Monounsaturated		31.9
$C_{18:1}$	Oleic	27.8
	Others	4.1
Polyunsaturated		2.9
$C_{18:2}$	Linoleic	1.4
$C_{18:3}$	Linolenic	1.5

Milk fat contains a very low proportion of polyunsaturated fatty acids (PUFAs) – less than 3 per cent.

Milk proteins

The proteins of milk consist of molecules which are, relatively speaking, so large that single molecules constitute colloidal particles dispersed through the aqueous phase of the emulsion (i.e. as a sol). The most important proteins in milk are casein (2.6 per cent by weight), which is precipitated under acid conditions and lactalbumin (0.12 per cent) and lactoglobulin (0.3 per cent) which are both whey proteins that remain in solution after acidification (see Cheese making, p. 83).

Casein is not a single substance, but a family of phosphorus-containing proteins that bind the calcium and other minerals present. The colloidal particles of casein are stabilized by a positive charge owing to the presence of bound calcium and magnesium ions. The charged particles are sensitive to changes of pH and to changes in concentration of surrounding ions. For example, during digestion, milk becomes solid owing to the coagulation or 'clotting' of casein. This is brought about by the enzyme rennin which, at the low pH prevailing in the stomach, converts casein into a coagulated form. The coagulated casein reacts with calcium ions to give a three-dimensional gel which is in the form of a tough clot called calcium caseinate.

The making of junket, a very old-fashioned dessert, is also an example of clotting. When milk is warmed to body temperature (37°C) and rennet added, it slowly coagulates into a white solid and exudes a slightly yellow liquid called whey. The change in the milk that occurs on making junket is the same as that which occurs in the stomach. Rennet is obtained from a calf's stomach but its essential constituent is rennin, which is responsible for the clotting of milk.

Lactalbumin and lactoglobulin are not coagulated by rennin but they are more easily coagulated by heat than casein. Thus, when milk is heated, lactalbumin and lactoglobulin coagulate and form a skin on the milk surface. This skin is responsible for the way in which milk so easily 'boils over', for expanding bubbles are trapped beneath the skin and build up a pressure which eventually lifts the scum and allows the milk to boil over the sides of the pan. The proteins of milk are among the common allergens which cause true food allergies in atopic individuals (contributing to asthma and eczema). Early exposure to cow's milk has also been linked to intestinal bleeding, and to development of type 1 diabetes in susceptible children.

Milk carbohydrate

The carbohydrate of milk consists of the disaccharide lactose, formed from the monosaccharides glucose and galactose, and is also called milk sugar. Lactose is the only sugar manufactured by mammals and is distinguished by its relative lack of sweetness compared with other sugars. The absorption of lactose depends on the presence of an enzyme in the small intestine, lactase, which catalyses the hydrolysis of lactose, which is itself not absorbable into glucose and galactose, which are. People vary in the amount of lactose present, which defines the amount of lactase absorbed. Babies need a great deal of lactase, but the amount declines with age. People originating from the Middle East and China often have virtually no lactose in adulthood and consequently become intolerant of milk – which causes diarrhoea. A solution, adopted empirically, is to convert the lactose by bacterial action before consumption, as yoghurt. During illness, and particularly if food consumption is markedly reduced, lactase levels in the gut decline and this can result in temporary lactose intolerance during the recovery period.

As is well known, milk readily becomes sour when it is stored. This is because milk contains bacteria, called lactic bacilli, in which are enzymes that bring about the breakdown of lactose into the sour-tasting lactic acid:

$$C_{12}H_{22}O + H_2O \xrightarrow[\text{bacilli}]{\text{lactic}} 4CH_3CH(OH)COOH$$

Lactose   Lactic acid

The pH of fresh milk is 7.4–7.7, the value being maintained within this narrow range by proteins, phosphate and citrate, which act as buffers. As milk turns sour the pH drops, and when it reaches 5.2 the milk curdles and the casein is precipitated in the form of flocculent curds. It will be noted that curdling and clotting are not the same chemically, as in curdling casein is merely precipitated whereas in clotting a tough mass of calcium caseinate is formed. Although milk which has been kept for a period curdles naturally because of the presence of lactic acid, any acid will produce the same effect. Curdling is hastened by warmth and it is for this reason that care must be taken when preparing dishes such as tomato soup where the acidity of the tomato juice may be sufficient to curdle the hot milk. If conditions are sufficiently acid, curdling may occur in the cold, for example, when milk is added to acid fruit, such as rhubarb.

Mineral elements of milk

The mineral elements of milk are either in the form of mineral salts or occur as constituents of the organic nutrients. Some are in solution and some are colloidally dispersed either as sol particles or combined with protein. As milk is the sole food of a young calf, it contains all the mineral elements required by the animal for growth. It is particularly rich in calcium and phosphorus, both of which are needed to build bone and teeth. These mineral elements are found in milk combined together in the form of calcium phosphate, which is not soluble but is held in suspension in the form of fine particles. Combined phosphorus is also found in casein and in phospholipids such as lecithin.

Many other mineral elements are present in small quantities; chlorine and iodine, for example, occur as soluble chlorides and iodides. Milk is an important source of iodine because in winter iodine is added to cattle feed to prevent goitre and stillbirth. Winter milk contains about 40 μg iodine/100 g milk while in summer, when cattle are grazing, milk contains only about 5 μg iodine/100 g milk. Iron is present in milk, but in such small quantities as to make it the one important mineral element in which milk is seriously deficient for human nutrition.

Whole milk has a sodium content of around 50 mg/100 g or 33 mmol/1000 kcal. This means that milk and dairy products are high sodium foods. The kidneys of young babies unable to excrete the sodium adequately if they are fed large amounts of cow's milk, and serious hypernatraemia can occur. In contrast, human milk has a sodium content of 15 mg/100 mL. This is the main reason for advice to avoid cow's milk until at least 1 year of age.

Vitamins in milk

The vitamins of milk are found either dissolved in fat globules or in aqueous solution. Vitamins A and D are both found in milk fat, the former in appreciable amounts, the latter in very much smaller quantities. The amount of both vitamins present in milk is greatest in summer when the cows are feeding on grass and receiving what sunshine our summers afford. The vitamin A value of milk is in part due to carotene and it is this substance which gives to milk its creamy colour.

Milk is a valuable source of riboflavin (see Table 7.1). It also contains useful amounts of thiamin and ascorbic acid and a small amount of niacin. The actual amounts of these vitamins in milk when it reaches the consumer depends upon the treatment it has received. Both ascorbic acid and thiamin are destroyed by heat treatment, while exposure to light destroys ascorbic acid and riboflavin.

Types of fresh milk

The nutrient composition of whole milk is given in Table 7.1. By law, it must contain at least 3 per cent fat (by weight). Such 'ordinary' milk is distinguished from milk from Jersey, Guernsey and South Devon breeds of cow, which has a higher fat content (an average of 4.8 per cent) than 'ordinary' milk. By law, milk from special varieties of cattle must contain at least 4 per cent fat.

Average milk consumption in Britain has declined over the last 50 years and is now about half a pint (284 mL) per day. An increasing proportion is in the form of skimmed or semi-skimmed milks from which a proportion of fat has been removed. The nutritional value of skimmed milk is as good as that of whole milk, except for the loss of fat and the fat-soluble vitamins A and D, which occurs when the cream is skimmed off. By law, skimmed milk must contain less than 0.3 per cent fat; in practice it contains, on average, only 0.1 per cent fat. Semi-skimmed milk must by law contain 1.5–1.8 per cent fat. The use of skimmed or semi-skimmed milk is helpful for those who wish to reduce their fat intake but such milks are unsuitable, because of their reduced vitamin content, for children under 2 years old. More specific fat contents, e.g. 1 or 2 per cent, are available in other countries.

Heat treatment of milk

Milk is such a rich source of nutrients that it is an ideal medium for the growth of microorganisms. Although milk should contain very low levels of bacteria when it is obtained from a clean and healthy cow, there are always some bacteria present and they soon multiply. Bacteria from the cow's skin, from the milk container, from the milker or milking machine and from the air pass into the milk, where they find congenial conditions in which to flourish. In addition to this normal contamination, unhealthy cows may contribute disease-bearing bacteria to the milk, the most dangerous of which is the tubercle bacillus. In the past this microorganism has caused thousands of deaths annually in both cattle and humans. In the UK in 1931, 2000 people died from tuberculosis contracted from milk. Other organisms such as *Brucella abortus*, which causes the disease brucellosis or undulant fever, and *Streptococcus pyogenes*, which causes sore throats and scarlet fever, may also pass from infected cows to man via untreated milk.

Most milk in Britain is now heat treated to ensure that harmful organisms are destroyed before it is consumed. As well as preventing the spread of disease, heat treatment of milk also considerably improves its keeping properties since lactic bacilli which cause milk to become sour are also killed.

Pasteurization of milk

Milk is pasteurized by heating it to at least 72°C for not less than 15 seconds, after which it is rapidly cooled to less than 10°C. The continuous process in which the milk is passed through a heat exchanger is known as HTST (high temperature short time). Over 99 per cent of the bacteria present are killed and although the product is not completely sterile, all harmful organisms are destroyed. The organisms which are not killed, together with any heat-resistant bacterial spores, are inactivated by the rapid cooling which follows pasteurization.

The temperatures used in pasteurization are not high enough to cause any significant physical or chemical changes in the milk, so that there is no noticeable change in palatability resulting from pasteurization. In some cases pasteurized milk has a flavour different from that of fresh milk, but this is caused by faulty pasteurization; either the milk has been heated to a temperature higher than normal or the process has been carried out in unsuitable equipment and the milk has thereby become tainted.

Pasteurization causes some slight decrease in nutritional value but, unless the recommended temperature and time of pasteurization are exceeded, only ascorbic acid and thiamin are appreciably affected, some 10–20 per cent of each being lost. Milk is not an important source of these vitamins, however, and even if this loss did not occur, it would only supply a small proportion of the body's needs. In addition, ascorbic acid is destroyed by storage in direct light, especially sunlight, so that even non-pasteurized milk is a doubtful source of this vitamin.

Sterilized milk

Sterilized milk is milk that has been homogenized, filtered and subjected to heat treatment so it will remain in good condition in an unopened bottle for at least a week and usually for several weeks. After homogenization, the milk is filtered, sealed into narrow-necked bottles and heated to at least 100°C and maintained at this temperature for up to an hour. In practice, higher temperatures and shorter heating times are used, a typical example being 112°C for 15 minutes.

Most sterilized milk in the UK is mow produced by ultra-high temperature (UHT) sterilization. This is carried out before the milk is bottled. The milk is homogenized and then heated to not less than 135°C for 1–3 seconds by flowing over a heated surface. A completely sterile product is thus obtained which, after cooling, is packed in sterile containers.

Sterilization causes a change in the flavour and physical composition of the milk and also causes a slight decrease in nutritional value owing to loss of vitamins. Lactalbumin and lactoglobulin are coagulated, some calcium phosphate is precipitated and about 30 per cent thiamin and 50 per cent ascorbic acid are destroyed. Milk sterilized by the UHT process resembles pasteurized milk much more closely, both in flavour and vitamin retention, but still has a 'cooked' flavour that some consumers dislike. The main virtues of sterilized milk are that its cream content is uniformly distributed, it is safe and it can be kept for considerable periods.

Preserved forms of milk

Milk is a nutritious food but, as we have already seen, it is perishable and even after pasteurizing needs rapid distribution and careful handling. It is also bulky and expensive to transport. For these reasons, and because seasonal surpluses of milk occur, effective methods of preserving milk in concentrated form are most desirable. Milk may be concentrated by removing a proportion of its water and it may be rendered safe by suitable heat treatment. The water is removed by evaporation, this being carried out in closed vacuum pans under reduced pressure. The temperature is kept below 70°C, so that the proteins are not coagulated and the production of a cooked flavour is avoided. Evaporated milk, also called unsweetened condensed milk in the UK, is pasteurized milk which after evaporation is homogenized and then sterilized in sealed cans. Condensed sweetened milk is made in a similar way, except that sugar is added and homogenization omitted. After evaporation further heat treatment is not necessary, because of the preservative action of the sugar.

Evaporated milk still contains about 68 per cent water and a much greater proportion of the water in fresh milk may be removed by drying it, usually by spray-drying. In this process the milk is first concentrated under vacuum at a low temperature and it is then dried by spraying it in the form of minute droplets into a flow of hot air. The product is almost 100 per cent soluble in water and is nutritionally only slightly inferior to pasteurized milk. Dried full-cream milk can be stored for fairly long periods but develops a tallowy taste after being stored for 9–24 months, owing to oxidative changes. Such changes can be prevented by packing the dried milk in sealed containers in which the air has been replaced by nitrogen. Properly stored spray-dried milk does not deteriorate as a result of the growth of microorganisms because its water activity is too low. Very few microorganisms survive the spray-drying process and those that do gradually die.

Although spray-dried milk is completely soluble in water, it is not easily wetted by water and this causes difficulty in reconstituting it in such a way that no lumps form. 'Instant' milk powders which can be reconstituted with ease are made from spray-dried skim milk by rewetting the particles in warm moist air and allowing them to clump together into porous spongy aggregates which are subsequently redried.

CREAM

Cream, like milk, is an oil-in-water emulsion. The way in which it is manufactured from milk is illustrated in Fig. 7.1. The milk is first heated to 50°C. This makes easier subsequent separation by centrifugal action into an upper cream layer and a lower layer of skimmed milk. The fat content of the cream produced can be adjusted by means of a pressure valve up to a maximum of 70 per cent fat.

The fat content of different creams is regulated by law, the minimum values for fat content being as follows: half cream, 12 per cent; single cream, 18 per cent; whipping cream, 35 per cent; double cream, 48 per cent; clotted cream, 55 per cent. The nutrient content of different types of cream is shown in Table 7.3.

Cream can be heat treated in a number of different ways including pasteurization, sterilization or ultra-heat treatment. Pasteurized frozen creams and UHT aerosol creams are available.

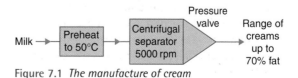

Figure 7.1 *The manufacture of cream*

Table 7.3 The nutrient composition of milks and creams per 100 g

Type	Energy (kJ)	Protein (g)	Fat (g)	Carbohydrate (g)	Sodium (mg)	Calcium (mg)
Half cream	568	2.8	12.3	4.1	55	96
Single cream	813	2.6	19.1	3.9	50	91
Whipping cream	1536	2.0	39.3	3.0	42	62
Double cream	1847	1.7	48.0	2.6	39	50
Whole milk	274	3.3	3.9	4.6	43	118
Semi-skimmed milk	195	3.5	1.7	4.7	43	120

Table 7.4 Nutrient content of low-fat yoghurts per 100 g

Nutrient	Plain	Fruit
Water (g)	85.7	74.9
Lactose (g)	4.6	3.3
Other sugars (g)	1.6[a]	14.6[b]
Protein (g)	5.0	4.8
Fat (g)	1.0	1.0
Minerals (g)	0.8	0.8
Energy (kJ)	216	405

[a]Galactose; [b]mainly sucrose.

YOGHURT

Yoghurt is made from heat treated, homogenized milk which is inoculated with a culture containing equal amounts of *Streptococcus thermophilus* and *Lactobacillus bulgaricus* bacteria. The essential change produced by these bacteria is that the lactose in the milk is converted into lactic acid. In the initial stages of the fermentation the streptococci are most active, converting lactose into lactic acid and also producing diacetyl until the acidity increases to pH 5.5. Thereafter, the lactobacilli continue the production of lactic acid until the acidity increases further to pH 3.7–4.3. At the same time acetaldehyde is produced and this gives yoghurt its characteristic flavour.

The fermentation process is continued until 0.8–1.8 per cent lactic acid is present and the product thickens. At this stage, if desired, flavours or fruit and sugar may be added. All such yoghurt contains live bacteria unless it is heat treated after fermentation, in which case this will be mentioned on the carton label. The nutrient content of various yoghurts is shown in Table 7.4. Yoghurt is a nutritious and easily digested food, though it does not have the somewhat magical health properties suggested for it at the beginning of this century and still believed by some people. In general, the nutrient value of yoghurt is that of the milk it contains and of any substances added to it during manufacture.

BUTTER

Butter, no less than milk, is a complex colloidal system and although the conversion of cream into butter is an ancient art, complete understanding of the mechanism of the process is still wanting. Butter is made from cream by churning. The cream used contains 35–42 per cent milk fat and may be used fresh or allowed to go sour, a process known as ripening, in which lactose is converted into lactic acid and flavour developed. After pasteurization the cream is chilled and agitated or churned. During churning the cream becomes increasingly viscous and eventually granules of solid butter appear. In modern creameries churning is carried out in a continuous butter-maker as shown in Fig. 7.2.

The conversion of cream into butter involves 'breaking' the oil/water (o/w) cream emulsion and turning it into an water/oil (w/o) emulsion, a process which is known as inversion. The detailed mechanism of this change is not known, but a simple outline can be given. At an early stage in churning air becomes trapped in the cream emulsion and a foam is formed. As already noted, natural emulsifiers present in cream stabilize the emulsion by being adsorbed at the oil–air interface. When air is trapped in the emulsion these emulsifiers become desorbed and spread out onto the surface of the air bubbles. The

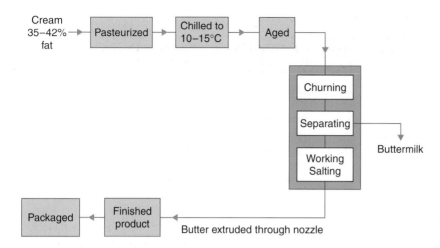

Figure 7.2 *Flow diagram of butter production*

oil droplets lose their stability and coalesce into larger drops. Continued churning brings about collapse of the foam structure, and the coalescing fat particles appear as visible granules and separate out from the aqueous phase.

Although both o/w emulsion and foam structures have collapsed, further churning brings about dispersion of a small amount of water in the fat and a w/o emulsion is formed. The nature of the final product is affected by the proportion of solid to liquid triglycerides present in the fat phase. Some liquid oil droplets are dispersed in the continuous fat phase, although continued churning reduces the proportion of such dispersed oil. If the temperature of churning is lowered, the proportion of crystalline triglycerides in the fat increases and a correspondingly harder butter is formed.

The composition of butter is variable. An average butter contains the following: 82 per cent fat, 0.4 per cent protein, 15 per cent water, 2 per cent salt, and vitamins A and D, particularly the former. The actual vitamin content varies considerably, being much higher in summer when the cows feed on grass than in winter when no fresh food is available. Summer butter may contain up to 1300 mg vitamin A (as retinol equivalent), whereas the average vitamin A content of butter is about 1000 mg/100 g. Summer butter contains about 0.8 mg vitamin D/100 g and about half this in winter. By law, butter must contain a minimum of 80 per cent fat and a maximum of 16 per cent water (European Council 1994).

Although some butter is sold unsalted, most types have salt added for flavour and preservation.

The high salt content of the aqueous phase helps to prevent the action of bacteria and enzymes that would cause hydrolytic rancidity (see Chapter 6).

CHEESE

Although there are more than 400 different named cheeses, the basic principles governing their manufacture are the same. Milk is coagulated and the solid formed is cut into small pieces to allow the whey to drain off. The solid curd is dried, salt is added and the cheese pressed or moulded and allowed to ripen. Cheddar cheese, which is a typical and popular hard cheese, will serve as a convenient example for discussing the main stages of cheese manufacture which are summarized in Table 7.5.

The essence of cheese making is the coagulation of milk and its conversion from a colloidal dispersion into a gel known as curd, and the subsequent release of water in the form of whey. The loss of moisture from a gel is known as synaeresis and results in a reduction in water content from 87 per cent in milk to less than 40 per cent in mature Cheddar cheese. The control of this water loss constitutes a major part of the art of cheese making. The rate at which water is lost depends upon three factors, namely temperature, pH and the way the curd is cut; in practice all three are controlled so as to give rapid synaeresis. Reduction of water content is most important as it determines the hardness and keeping quality of the cheese. The changes in water content and pH during cheese making are shown in Fig. 7.3.

Table 7.5 Stages in making Cheddar cheese

Stage	Description of physical and chemical changes
1. Pasteurization	Whole milk is pasteurized
2. Ripening or souring	Lactic acid bacteria starter added. Lactose is converted into lactic acid with consequent fall in pH
3. Clotting or coagulation	Rennet added to sour milk at 30°C. Casein is precipitated as a tough gel or clot of calcium caseinate known as curd
4. Cutting	Curd is cut into small pieces
5. Scalding and pitching	The temperature is raised to about 40°C, pH continues to fall and cutting is continued. Pieces of curd matt together and whey is run off
6. Cheddaring and piling	Curd is cut into blocks and piled up. Whey drains off and curd forms solid mass with a firm, soft texture
7. Milling and salting	The dry curd is milled into small pieces and salt is added. More whey is lost
8. Pressing	The soft cheese is put into moulds, pressure is applied and more whey is expressed
9. Maturing	After removal from the mould, the cheese is allowed to mature for 3 months or longer

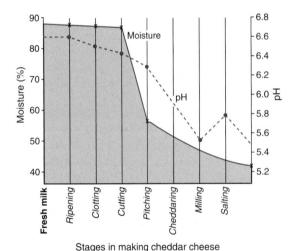

Figure 7.3 *The variation of water content and pH during cheese making*

The chemical changes that occur during maturing of cheese are still not completely understood, but are certainly brought about by enzymes. Lactic acid bacteria thrive in the immature acid cheese and the enzymes present in them bring about a number of chemical reactions which are responsible for the development of flavour and aroma. A week after manufacture is started, all the lactose has disappeared, having been converted into lactic acid. Apart from lactose breakdown, maturing mainly involves breakdown of protein and fat. Protein is broken down by enzymatic hydrolysis brought about by rennin and other peptidases. Proteins are progressively broken down into smaller molecules such as peptones and ultimately into amino acids. Such soluble and low molecular weight nitrogen compounds certainly contribute to cheese flavour and in addition bring about physical changes in the cheese, causing it to become softer and creamier. Fat, like protein, is broken down by enzymatic hydrolysis and is converted into glycerol and free fatty acids. Milk fat is relatively rich in low molecular weight fatty acids such as butyric, caproic and capric, which are released on hydrolysis and, being volatile and strong-smelling, contribute to cheese flavour.

Amino acids and fatty acids produced by breakdown of protein and fat may be further broken down by enzymes, yielding low molecular weight molecules such as amines, aldehydes and ketones which are volatile and strong-smelling, and thus contribute to the flavour of mature cheese.

Table 7.6 Some types and varieties of cheese

Type	Variety	Milk used	Water (%)	Nature
Very hard	Parmesan	Skimmed ripened milk	<25	Dry cheese excellent keeping qualities, matured >1 year
Hard	Cheddar	Whole ripened milk	35	Mature, non-crumbly
	Cheshire	Whole ripened milk	38	Immature, crumbly, mild flavour
	Edam	Unripened skimmed milk	35–40	Mild, firm, red colour (Dutch)
Soft	Cambridge	Unripened whole milk	>40	Immature cheese, curd is not cut
Cream	Cream	Ripened cream	45–50	Soft, mild, rich flavour
Internal mould	Stilton	Ripened whole milk	33–35	Blue mould, mellow flavour, cured 4–6 months
External mould	Camembert	Ripened whole milk	45–55	Soft, creamy consistency (French)

Table 7.7 A comparison of the composition of cheese and summer milk

Name	Energy (kJ) per 100 g	Nutrients per 100 g					
		Protein (g)	Fat (g)	Carbohydrate (g)	Calcium (mg)	Vitamin A (μg)	Vitamin D (μg)
Cheddar	1680	26.0	34.0	0	800	363	0.30
Stilton	1930	26.0	40.0	0	350	450	0.30
Cream cheese	1840	3.0	47.0	0	100	450	0.30
Summer milk	272	3.3	3.8	4.7	103	56	0.03

It is evident that the flavour of cheese results from a very large number of different substances and much more research is needed before they all become known. After Cheddar cheese has been stored for about 3 months it has developed its full flavour, although it may be stored for a year or longer.

The very large number of cheeses available makes it impracticable to do more than describe the main types and varieties, and this is done in Table 7.6. The main distinction is between soft cheeses, which are not pressed and therefore have a high moisture content, and hard cheeses, which are pressed and therefore have a lower moisture content and better keeping qualities. Soft cheeses have an open texture and provide suitable conditions for development of moulds, which require air for successful growth. The best known of the British mould-ripened cheese is Stilton, the blue-green veins of which are caused by moulds. White Stilton is merely ordinary Stilton which has not been matured long enough for mould to develop.

NUTRITIONAL VALUE OF MILK AND DAIRY PRODUCTS

As mentioned earlier, milk contains most of the essential nutrients in reasonably balanced amounts. Indeed, the presence of a nutrient in milk is often taken as (weak) evidence for its essentiality. Why else would nature have put it there?

Cheese has a high nutritional value, as would be expected from the fact that a pint (568 mL) of milk produces only about 56 g cheese. Certain water-soluble nutrients of milk are lost in the whey, but most of them are retained in the curd. A hard cheese, such as Cheddar, consists of roughly one-quarter protein, one-third fat and one-third water. It is a rich source of calcium, phosphorus and vitamin A, and also contains useful quantities of other nutrients, as shown in Table 7.7. It is a much more concentrated food than milk but is less complete because of its lack of carbohydrate. Soft cheeses retain a higher percentage of moisture than hard ones and, therefore, have a lower percentage of other nutrients. Cream cheeses, which are made from cream, are rich in fat but contain much less calcium, phosphorus and vitamin A than Cheddar. The amount of water is regulated by law and Cheddar cheese, for example, must not contain more than 39 per cent water. The actual vitamin content of a cheese is very variable depending upon the quality of milk used in its production. Thus, Cheddar cheese which is rich in vitamin A contains on average 363 µg/100 g of cheese, although the amount in a particular sample may differ greatly from this figure.

Hard cheeses are largely free of additives, except for the use of the vegetable dye annatto used to colour some varieties such as Red Leicester. Processed cheese, on the other hand, contains a variety of additives such as dried milk powder, emulsifiers and flavours. A preservative such as sodium nitrite may also be used.

Key points

- Milk is the optimal food for baby cows
- Milk contains a full range of essential nutrients for humans, but not all in the best proportions (too much sodium and saturated fatty acids)
- Lactose in milk is variably absorbed in the small intestine, and functions like dietary fibre as a nutrient for normal large-bowel bacteria. This can result in diarrhoea and intolerance for some people
- Lactose is fermented to lactic acid in yoghurts and some cheeses

---

Chapter summary

Milk is a very major commercial food. It is often considered a 'natural' food, but requires substantial application of food technology to overcome bacterial contamination (pasteurization), fat separation (homogenization), oxidisability and rancidity (sterilization) and storage problems (evaporation, spray-drying).

FURTHER READING

EUROPEAN COUNCIL REGULATION (1994). No 2991/94 of 5 December 1994. Laying down standards for spreadable fats. *Official Journal* L 316, 09/12/1994 p. 2–7.

ALFA-LAVAL (1980). *Dairy Handbook*. London: Alpha-Laval Co.

BRITISH NUTRITION FOUNDATION (1987). Report of the Task Force on *Trans Fatty Acids*. London: BNF.

BRITISH NUTRITION FOUNDATION (1992). Report of the Task Force on *Unsaturated Fatty Acids – Nutritional and Physiological Significance*. London: BNF.

CURR, M. (Ed.) (1991). *Polyunsaturates: Their Role in Health and Nutrition*. London: The Butter Council.

CHRISTIAN, G. (1977). *Cheese and Cheesemaking*. London: Macdonald Educational.

DEPARTMENT OF HEALTH (1994). *Nutritional aspects of Cardiovascular Disease*. London: HMSO.

DEPARTMENT OF HEALTH AND SOCIAL SECURITY (1984). Committee on Medical Aspects of Food Policy (COMA), *Diet and Cardiovascular Disease*. London: HMSO.

EVERETT, D.H. (Ed.) (1988) *Basic Principles of Colloid Science*. London: Royal Society of Chemistry.

FAO/WHO (1980). *Dietary Fats and Oils in Human Nutrition*. London: HMSO.

GURR. M.I. (1984). *Role of Fats in Food and Nutrition*. Amsterdam: Elsevier.

HYDE, K.A. AND ROTHWELL, J. (1973). *Ice-cream*. Edinburgh: Churchill Livingstone.

KON, S.K. (1972). *Milk and Milk Products in Human Nutrition*, 2nd edition. Rome: FAO.

MEYER, A. (1973). *Processed Cheese Manufacture*. Orpington: Food Trade Press.

NATIONAL ADVISORY COMMITTEE ON NUTRITION EDUCATION (NACNE) (1983). *Proposals for Nutritional Guidelines for Health Education in Britain*. London: Health Education Council.

NATIONAL DAIRY COUNCIL (1988). *From Farm to Doorstep … A Guide to Milk and Dairy Products*. London: NDC.

NATIONAL DAIRY COUNCIL (1991). *Coronary Heart Disease I*. Fact File No. 7. London: NDC.

NATIONAL DAIRY COUNCIL (1992). *Liquid Milk Report*. London: NDC.

NATIONAL DAIRY COUNCIL (1992). *Coronary Heart Disease II*. Fact File No. 8. London: NDC.

NATIONAL DAIRY COUNCIL (1994). *A–Z of Dairy Products*. London: NDC.

NATIONAL DAIRY COUNCIL (1994). *Trans Fatty Acids*. Topical Update 1, London: NDC.

PORTER, J.W.G. (1975). *Milk and Dairy Foods*. Oxford: Oxford University Press.

RANCE, P. (1983). *The Great British Cheese Book*. London: Papermac.

ROBINSON, R.K. (Ed.) (1986). *Dairy Microbiology* (2 vols). Barking: Applied Science.

SCHMIDT, G.H. AND VAN VLECK, L.D. (1974). *Principles of Dairy Science*. USA: Freeman.

SCOTT, R. (1986) *Cheesemaking Practice*. Barking: Applied Science.

SHAPER, A.G. (1988). *Coronary Heart Disease: Risks and Reasons*. London: Current Medical Literature Ltd.

WALKER, A.F. AND WOOD, E. (1991). *Cholesterol: Its Role in Health and Disease*. London: The Butter Council.

WEBB, B.H. *et al.* (1974). *Fundamentals of Dairy Chemistry*, 2nd edition. USA: Avi.

WRIGHT, G. (1987). *Milk and the Consumer*. Bradford: University of Bradford, Food Policy Research Unit.

WILLIAMS, K. (Ed.) (1992). *The Community Prevention of Coronary Heart Disease*. London: HMSO.

8

Carbohydrates

Carbohydrates constitute one of the three main classes of 'macro-nutrients'. They occur in food as sugars and starches, which are a major source of energy in the diet, and as cellulose which is the main non-starch polysaccharide.

Sugars are produced in plants as the end product of photosynthesis, from carbon dioxide and water. At the same time oxygen is evolved, as shown in the equation for the formation of the simple carbohydrate glucose:

$$6CO_2 + 12H_2O \rightarrow C_6H_{12}O_6 + 6O_2 + 6H_2O$$
$$\text{Glucose}$$

Water appears on both sides of this equation because it has been shown that all the oxygen evolved originates from the water. The oxygen atoms in the glucose and water molecules on the right-hand side of the equation are those which were originally combined with carbon in the carbon dioxide. The equation is a comparatively simple one, but it shows only the starting materials and final products of a series of complex reactions.

The building-up of carbohydrate molecules by plants is accomplished by photosynthesis. Energy is required to transform the carbon dioxide and water into carbohydrates and this is supplied by the action of sunlight on chlorophyll in the leaves. Consequently, photosynthesis does not take place in the dark. Animals, including man, are unable to synthesize carbohydrates, and this is one of the fundamental differences between animals and plants. The sugars formed by photosynthesis are transported within the plant as sucrose, which is soluble in water. Sucrose is subsequently converted by the plant to polysaccharides, the most important of which are starch and cellulose. Starch is the principal energy reserve of most plants stored in tubers and elsewhere, whereas cellulose, which is the main component of plant walls, provides structural support and synthesized in growing plants of plants.

The solar energy used in photosynthesis is stored as chemical energy and this may later be drawn upon by the plant, which, by oxidizing the carbohydrate back to carbon dioxide and water, is able to make use of the energy liberated. Alternatively, animals, by eating the plant, may utilize the chemical energy stored in the carbohydrate molecules.

Carbohydrates contain only carbon, hydrogen and oxygen and, except in rare cases, there are always two atoms of hydrogen for every one of oxygen. Accordingly, carbohydrates have the general formula $C_x(H_2O)_y$ where x and y are whole numbers, and it is from this formal representation as hydrates of carbon that the name carbohydrate is derived. There are, of course, no water molecules as such present within the molecule of a carbohydrate. However, starch usually exists in nature is usually in hydrated form (i.e. associated with water molecules); for example, the storage of carbohydrate and glycogen always involves increased weight from water.

Many of the carbohydrates known, particularly the simple ones, do not occur naturally but have been obtained by synthesis in the laboratory. The naturally occurring carbohydrates containing six, or multiples of six, carbon atoms are particularly important. Familiar examples are glucose $C_6H_{12}O_6$, sucrose $C_{12}H_{22}O_{11}$ and starch, the very large molecules which are represented by the formula $(C_6H_{10}O_5)_n$.

SUGARS

The simpler carbohydrates, called sugars, are crystalline solids which dissolve in water to give sweet solutions. The simplest of these, such as glucose and fructose, are called monosaccharides and they are of great importance as the units or building blocks from which the more complex carbohydrates are built. Disaccharides, for example sucrose, maltose and lactose, contain two connected monosaccharide units which may be alike or different. Similar to the monosaccharides, disaccharides dissolve in water to give sweet solutions and so are classified as sugars. Disaccharides can be hydrolysed with dilute acids, or by enzymes, to give the monosaccharides from which they are built up. For example, sucrose on hydrolysis gives equal parts of glucose and fructose. Disaccharides and starches must be hydrolysed to monosaccharides for absorption from the gut. Non-starch polysaccharides, such as cellulose, are not digestible and pass through the small intestine to be fermented by large-bowel bacteria.

Monosaccharides

D-Glucose, dextrose or grape sugar, $C_6H_{12}O_6$

These are all names for the same sugar which is found in grapes (up to 7 per cent) by weight and other sweet fruits. Onions and tomatoes also contain about 1–2 per cent glucose, but honey, which contains about 30 per cent by weight is the richest natural source of the sugar. It plays an essential part in the metabolism of plants and animals and is the main product of photosynthesis in plants. In animals, it is produced during digestion of starch and other carbohydrates and it is a normal component of the blood of living animals. Human blood contains about

80–120 mg/100 mL and it is the only sugar which plays a significant part in human metabolism.

Glucose is a white solid; like all sugars, it is sweet-tasting but it is less sweet than sucrose. Its alternative name, dextrose, is derived from the Latin word *dextra* meaning 'right'. If a beam of polarized light is passed through a solution of glucose its plane of polarization is rotated to the right. We need not trouble ourselves unduly about the nature of polarized light, it will be sufficient to regard it as light which has been such treated that the wave vibrations all occur in one plane, which is called the plane of polarization. Substances such as glucose which rotate the plane of polarization of polarized light in this way are said to be optically active, and glucose, which rotates it to the right, is said to be dextro-rotatory. The effect of optically active substances on polarized light is a consequence of the precise spatial arrangement of groups of atoms in the molecule.

Five of the carbon atoms and one of the oxygen atoms in a glucose molecule are connected together to form a six-membered or hexagonal ring structure. D-Glucose exists in two isomeric forms which differ very slightly. Ordinary D-glucose is the α-isomer. Semi-pictorial formulae which give an idea of the way in which the atoms are arranged are given in Fig. 8.1: the carbon atoms are numbered to make it easier to refer to them later in this chapter when some important polysaccharides are considered.

The plane of the rings in Fig. 8.1 should be imagined to be projecting forward from the plane of the paper with the thick edge towards the reader and the substituent H, OH and CH_2OH lying above and below the plane of the ring. However, the situation is far more complex than this as the ring is not planar and it can fold or buckle to take up various shapes, which are referred to as configurations.

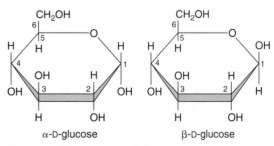

Figure 8.1 *The structure of glucose*

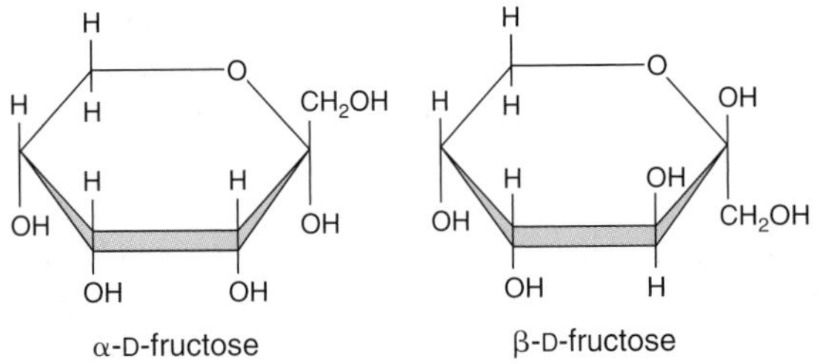

Figure 8.2 *The structure of fructose*

D-*Fructose, laevulose or fruit sugar, $C_6H_{12}O_6$*

The sugar fructose is mainly found with glucose in sucrose, but in some foods the sucrose is 'inverted' to glucose and fructose. This occurs naturally in the nectar of flowers, because fructose is very sweet. Thus, fructose is abundant in honey, which contains about 35 per cent, and in sweet fruit juices. Fructose is not a major dietary component in its own right in most normal diets, although its use as an added sweetener can result in some people having large intakes. It is produced in the body by hydrolysis whenever food containing sucrose is eaten. It is a laevorotatory sugar, which means that when a beam of polarized light is passed through a solution of fructose the plane of polarization is rotated to the left. This is the origin of its alternative name laevulose.

Fructose is a C_6 sugar similar to glucose and it shares the same molecular formula, $C_6H_{12}O_6$. Five of its carbon atoms and an oxygen atom form a six-membered ring with the other groups of atoms disposed about it, as shown in Fig. 8.2.

Fructose and glucose have very similar molecular structures (Figs 8.1 and 8.2). At first, the structure of fructose may appear to be identical with that already given for glucose in Fig. 8.1, but close comparison will show that this is not so. The differences between them, although slight, are detected with ease by biological systems such as our bodies. For example, they differ in sweetness because they have different effects on taste receptors. Fructose is more readily converted to fat (triglyceride) than glucose in the liver. Fructose is about twice as sweet as sucrose (ordinary table sugar) but it has the same energy value, about 17 kJ/g. This means that the same sweetening effect is produced by about half the weight of fructose if it is substituted for sucrose.

Until fairly recently, fructose was not available cheaply but it is now made from commercial glucose (glucose syrup or corn syrup, see p. 107) by treating it with an enzyme which is able to isomerize glucose to fructose. Fructose is widely used in sweetened drinks and confectionery. It tends to be used more in slimming foods because of the caloric saving compared with a greater amount of glucose needed to reach the same sweetness. Evidence is lacking that this has any significant impact for weight management, perhaps because the taste for very sweet food is perpetuated.

Pentose sugars (with five carbon atoms) also exist e.g. D-ribose and D-xylose. They are not major component in foods but ribose is important in metabolism as part of ATP and of nuclear material such as DNA and RNA.

Disaccharides

Disaccharides are formed by the union of two monosaccharide molecules. with the loss of a molecule of water. This is known as a condensation reaction (see equation below).

It is not possible to prepare disaccharides from monosaccharides in the laboratory by this process despite its apparent simplicity. Nature, however, accomplishes it without difficulty. Disaccharides are easily split into their component monosaccharides by enzymes or by boiling with dilute acids. Many disaccharides are known, but the most important, and the only natural ones of interest in food science, are sucrose, maltose and lactose.

Sucrose, cane sugar or beet sugar, $C_{12}H_{22}O_{11}$

Ordinary sugar, whether obtained from sugar cane or sugar beet, is substantially pure sucrose. It is a white

$$(C_6H_{11}O_5)O\,\vdots\,H + HO\,\vdots\,(C_6H_{11}O_5) \rightarrow (C_6H_{11}O_5)—O—(C_6H_{11}O_5) + H_2O$$

Two monosaccharide molecules   A disaccharide molecule

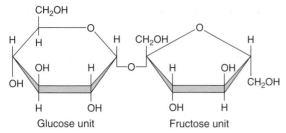

Glucose unit   Fructose unit

Figure 8.3 *The structure of sucrose*

crystalline solid which dissolves in water to give a dextrorotatory solution. Sucrose is widely distributed in the vegetable kingdom in many fruits, grasses and roots and in the sap of certain trees. It is produced and consumed in far larger quantities than any other sugar. Over two million tonnes of sucrose are used annually in this country (which is roughly 41 kg per person per year) and of this about one-half comes from home-grown sugar beet. Home consumption of table sugar is decreasing, having been 9.5 kg per head in 1989 but less than 6 kg per head in 2001–2002. This does not include the sugar that is added to cereals, confectionery and soft drinks, so people are probably not consuming less sugar but obtaining it from different sources.

Sucrose can be hydrolysed by heating with dilute acid or by using the enzyme sucrase. When this is done, equal quantities of glucose and fructose are obtained because the sucrose molecule is composed of a glucose unit and a fructose unit combined. The fructose unit does not have a six-membered ring but a five-membered ring, as shown in Fig. 8.3. The mixture obtained on hydrolysis is called invert sugar and it is laevorotatory because fructose is more strongly laevorotatory than glucose is dextrorotatory. This change of sign of rotation is called an inversion, producing inversion products.

The mixture of glucose and fructose produced by the inversion is called invert sugar and has been known in the form of honey for many centuries. Bees collect nectar, which is essentially sucrose, from flowers and it is inverted by enzymes during passage through their bodies. Honey is not pure invert sugar because it contains, in addition to glucose and fructose, some sucrose, about 20 per cent water and small quantities of extracted flavours peculiar to the flowers from which it was obtained. When sucrose is used in the preparation of acidic foodstuffs, a certain

amount of inversion invariably takes place. For example, if sucrose is used for sweetening fruit drinks, it is completely inverted within a few hours. Jams and sweets also contain invert sugar.

Sucrose is obtained commercially from sugar cane, which can only be grown in tropical countries, and sugar beet, which can be grown in any temperate climate. Whichever is used, the same product is obtained: there is no difference between the sugar obtained from sugar beet and that obtained from sugar cane.

Maltose or malt sugar, $C_{12}H_{22}O_{11}$

The sugar maltose is obtained when starchy materials are hydrolysed by the enzyme diastase. Maltose can be further hydrolysed by the enzyme maltase or by heating with dilute acid. D-Glucose is the only monosaccharide formed during these hydrolyses and this indicates that maltose contains two connected glucose units.

Lactose or milk sugar, $C_{12}H_{22}O_{11}$

Lactose, a white crystalline solid which is somewhat gritty in appearance, is the principal sugar present in milk. Cow's milk contains about 4–5 per cent lactose and human milk about 6–8 per cent. Lactose provides about 40 per cent of an infant's energy requirements and it enhances the growth of lactobacilli in the gut.

On hydrolysis of lactose, equal quantities of the two monosaccharides, glucose and galactose, are obtained. This demonstrates that the lactose molecule consists of these two monosaccharide units linked together.

Oligosaccharides

Oligosaccharides are carbohydrates with 3 to 10 monosaccharide units. Examples are the trisaccharide raffinose (Gal-Glc-Fuc) and the tetrasaccharide stachyose (Gal-Gal-Glc-Fuc), both found in legumes. Because of their non-digestibility in the small bowel, they provide substrates for bacterial fermentation in the large intestine and in particular gas formation (flatulence). Their most important property, which may be unique, is to selectively stimulate bifidobacterial growth while suppressing the growth of some other species such as *Clostridium perfringens*.

Sweetness and sweeteners

Why is sugar sweet? A simple question but, as with so many simple questions, the answer is complex. It is even difficult to say with any degree of precision what we mean by sweetness. The term can only be defined in subjective terms and the property is measurable only by tasting and not, as with most other properties, by using an appropriate instrument. Although it is difficult to define sweetness and impossible to measure it in any absolute way, it is possible to compare the relative sweetness of different substances. In practice, relative sweetness is determined by human beings using that well-tried and exceedingly sensitive organ the human tongue, the tip of which is believed to be the area concerned with the sensation of sweetness. By carrying out large numbers of tasting tests with sugars and other substances and adjusting their concentrations until they are of apparently equal sweetness, or by finding the lowest concentration at which sweetness can be detected, it is possible to draw up a table of relative sweetness, such as Table 8.1.

Most of the substances listed in Table 8.1 are compounds we have not yet discussed, but all of them (except cyclamate) are approved for use as sweeteners in food (see p. 301). Sorbitol, mannitol and xylitol are not sugars, but sugar alcohols obtained by reduction of the sugars sorbose, mannose (both hexoses) and xylose (a pentose sugar), respectively. Xylitol is produced commercially from birch wood. It has the same energy value as sucrose and hence is of no use as a sugar substitute for slimmers. It is not fermented to acids by bacteria present in the mouth (see p. 114) and hence, unlike sucrose, it does not promote cavities in teeth, i.e. it is not cariogenic. Xylitol does not require insulin for its metabolism.

Assessment of relative sweetness is subjective and as perceived by an individual may differ from time to time. A solution which appears to be 'less sweet' on one occasion may appear to be 'more sweet' on another. There is influence from recent food consumption and by long-term habitual exposure. Moreover, perception of relative sweetness may differ if the sweetness of solid substances rather than the sweetness of solutions of them is compared. It is not surprising, therefore, that the estimations of relative sweetness published by different groups of investigators are far from consistent. For this reason, the values given in Table 8.1 should be regarded as representative and treated with caution.

A great deal of work has been done to see whether there is any link between the sweetness of a compound and its chemical structure. Some progress has been made and it has been suggested by one group of workers that in all sweet substances a 'sweetness-producing' structural feature called a 'saporous unit' could be identified. The saporous unit, which contains two adjacent electronegative atoms, is thought to interact by hydrogen bonding with suitable receptor units in the tongue. Interestingly, proteins which bind sweet-tasting substances in proportion to their sweetness have been isolated from the taste buds of a cow's tongue. Whether a cow's perception of sweetness is the same as that of a human being, however, is purely a matter of speculation.

Sweetness is perceived by infants at birth as one of our basic tastes. It is believed to help guide infants to human breast milk, which is very sweet.

POLYSACCHARIDES

Polysaccharides are carbohydrates of high molecular weight which differ from the sugars in being non-crystalline, generally insoluble in water and tasteless unless hydrolysed by amylase in salivary fluid. A piece of bread will begin to taste sweet after chewing as the starch begins to be converted to glucose. A polysaccharide is built up from a large number of connected monosaccharide units which may be alike or different. As in the case of disaccharides, one molecule of water is lost in the union between one monosaccharide molecule and the next. The polysaccharides which are of importance in food chemistry are all built up from monosaccharides containing six

Table 8.1 Relative sweetness

Sweetener			
Sucrose	1.0	Acesulfame-K	150
Glucose	0.5	Aspartame	200
Fructose	1.7	Saccharin	300
Lactose	0.4	Thaumatin	3000
Sorbitol	0.5	Cyclamate	30
Mannitol	0.7	Splenda	600
Xylitol	1.0		

carbon atoms and are best formulated $(C_6H_{10}O_5)n$. The value of n varies, but in most cases is quite large. A single cellulose molecule, for example, can contain several thousand connected glucose units. Hydrolysis breaks down a polysaccharide molecule into smaller portions containing various numbers of monosaccharide units and may, if sufficiently drastic, convert the polysaccharide completely to monosaccharide:

$$(C_6H_{10}O_5)n + nH_2O \rightarrow nC_6H_{12}O_6$$

Like the sugars, polysaccharides are built up by plants from carbon dioxide and water and it is probable that the sugars represent an intermediate stage in the photosynthesis of polysaccharides. It has already been mentioned that animals are unable to build up carbohydrates by photosynthesis and for this reason polysaccharides are found predominantly in plants. The polysaccharide glycogen, however, is elaborated by man from glucose, and several similar examples of animals synthesizing polysaccharides from monosaccharides are known. In man, glycogen constitutes a store of carbohydrate; starch performs a similar function in plants and glycogen is sometimes called animal starch. In plants, polysaccharides also serve as skeletal material – a function not paralleled in animals.

Starch

Starch is the chief energy and nutritional reserve of all higher plants and it is converted by the plant, as required, into sugars. It may be stored in the stems, as in the sago palm, or in the tubers, as in potatoes and cassava, from which tapioca is made. Unripe fruits contain appreciable amounts of starch which is converted to glucose as the fruit ripens. It is especially abundant in seeds such as cereal grains and the pulses.

On microscopic examination, starch from various plant sources is found to consist of small particles called granules, the shape and size of which are peculiar to the plant from which they have been obtained. Starch granules are very small and cannot be seen by the naked eye, but they are clearly visible on microscopic examination. They vary in size and the granules of a particular type of starch need not all be of one size. The granules of potato starch, for example, vary in size from 0.0015 cm to 0.01 cm: in other words, the largest granules are about seven times as big as the smallest. There are two distinct types of granules in starch obtained from cereal grains such as wheat, barley and rye. Larger granules, which are lenticular in shape (i.e. shaped like lentils or double-convex lenses) and about four-millionths of a centimetre in diameter, are accompanied by smaller spherical granules which are only about a quarter as large. The smaller granules outnumber the larger ones by about ten to one, but only account for about 30 per cent of the weight of the starch.

Uncooked starchy foods are not easy to digest because the starch granules are contained within the cell walls of the plant which the digestive juices cannot easily penetrate. Cooking softens the cell walls and allows water to enter the starch granules causing them to disintegrate and gelatinize as shown in Fig. 8.4.

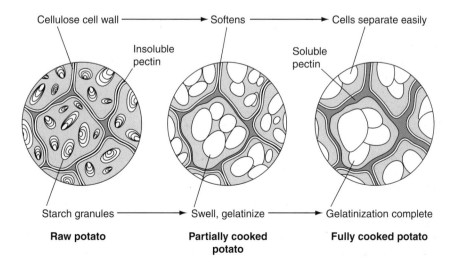

Figure 8.4 *Section of a potato as seen through a microscope*

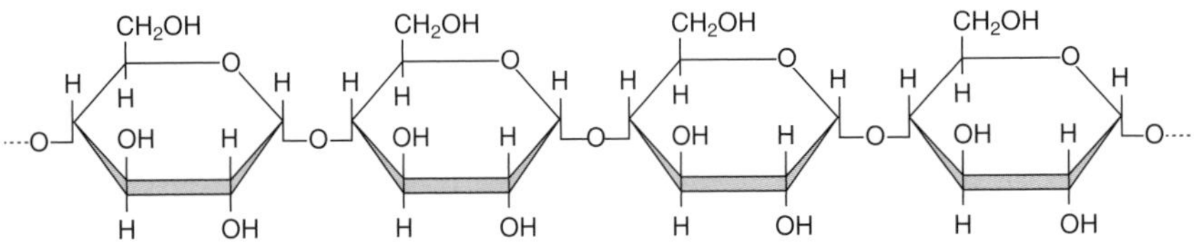

Figure 8.5 *Part of an amylose molecule showing 1–4 connected α-D-glucose units*

However, heating can also result in structural changes to starch known as retrograding, such that it escapes digestion by amylase in the small intestine, so is not absorbed as glucose and reaches the large bowel where it functions in the same way as non-starch polysaccharide (NSP). The proportion of retrograded starch is difficult to determine but is present in processed products and boiled and cooled potatoes. Overcooking may cause the cell walls to disintegrate completely, producing an unpalatable mush.

Structure of starch

When starch is hydrolysed, D-glucose is the only monosaccharide obtained. It was once thought that starch was composed, like cellulose, of strings of connected glucose units, the only difference between the two being that the glucose units in cellulose were the β-isomer and in starch the α-isomer. It is now known, however, that starch is mainly composed of two substances called amylose and amylopectin. Both of these are polysaccharides and there is usually about three to four times as much amylopectin as amylose.

Amylose is responsible for the blue colour produced when starch reacts with iodine. It can be separated from amylopectin by formation of an insoluble complex with a suitable liquid such as butyl alcohol. The enzyme β-amylase, which is present in cereals, hydrolyses amylose almost completely to maltose. Amylopectin, on the other hand, gives a reddish-brown colour with iodine and only about half of it is converted into maltose by β-amylase, the residue being referred to as a dextrin. Glucose syrup (p. 107) contains considerable quantities of dextrins, which are produced by incomplete hydrolysis of starchy materials. When dry starch is heated, so-called pyrodextrins are formed. These are brown in colour and soluble in water. Toast and bread-crust both derive some of their brown colour from pyrodextrins.

The molecular weight of amylose varies from about 10 000 to about 50 000 and this corresponds

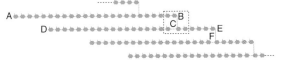

Figure 8.6 *Part of an amylopectin molecule*

to 70–350 glucose units. The glucose units are connected in a 1–4 manner to form a chain as in cellulose. Maltose is the only disaccharide obtained when amylose is hydrolysed and this shows that the glucose units are the α-isomer and not the β-isomer as in cellulose. The structure of amylose is shown in Fig. 8.5.

The structure of amylopectin is not as simple as that of amylose. To begin with, the molecule is larger and may contain several million glucose units. The amylopectin molecule is, in fact, one of the largest molecules found in natural products and it is made up of a large number of comparatively short interconnected chains of glucose units. A portion of an amylopectin molecule can be represented diagrammatically as in Fig. 8.6. In this diagram each hexagon represents a glucose unit and AB and DE are the short chains of about 24 glucose units connected at BC and EF. The links connecting the chains are from the reducing group at the end of one chain to a primary alcohol group on another (i.e. from C_1 to C_6). The section of Fig. 8.6 enclosed in a broken line is shown in detail in Fig. 8.7.

In a single amylopectin molecule there are large numbers of these chains each containing 20–30 glucose units, depending upon the source of the starch. In Fig. 8.7, only one 'branch' has been shown originating from each chain of glucose units. Most chains have more than one branching point, however, and a most complex three-dimensional bush-like structure can result.

Now that we know something of the structure of amylopectin it is possible to understand why β-amylase can only convert about half of it into

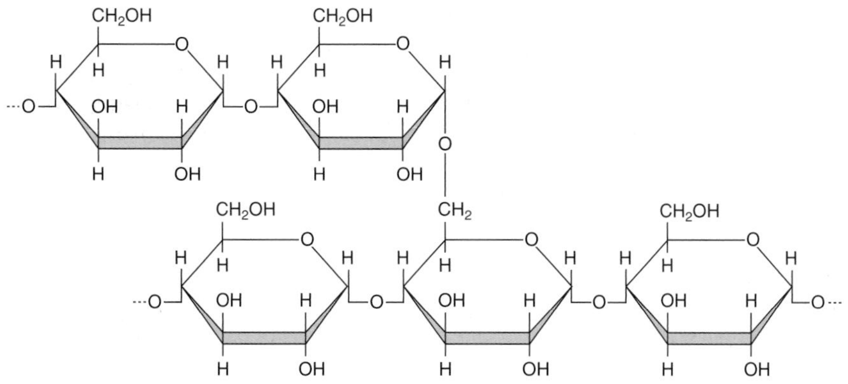

Figure 8.7 *Part of an amylopectin molecule (boxed section in Fig. 8.6)*

maltose. The reason is that amylase splits off pairs of glucose units, in the form of maltose, from the free end of the chains of glucose units in the amylopectin molecule (i.e. the left-hand ends in Fig. 8.6). When the chain has been degraded as far as a branching point the amylase is unable to split off further pairs of glucose units and the product is referred to as a β-limit-dextrin.

In addition to amylose and amylopectin, starch may contain small amounts of non-carbohydrate material such as phosphates and fats. The amount and composition of this extraneous material depend upon the source of the starch. Potato starch and wheat starch each contain about 0.5 per cent non-carbohydrate material and phosphates predominate. Wheat starch, on the other hand, contains about 0.75 per cent, made up largely of fats.

Gelatinization of starch

If powdered starch is shaken or stirred with cold water it does not dissolve but forms a milky suspension which settles out. When such a suspension is heated, water diffuses into the granules and causes them to swell. This begins at about 60°C and as the temperature increases the granules are progressively disrupted. When the temperature reaches about 85°C, a colloidal sol is obtained in which the amylose and amylopectin molecules are completely dispersed in the water. This sequence of events is known as gelatinization. When a starch sol is cooled, it congeals into a semi-liquid, semi-solid gel (see p. 56 for a discussion of sols and gels).

Starch resists cold water because the amylose and amylopectin molecules are closely packed in an orderly, almost crystalline, fashion, particularly at the surface of the granules. Hydrogen bonding between adjacent hydrogen and oxygen atoms helps to hold the molecules together and this gives cohesion to the starch particles and increases their resistance to penetration by water molecules. As the temperature increases, however, the molecules of water, amylose and amylopectin acquire additional vibrational energy until eventually the comparatively weak hydrogen bonds between the amylose and amylopectin molecules break down and water molecules are able to penetrate the granules. This starts at about 55–70°C (depending upon the type of starch), which is known as the initial gelatinization temperature.

As gelatinization proceeds, the granules swell and a dramatic increase in viscosity occurs. Eventually, the granules lose their separate identity and amylose molecules 'leak out' into the surrounding water to form a sol of somewhat lower viscosity. When the sol cools, the thermal energy of the water molecules (and, for that matter, the amylose and amylopectin molecules) decreases, hydrogen bonding is re-established between adjacent molecules and the mixture thickens to become a gel.

Amylose molecules are smaller than amylopectin molecules, but in suspension in water the molecules take up spiral shapes which provide ample opportunity for the formation of hydrogen bonds with adjacent amylose, amylopectin or water molecules. In this way a loose and irregular network is formed in which water molecules are immobilized both by entrapment in network voids and by the weak electrostatic forces of hydrogen bonding. The molecules of amylopectin, although much larger than those of amylose, are relatively more compact and the possibilities of network formation and extensive hydrogen bonding are less pronounced.

The formation of pastes or pasty liquids by heating starchy substances with water or water-containing fluids is of great culinary importance as it is the basis of many dessert, sauce and gravy recipes. Starch-based sauces such as Bechamel, Bordelaise and Espagnole are prepared by heating flour or some other starchy ingredient with butter (or another source of fat) for a few minutes to form a roux in which the starch granules are coated with fat. Milk, or a mixture of milk and stock, is then added and heating continued until the starch granules gelatinize. By varying the ingredients and/or their proportions a range of basic sauces, all of which are essentially gelatinized starch, can be prepared.

Several types of starch are used for thickening desserts, sauces and gravies. In Europe and North America, wheat starch, in the form of flour, is favoured but potato starch, cornflour and arrowroot are also used. Cornflour (known in North America as cornstarch) is made from maize and is a fairly pure form of starch which gives translucent and glossy sols and gels. Arrowroot, as is clear from its name, is a root starch. It is made from the underground stem or rhizome of a West Indian plant with the unmemorable name of *Maranta arundinacea*.

When a starch-thickened dish is prepared in the kitchen, it should be borne in mind that a hot concentrated starch sol becomes a gel when it cools and the near-liquid sol may change into a near-solid gel. This may be acceptable – even desirable – but if it is not the resulting gooey mess will do little to enhance the reputation of the cook. Sauces and desserts based on starch sols and gels should be freshly prepared. Sols may become thin and 'runny' on keeping, whereas pastes and gels may 'weep' water and become tough and rubbery. In both cases, the change in physical properties is caused by what is known as retrogradation, in which the amylose molecules clump together and separate from the sol or gel, thus destroying the semi-elastic network on which its properties depend. Starches with a very high amylose content undergo retrogradation less readily than those with a lower amylose content and such starches are commercially available to food manufacturers. Flour-thickened sauces or soups may also become thinner on keeping because of the breakdown of the starch by the enzyme α-amylase in the flour. This can be prevented in manufactured foods (e.g. in 'packet' soups) by the use of enzyme-inactivated flour (see p. 122).

Modified starch

Starch which has been chemically and/or physically treated so that it will form a gel with cold water or milk is used by food manufacturers under the name of modified starch. Among other things, it is used in the manufacture of a wide variety of 'instant' desserts, mousses, 'toppings' and whips which have been most successfully marketed by the food industry. These products also contain phosphates, such as disodium phosphate, Na_2HPO_4, which, in the presence of calcium ions from milk, form a gel with the modified starch and milk proteins. These concoctions also contain sucrose (the main ingredient), milk solids and a veritable catalogue of additives, including permitted gelling agents, emulsifiers, stabilizers, antioxidants, colours and flavourings.

Non-starch polysaccharides

Cellulose

Cellulose is the chief structural carbohydrate of plants and, as such, is very widely distributed. All forms of plant life, from the toughest tree-trunk to the softest cotton wool, contain cellulose and, indeed, the latter is almost pure cellulose. Whatever its source the constitution of cellulose is the same. Because it is so widely distributed in the vegetable kingdom, cellulose is found, to a greater or lesser extent, in all foods of vegetable origin.

Cellulose can be hydrolysed by heating it with hydrochloric or sulphuric acid. The only monosaccharide obtained in this process is D-glucose and it has been shown that the cellulose molecule consists of a large number of β-D-glucose molecules connected together at carbon atoms 1 and 4 to form very large chain-like molecules as shown in Fig. 8.8.

The number of glucose units connected in this way to form a cellulose molecule varies with the origin of the cellulose, but it is always large and may be as high as 12 000. Bundles of chains lying side-by-side are linked together by hydrogen bonds to give cellulose fibres.

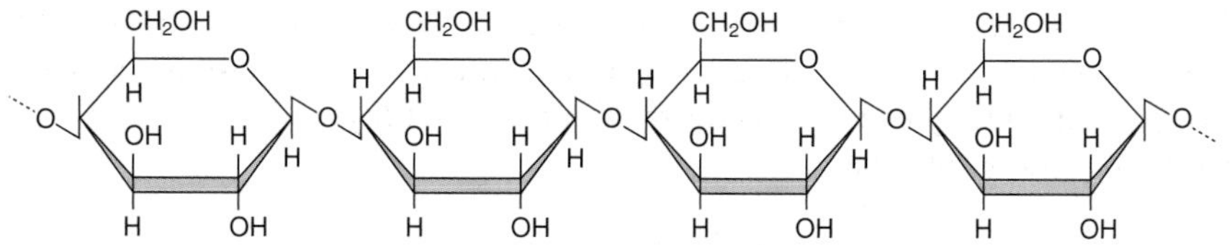

Figure 8.8 *Part of an cellulose molecule showing 1–4 connected β-D-glucose units*

Cellulose is totally insoluble in water. It can be digested by horses and ruminants such as cows. The latter have auxiliary stomachs containing microorganisms which produce enzymes capable of hydrolysing cellulose to glucose. Cellulose cannot be digested by man or most other carnivorous animals because the enzymes present in the intestines cannot rupture the β-1-4 links between the glucose units. This is unfortunate because cellulose is the most abundant natural product and if we were able to digest it and obtain nourishment from it, an unlimited additional supply of food would be readily available. Much cellulose is removed during food processing; for example, the husks of cereal grains, which are mainly cellulose, are usually removed. Cellulose serves a useful function in the diet as a non-starch polysaccharide (see p. 98) and removal of large amounts of it during food processing is nutritionally undesirable. Its presence in food promotes healthy bowel motility, helping to protect against bowel cancer. Most non-starch polysaccharides (and any starch which reaches the colon) can be metabolized by bacteria, and thus provide a fuel and nutritional resource for the normal bacteria of the large bowel (colon). This is a fermentation process which releases substantial amounts of short-chain fatty acids (as acetate, propionate and butyrate). All of these can be absorbed to provide a nutrient source for the colon itself and elsewhere. The metabolism of different NSPs varies. It is affected by cooking and by bowel absorption but on average NSP can provide up to 2–3 kcal/g.

Cellulose in plant tissues is usually accompanied by water-soluble polysaccharides called hemicelluloses which were formerly regarded as low molecular weight versions of cellulose. Despite their name, however, hemicelluloses are not chemically related to cellulose. They are composed, like cellulose, of chains of connected sugar units connected by β-1-4 links but the sugar units are the C_5-sugar xylose. Single sugar units, or sugar-related units, are attached at intervals to the main 'backbone' of connected xylose units.

Pectin

Pectin is the name given to a mixture of polysaccharides found in soft fruits and in the cell walls of all plants. Concentrated pectin extracts can be bought for use in jam making (see p. 112). They are made either from citrus fruit residues or from the pulp remaining after the expression of juice from apples. The pectin is extracted by pressure cooking with water or very dilute acid. The extract is filtered, vacuum concentrated, and the pectin precipitated by adding alcohol.

Pectin from various sources differs somewhat in composition and hence it is not possible to specify its structure precisely. However, all pectins consist essentially of the polysaccharide methyl pectate which has long chain-like molecules of several hundred connected units of α-D-galacturonic acid – an acid derived from the monosaccharide galactose. Some of the acid groups have been esterified and converted from free carboxyl (—COOH) groups to the methyl ester (—$COOCH_3$). Other sugars (or acids derived from them) may also be present in the chain. This sounds complicated (and it is) but fortunately the properties of pectin are of more interest to the practising food scientist than its exact chemical composition, and its use as a gelling agent is discussed in connection with jam making in the next chapter.

Pectin is present in unripe fruits and vegetables mainly in the form of its precursor protopectin. This is a water-insoluble compound in which most of the carboxyl groups are esterified. Protopectin is responsible for the hard texture of unripe fruits and vegetables: during ripening enzymes present in the plant convert it into pectin.

Glycogen

The polysaccharide glycogen acts as a reserve carbohydrate for man and other animals. Because its function in man parallels that of starch in plants it is sometimes referred to as animal starch. It is a very large molecule consisting of branched chains of α-D-glucose units and its structure is very similar to that of amylopectin but chain branching occurs, on the average, at about every 18–20 glucose units (compared with about 20–30 in amylopectin).

Glycogen is present in man and other animals in the muscles and in the liver; its function is to supply short-term local needs for glucose, for example during exercise. There may be several kilograms present in the body of a large animal such as a cow. Despite this, however, glycogen is not a normal constituent of the diet because it is mostly converted into lactic acid after an animal has been killed. In some special foods, e.g. fatty liver, in foie grass or pates and in fresh shellfish, there is significant glycogen present, which gives a sweet taste after hydrolysis in the mouth.

Non-starch polysaccharides: dietary fibre

Starch is the most important dietary polysaccharide, but other non-starch polysaccharides (referred to more conveniently as NSP) occur with starch in foods of plant origin. The NSP comes from the cell walls which form the structural support of the plant from which the food originated. Cell walls of a plant cell consist essentially of a rigid scaffolding of cellulose molecules embedded in a jelly-like matrix of water-soluble NSP composed of pectins, hemicelluloses (see p. 96) and a diverse mixture of gums. The fact that cellulose is insoluble in water whereas the other NSP are water-soluble is a distinction which, as we shall see, is of some importance from the point of view of their behaviour in the digestive system. Non-carbohydrate, high molecular-weight materials such as lignin (a constituent of wood) may also be present in food to a minor extent, but they are of little dietary significance.

Non-starch polysaccharides differ from starch, in that the link between the monosaccharide units of which they are composed is not an α-link (see p. 94). Because of this they are not broken down by the enzymes of the small intestine and they enter the large intestine, or bowel, unchanged.

Non-starch polysaccharides were formerly referred to, somewhat vaguely, as dietary fibre and, earlier still, as roughage. The term dietary fibre was a considerable

improvement on its predecessor, if only because it did not conjure up visions of intestinal abrasion associated with the term roughage. Nevertheless, it was a far from ideal term dating to the times when these substances were considered metabolically inert. To begin with, there are other 'fibrous' components of food – notably muscle fibre in proteins – which were not classed as dietary fibre because they are digested and absorbed. In addition, not all the dietary components regarded as dietary fibre were 'fibrous' in nature. Pectin, for example, is an amorphous substance which can hardly be regarded as fibrous. Even the cellulose component of dietary fibre is fibrous only at a molecular level and bears little physical resemblance to the cellulose fibres found, for example, in cotton wool. Foods rich in NSP are generally not noticeably fibrous in character: the presence of NSP does not confer coarseness or stringiness and it cannot normally be detected by the tongue.

The most important reason for adopting the term NSP in place of the more familiar 'dietary fibre', however, is the fact that the latter term was used somewhat indiscriminately to describe almost any type of 'indigestible' food component. Attempts at clarification by the use of such terms as 'raw fibre', 'crude fibre', 'soluble fibre' and 'insoluble fibre' did little to help. There was still an implication that their materials were inert. Many methods of analysis were used to determine how much of these various ill-defined types of dietary fibre was present in different foods and it became difficult to make meaningful comparisons of their dietary fibre content. About the only thing which can be said in favour of the term 'dietary fibre' is that is was well accepted by the general public who will, no doubt, take less readily to the more cumbersome term 'non-starch polysaccharides'.

To ensure consistency in the use of the term NSP and comparability of the results of chemical analysis a standard method of analysis has been adopted in the UK. This is the analytical technique developed by Englyst and Cummings, which is capable of differentiating between soluble and insoluble NSP. In the USA a different method, which determines 'total dietary fiber' (TDF), is more widely used. Fortunately, for most vegetables and fruits and many unprocessed cereal foods, the two methods give almost identical results. The TDF values for heat-processed cereal foods, however, are higher than NSP values for the same foods.

Sources of NSP

Cereal grains are rich in NSP and foods made from them are a major dietary source, especially if the whole grain is used. The NSP in wheat, maize and rice is mainly composed of cellulose and hence is largely insoluble. A significant proportion of the NSP in oats, barley and rye, on the other hand, is soluble. Vegetables contain more water than cereal grains and hence the NSP content is lower: the amounts of soluble and insoluble NSP are, in general, about equal. The ratio of soluble to insoluble NSP present in fruit and nuts varies widely but the soluble component is largely pectin which, as we have already seen, plays an important part in jam making. The NSP content of some foods is given in Table 8.2.

Table 8.2 Non-starch polysaccharide (NSP) content of some common foods

Foodstuff	NSP (g/100 g)		
	Soluble	Insoluble	Total
Apples	0.8	1.0	1.8
Baked beans	2.1	1.4	3.5
Bananas	0.7	0.4	1.1
Brown bread	1.1	2.3	3.4
Brown rice	0.0	1.9	1.9
Cabbage	1.2	1.2	2.4
Carrots	1.4	1.0	2.4
Haricot beans	2.7	3.4	6.1
Hazelnuts	2.5	4.0	6.5
All Bran	4.1	20.4	24.5
Cornflakes	0.4	0.5	0.9
Rice Krispies	0.1	0.4	0.5
Kidney beans	3.0	3.3	6.3
Nabisco Shredded Wheat	2.0	7.8	9.8
Peanuts	1.9	4.3	6.2
Potatoes	0.7	0.5	1.2
Raisins	1.0	1.0	2.0
Rolled oats	4.0	2.8	6.8
Runner beans	0.8	1.2	2.0
Spaghetti	1.5	1.4	2.9
Spaghetti (wholewheat)	2.0	6.4	8.4
Weetabix	3.1	6.6	9.7
White bread	0.9	0.6	1.5
White rice easy cook raw	0.0	0.4	0.4
Wholemeal bread	1.6	4.2	5.8

Dietary intakes of NSP in Britain average 11–13 g per day (about half of which is soluble NSP) but individual consumption varies widely between 2 g and 25 g per day. About half the NSP is provided by fruit and vegetables and the remainder mainly by cereal products.

Effects of NSP

At one time it was believed that the presence of 'roughage' in the diet was of value only as a means of easing or preventing constipation. It certainly does this, and thereby probably helps to prevent colorectal cancer. Thus, the main selling-point for bran-rich breakfast cereals was their efficiency in promoting regular bowel movements. This is partly a physical consequence of the absorption of water by NSP in the small intestine leading to speedier transit of food through gut and the formation of softer and larger stools. The 'transit time' for a typical British diet may be as long as 100 hours compared with as little as 35 hours or less if a diet with a high NSP content is eaten.

The prevention of constipation may not be of earth-shattering importance, except perhaps to a sufferer. Eating enough NSP has other, more important, beneficial effects, however, and there is substantial evidence to show that it helps to prevent many bowel diseases. Appendicitis, diverticular disease (in which distended pockets are formed in the bowel walls) and haemorrhoids are all less likely to occur if the NSP content of the diet is high.

Diets high in soluble NSP have also proved to be of value to sufferers from the disease diabetes mellitus in which the concentration of glucose and fats in the blood exceeds the normal levels. Diets with a high-fibre content and, in particular those rich in soluble NSP, are able to slow down the release of glucose to the bloodstream and in this way the metabolic consequences of the disease are minimized. Post-prandial blood lipids and glucose are reduced, so lowering the risk of coronary heart disease (CHD). Dietary NSP provides fuel for bacterial metabolism, so 'high fibre' diets increase colonic bacterial mass and lower the pH, both increasing bowel motility.

Diets rich in water-soluble NSP help to lower blood-cholesterol levels. This may account for the statistical link which has been found to exist between diets rich in NSP and a lower incidence of

CHD (see Chapter 3). However NSP is only one, and a relatively minor factor in prevention of CHD. A valuable consequence of the action of NSP is that a high intake of soluble NSP allows people to eat diets light in carbohydrates and so lower in fat. Without soluble NSP, blood sugar and insulin tend to rise rapidly after eating.

The NSP found in cereals, especially wheat, is associated with phytates and phytic acid (see pp. 122, 128 and 195) which can form complexes with minerals present in the diet and interfere with their absorption. Thus, a diet with a high NSP content, especially unprocessed wheat bran, may lead to mineral deficiency in individuals, such as elderly people whose diet is only marginally adequate in minerals.

Non-starch polysaccharide is unaffected by the enzymes of the digestive system and passes more-or-less unchanged to the large intestine. Once there, however, it is attacked and broken down by the harmless bacteria which inhabit the bowel and partly converted to short chain fatty acids, carbon dioxide, hydrogen and methane. The short chain fatty acids – mainly acetic, propionic and butyric (i.e. C_2, C_3 and C_4 acids) are absorbed into the bloodstream and hence contribute to the body's energy intake.

The hydrogen formed when bacteria break down NSP in the bowel is absorbed and subsequently expired in the breath. The carbon dioxide and methane are not absorbed, however, and, although harmless, may be a source of embarrassment, but many who have switched to a diet high in NSP for weight reduction purposes have found over time, bacterial profiles adapt, so that gas production is less problematic.

Dietary targets for NSP intake

Non-starch polysaccharide is so varied in composition and individual reaction to it is so unpredictable that it is not practicable to give precise dietary reference values. It is possible, however, to set daily target figures. Daily intake (as measured by the Englyst and Cummings method) is about 11–13 g. In the 1991 Committee on Medical Aspects of Food Policy (COMA) Report on Dietary Reference Values it is proposed that the 'target figure' should be in the range of 12–24 g, with an average of about 18 g per day for adults and proportionately smaller amounts for children. This can be most readily achieved by eating a range of foods rich in NSP, namely cereals, fruit and vegetables and legumes. It is normal with Mediterranean diets.

Foods rich in NSP tend to be bulky and there is a small risk that children's diets which contain excessive amounts of NSP may be inadequate in nutrient and energy content. Diets with a high NSP content may also have a high phytate content, if the NSP is derived largely from cereals, which may interfere with the absorption of minerals (see p. 128). Consequently, it is possible that people with marginally satisfactory diets may be under-provided with minerals if they consume too much NSP. This is unlikely to occur with a normal diet, but problems may arise if the NSP content of a diet is artificially increased by the addition of bran for slimming or laxative purposes.

Some of the starch in the diet may behave like NSP by resisting enzymatic hydrolysis to glucose in the stomach and small intestine and passing through to the large intestine, or bowel, unchanged. Such resistant starch probably owes its ability to withstand the action of digestive enzymes to the presence of tough cell walls around the starch granules which have not been completely broken down during grinding of cereal grains or during chewing. Starch which has undergone retrogradation (see p. 96) may also be resistant to enzymatic hydrolysis.

Undigested starch which finds its way into the large intestine will be fermented in the same way as NSP and will contribute to the body's energy intake via the short-chain fatty acids formed.

CARBOHYDRATES IN THE DIET

How much carbohydrate should there be in a healthy diet? We know that foods rich in carbohydrates are of value primarily as a source of energy but, weight for weight, proteins provide roughly the same amount of energy as carbohydrates and fats over twice as much. Of the three, however, carbohydrates are by far the cheapest and the most easily digested and absorbed. In the absence of sufficient carbohydrate the energy needs of the body can be met by protein and fat, and although it is possible to live on a diet containing little carbohydrate, this is not normally a good thing to do. Carbohydrate is usually considered an obligatory fuel for brain, and it is necessary to replenish glycogen stores in muscle, to be available for rapid high-energy exertions (which employ glycolytic type 2 muscle fibres). Lack of glycogen causes extreme tiredness although muscles can adapt to use fats as their main fuel. It is well known that Inuits, for example, traditionally lived almost exclusively on protein and fat but, in general, if too little carbohydrate is eaten fats also present in the diet may not be fully oxidized and ketosis may occur (see p. 67). If there is not enough carbohydrate to supply the energy needs of the body, dietary protein will be used to make up the deficit rather than for its primary purpose of tissue growth and repair. A further consequence of a low carbohydrate intake is that the proportion of the body's energy intake supplied by fat will be higher and may exceed the 'target figure' of 35 per cent.

Clearly, a low level of carbohydrate intake is not to be recommended. Are there likely to be similar objections to diets containing large amounts, such as the traditional Japanese diet, where about 80 per cent of the total energy intake is supplied by carbohydrate? A high intake of carbohydrate is not in itself harmful (though the presence of too much extrinsic sugar is not good for dental health: see p. 114) unless the diet is overloaded with calories, in which case an unhealthy weight gain may result. There is an obvious risk, however, that if the appetite is satisfied by a high carbohydrate intake other nutrients may not be eaten in sufficient quantity for the maintenance of good health.

However, a high intake of starch or sugars provide a high glycaemic index load which has effects on blood lipids and blood glucose. The COMA Panel on Dietary Reference Values propose that starches and intrinsic and milk sugars should make up the balance of the appropriate level of dietary food energy not provided by protein, fat, non-milk extrinsic sugars and alcohol. This means that in an average adult diet, about 37 per cent of the food energy intake should be provided by starches, intrinsic and milk sugars. The panel considered that consumption of non-milk extrinsic sugars should be limited to about 10 per cent of the body's total energy requirements. On average, for the population as a whole, this amounts to about 60 g of non-milk extrinsic sugars per day. This may sound rather complicated but, in essence, it means that, ideally, on average for the population as a whole, about half of dietary energy should be provided by carbohydrates and not more than about one-fifth of that amount (10 per cent of total energy) should come from non-milk extrinsic sugars. This represents a halfway house between traditional diets and the western diet profile.

CARBOHYDRATES IN THE BODY

During digestion the carbohydrates contained in food (with the exception of NSP) are hydrolysed by enzymes to their component monosaccharides. The process starts in the mouth, where saliva, which contains salivary amylase, is intimately mixed with the food and begins to hydrolyse the starch to maltose. The hydrolysis continues in the stomach until the food is acidified by mixture with the gastric juice. The food passes from the stomach to the small intestine, where pancreatic amylase continues the conversion of starch to maltose. Maltase present in the intestinal juices hydrolyses the maltose so formed to glucose. Lactase and sucrase, which are also present, convert lactose and sucrose to glucose, galactose and fructose. The monosaccharides pass from the small intestine into the bloodstream and are carried to the liver (where fructose and galactose are enzymically converted to glucose) and to the muscles.

The liver and muscles are able to convert glucose to glycogen, which serves as a reserve of carbohydrate for the body. Glycogen is reconverted to glucose, as required, according to the energy needs of the muscles and other tissues. Glucose is the main source of energy available to the body and it can be used by all cells. If there is insufficient carbohydrate in the diet, the body can make up to about 130 g of glucose per day from protein. Fats can also meet most of the body's energy needs but glucose is essential for proper functioning of the brain and nervous system. The body of a well-nourished man may contain several hundred grams of glycogen, about one-quarter of which is stored in his liver. When the muscles and liver can accommodate no more glycogen, the surplus glucose is converted by the liver into fat which is stored in fat depots as the body's second line of defence against food shortage. A small amount of glucose circulates in the blood for transport to tissues, drawing upon the liver's carbohydrate stocks or for transport to the liver to be converted to glycogen.

Within minutes of eating a meal, glucose enters the bloodstream from the small intestine, at different rates according to the glycaemic index of the food. Table 8.3 shows a ranking of foods by glycaemic index. The reference food for rapidly available carbohydrates is usually glucose itself or white bread, mashed potato also gives a very rapid rise in blood glucose after eating. The hydrolyses of starch in white bread or potato is then very rapid, and absorption is

Table 8.3 The glycaemic index of some common foods using glucose as standard

Glycaemic index of common foods	
Foods with a low GI factor (GI less than 55)	
Noodles and pasta	*Lentils*
Apples/apple juice	*Pears*
Oranges/orange juice	*Grapes*
Low fat yoghurt	*Fruit bread*
Baked beans	*Chocolate*
Foods with an intermediate GI factor (GI 55–70)	
Basmati rice	*Banana*
Rolled oats	*Soft drinks*
Sweetcorn	*Pineapple*
White sugar	
Foods with a high GI factor (GI > 70)	
Bread (white or wholemeal)	*Baked potato*
Cornflakes	*French fries*
Honey	*Mashed potatoes*
White rice (low amylase or sticky rice)	

Foster-Powell K, Holt SHA, Brand-Miller JC (2002). International tables of glycemic index and glycemic load values. *Am J Clin Nutr*, 76: 5–56. Foster-Powell K and Brand-Miller JC (1995). International tables of glycaemic index. *Am J Clin Nutr*, 62 (supp): 871–93. Reproduced with permission.

limited by bowel motility and osmotic rearrangement, to the same degree as glucose itself. For other foods, lower glycaemic indices reflect their physical structure, the presence of other nutrients such as NSP and fat and in some cases the degree of retrograding of starch by cooking. Low glycaemic index foods are encouraged in a healthy diet, to reduce the elevation of insulin and lipids after a meal. After it reaches the bloodstream, some glucose is used immediately for metabolism of brain and muscles but most enters the body's energy stores, from which it provides fuel until the next meal. The first store to be used is glycogen, in liver and muscle. If this capacity is exceeded then the glucose must be converted to fat for storage and this increases some energy usage. The blood may contain up to 8 mmol/L (about 0.14 per cent) glucose but this figure falls to about 4 mmol/L (about 0.08 per cent) some 2 hours or so after eating. This is quite a small amount and is equivalent to only about 5 g of glucose in circulation at any time.

If the glucose concentration in the blood is halved (hypoglycaemia) then there is insufficient for the brain to function normally. As brain glucose content falls, increasingly unpleasant symptoms develop, including dizziness, disturbances of vision, nausea, sleepiness, headache, confusion, and ultimately even loss of consciousness and epileptic seizures.

There are many normal mechanisms to prevent hypoglycaemia, including hormones such as cortisol, adrenaline and glucogen. Serious hypoglycaemia ('hypos') only occur with insulin overdosage. Most other people who think they are hypoglycaemic are not.

The oxidation of glucose

The body obtains energy by converting fats, proteins and carbohydrates to glucose and oxidizing that to simpler molecules and ultimately to carbon dioxide and water. The overall process may be likened to the release of energy from fossil fuels by burning them in a power station or boiler. Metabolic oxidation is infinitely more subtle and impressive, however, and man's most sophisticated fuel burning appliances are primitive compared with nature's delicately balanced and controlled complex of interdependent reactions.

The living cell has to function in an aqueous environment at a constant pH and at a comparatively low and essentially constant temperature. It cannot use heat energy to do work and, bearing in mind the limitations mentioned, it may seem surprising that any energy is made available at all. However, as we shall see below, almost half the energy locked up in the glucose molecule is captured by the body and this is a better conversion rate than that achieved by the most modern fuel-burning power station.

When glucose is completely oxidized to carbon dioxide and water by burning in oxygen a large amount of heat is evolved:

$$C_6H_{12}O_6 + 6O_2 \rightarrow 6CO_2 + 6H_2O + 2820 \text{ kJ}$$

In the body, however, oxidation does not take place in one step but by a complicated and elegant series of nearly 30 reactions, each of which releases only a fraction of the energy which would be made available by complete oxidation of the glucose molecule. Many of the oxidative steps in this sequence of reactions do not involve direct reaction with oxygen at

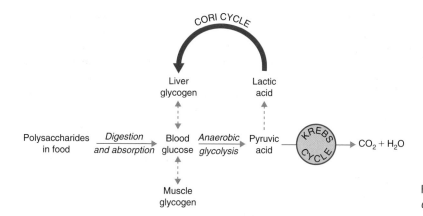

Figure 8.9 *Digestion, absorption and oxidation of carbohydrates*

all, but are simple dehydrogenation reactions which can be represented by a general equation:

$$AH_2 \xrightarrow{-2[H]} A$$

In many of these reactions the two hydrogen atoms removed are transferred to a coenzyme, for example, Coenzyme 1 (nicotinamide adenine dinucleotide, or NAD) or coenzyme II (nicotinamide adenine dinucleotide phosphate, or NADP), which act as hydrogen acceptors. The transfer is catalysed by oxidases which are highly specific in the sense that a particular oxidase will only work with one substrate – coenzyme pair.

There are two main stages in the oxidation of glucose by the body. In the first stage it is converted by a series of reactions to pyruvic acid:

$$C_6H_{12}O_6 \xrightarrow{-4[H]} 2CH_3COCOOH$$

No oxygen required

In the second stage the pyruvic acid is oxidized by a further series of reactions to carbon dioxide and water:

$$CH_3COCOOH \xrightarrow{+5[O]} 3CO_2 + 2H_2O$$

Oxygen required

The first stage is called glycolysis or, more precisely, since it takes place in the absence of oxygen, anaerobic glycolysis. The amount of energy made available by glycolysis is small compared with that released during the second stage. Energy for violent physical exercise – such as running to catch a bus – is required instantly, and as the bloodstream may be unable to supply oxygen sufficiently quickly to permit complete oxidation of glucose, anaerobic glycolysis takes place preferentially. The pyruvic acid produced is reduced to lactic acid and this is carried by the bloodstream to the liver where part of it is oxidized to provide energy for reconversion of the remainder to glycogen and glucose.

The cyclic conversion of glucose to pyruvic acid, lactic acid and back to glucose is known as the Cori cycle after its discoverers, Carl and Gerty Cori. When energy is not required so quickly, it is obtained by complete oxidation of glucose to carbon dioxide and water via pyruvic acid and about 75 per cent of the cell's energy requirements is provided by the second stage. Conversion of pyruvic acid to carbon dioxide and water occurs by a cyclic process involving citric acid which is often referred to as the citric acid or Krebs cycle, after Sir Hans Krebs, who worked out the details of the process, the Krebs cycle. Figure 8.9 summarizes the changes which occur during the digestion, absorption and oxidation of carbohydrates by the body.

The biochemical oxidation of glucose is a complex and involved process, and it took many years to work out exactly how it occurs. All the separate reactions are enzyme-controlled, 10 enzymes being required for the conversion to pyruvic acid and another 10 for the second stage of oxidation to carbon dioxide and water. The whole sequence is of great importance and beauty, but readers may be relieved to learn that we do not intend to give complete details of it here. However, one aspect of the oxidation process, which is common to both the first and second stages, and is indeed a feature of many other biochemical energy transformations, deserves further attention. This is the way in which adenosine triphosphate (or ATP) can behave as an energy bank or energy storehouse for the body. Adenosine triphosphate is built up from one molecule of the purine derivative adenine, one molecule of the sugar ribose (which together form the nucleotide adenosine) and three molecules of phosphoric acid.

In the body the phosphate groups may be split off successively from an ATP molecule to yield first adenosine diphosphate (ADP), then adenosine monophosphate (AMP), and finally adenosine itself. The adenosine part of the molecule is unchanged in this series of reactions and if we represent it by Ⓐ we can represent the series of reactions as follows:

$$Ⓐ - \overset{\overset{O}{\|}}{\underset{\underset{OH}{|}}{P}} - O - \overset{\overset{O}{\|}}{\underset{\underset{OH}{|}}{P}} - O - \overset{\overset{O}{\|}}{\underset{\underset{OH}{|}}{P}} - OH \xrightarrow{H_2O}$$

(ATP)

$$Ⓐ - \overset{\overset{O}{\|}}{\underset{\underset{OH}{|}}{P}} - O - \overset{\overset{O}{\|}}{\underset{\underset{OH}{|}}{P}} - OH \xrightarrow{H_2O}$$

(ATP)
+ H$_3$PO$_4$

$$Ⓐ - \overset{\overset{O}{\|}}{\underset{\underset{OH}{|}}{P}} - OH \xrightarrow{H_2O} Ⓐ$$

(AMP)
+ H$_3$PO$_4$ + H$_3$PO$_4$

The importance of this series of reactions is the fact that the two terminal phosphate groups are attached by high-energy phosphate bonds (shown in dark print in the equations) and conversion of one mole of ATP to ADP or one mole of ADP to AMP is accompanied by the release of 33 kJ. Conversion of AMP to adenosine, on the other hand, only yields 12.6 kJ. In the reverse reactions the same amounts of energy are absorbed:

Energy evolved available for synthesis or work

$$\text{ATP} \underset{\text{33 kJ absorbed}}{\overset{\text{33 kJ evolved}}{\rightleftarrows}} \text{ADP} \underset{\text{33 kJ absorbed}}{\overset{\text{33 kJ evolved}}{\rightleftarrows}} \text{AMP} \underset{\text{12.6 kJ absorbed}}{\overset{\text{12.6 kJ evolved}}{\rightleftarrows}} \text{A}$$

Energy absorbed from oxidation of glucose

The energy-rich phosphate bonds function as energy stockpiles for energy released during oxidation of glucose in the cell. The energy is available for

reuse on demand, for muscular contraction or to make possible the synthesis of some other molecule by the body, or for any other purpose. When this occurs, ATP is converted to ADP or AMP which are then available for reconversion to ATP at a time when surplus energy is available.

During the complete oxidation of one mole of glucose by the body 36 moles of ATP (or their equivalent in related compounds) are formed from ADP and the energy absorbed in this process (and hence available for further use) is $36 \times 33 = 1188$ kJ. This compares with the 2820 kJ evolved when glucose is burned in oxygen and from this we see that the body is able to capture about 43 per cent of the energy of the glucose molecule. The residue is either used up in making other molecules during the oxidation process or is dissipated as heat. This is why we get hot and perspire freely when involved in strenuous physical activity.

The complicated series of reactions involved in the assimilation and utilization of glucose by the body are controlled by several hormones, the best known of which is insulin, which is secreted by the pancreas. In the disease diabetes mellitus insufficient insulin is produced by the pancreas; as a result glucose circulates in the blood in abnormally large amounts and is not taken up by the liver or muscles for conversion to glycogen or for oxidation. The body is thus unable to utilize carbohydrate foods and has to resort instead to fats and proteins to make up its energy deficiencies. Unfortunately, increased utilization of fat in this way leads to accumulation of certain poisonous products of fat metabolism in the liver and the bloodstream and this can have serious consequences (see ketosis, p. 67).

Key points

- Carbohydrates are macronutrients with low energy-density (3.75 kcal/g) providing about 40–50 per cent of energy in normal diets
- Starch (in plants) and glycogen (in animals) and storage polymers (polysaccharides) of glucose (sugar) which can only be made by plants (photosynthesis)
- Dietary fibre is a group of polysaccharides which escapes digestion in the small intestine and functions as the energy supply for metabolism by colonic bacteria

Chapter summary

The term carbohydrates, describing the chemical structure of this nutrient class, is not well understood by lay people. Carbohydrates are often wrongly equated with sugar, or sweeteners, and linked to obesity. Diets with higher proportion of energy from carbohydrate are usually protective against obesity, and low-carbohydrate diets are not helpful in combating obesity although avoiding sugars (mono and di-saccharides) can be.

FURTHER READING

CUMMINGS JH, ROBERFROID MB, ANDERSSON H, BARTH C, FERRO-LUZZI A, *et al* (1997). A new look at dietary carbohydrate: chemistry, physiology and health. *Eur J Clin Nutr* **51**:417–423.

DEPARTMENT OF HEALTH (1991). Dietary reference values for food energy and nutrients for the UK. Report of the Panel on Dietary Reference Values of the Committee on Medical Aspects of Food Policy No. 41. London: HMSO. www.nutrition-matters.co.uk/misc/1991COMAreport.htm

EXPENDITURE AND FOOD SURVEY 2001/2002. National Statistics publication. 2003.

KIRK RS, RONALD SAWYOR R (1990). *Pearson's Composition and Analysis of Foods*. Harlow: Longman.

MAFF (2000). *National Food Survey*. London: HMSO.

SUSTAINABLE DEVELOPMENT COMMISSION (2004). Sustainability of Sugar Supply Chains. Executive Summary Report http://www.sd-commission.gov.uk/pubs/sugar/02.htm

9

Carbohydrate-rich foods

With the exception of lactose, which is present as 24 per cent of energy in cow's milk, carbohydrate foods are of plant origin. The amount of glycogen in liver – its most abundant source is only registered as a trace in tables of food composition. A substantial amount of energy is required to enable the plant to transform the simple molecules of carbon dioxide and water to the more complex carbohydrate molecules and this is obtained from sunlight. When we eat carbohydrates this process is, in effect, put into reverse to release energy for use by our bodies. The way in which this is done has already been discussed in Chapter 8.

About one-third of the total dietary intake of carbohydrates in Britain consists of sucrose or glucose syrup, about one-twentieth is lactose and the remainder is starch and dietary fibre (non-starch polysaccharides, NSPs). These proportions may vary between individuals. Some children obtain almost half their calories from sugars.

The carbohydrate content of some foods is shown in Table 9.1. They are ranked by per cent weight as carbohydrates. The range, is large, even for quite similar foods and the difference is mainly from variations in water content. To evaluate these foods in terms of nutrition, their carbohydrate contents are also shown in terms of per cent energy content. The range is again large, but in this case depends on the variable content of proteins and fat, which also contribute energy (measured in kJ or kcal). A fuller list can be found in McCance and Widdowson, *The Composition of Foods*.

Table 9.1 The carbohydrate content of some foods ranked by per cent weight

Food	% By weight	% Energy from carbohydrate
Cornflakes	90	89
Rice (raw)	86	84
Honey	76	99
Weetabix	76	81
Spaghetti (raw)	74	81
Jam	69	99
Milk chocolate	57	42
Lentils (dry)	56	67
Potato crisps	53	39
Bread (white)	46	79
Bread (wholemeal)	42	73
Fried chipped potatoes	30–40	47
Bananas	23	92
Dairy ice cream	20	43
Boiled potatoes	18	90
Grapes	15	96
Baked beans	15	69
Peanut butter	13	8
Apples	12	95
Peas (cooked)	10	46
Porridge (made with water)	8	66
Yoghurt (whole, plain)	8	37
Milk (whole)	5	26
Green beans (cooked)	5	70
Lettuce	2	46
Liver (lamb raw)	0	0
Beef (lean)	0	0

SOURCES OF SUGARS

Monosaccharides

Glucose and fructose are the only monosaccharides present to any extent in an average diet. They occur naturally in honey in roughly equal amounts and as industrially inverted products of sucrose or hydrolysed starch in 'glucose syrup' or purified fructose which are extensively used by food manufacturers for sweetening their products.

Honey

The nectar of flowers from which bees make honey consists largely of sucrose. During its passage through the bee's honey sac, and during further activity by bees in the hive, the sucrose is hydrolysed by enzymes into glucose and fructose and the product – honey – consists of about 20 per cent water and about 76 per cent glucose and fructose. The balance is made up of a small amount of unconverted sucrose, some other minor disaccharides and trivial quantities of minerals, acids, vitamins and flavour-producing substances.

The very variable flavour of honey depends essentially on the flowers from which the nectar was collected. Honey contains over 200 different substances but honey lovers are able to distinguish honey derived mainly from clover, for example, from that originating from other flowers.

Although honey is now mainly eaten as a spread like jam it has been used as a sweetener since ancient times and it was the only sweetening agent used until sucrose became available from sugar cane, and later sugar beet. It was also used for making the alcoholic drink mead, which is made by fermenting diluted honey with yeast. Honey keeps well because the water content is too low (i.e. its osmotic load too high) to permit growth of bacteria or fungi.

The nutritive and curative properties of honey are often grossly exaggerated. It is really no more than a flavoured, concentrated solution of glucose and fructose. There is no evidence that honey has special nutritional or medicinal properties or that it can function as an aphrodisiac or delay the onset of old age. Like other sugars, its nutritional function is solely to act as a source of energy but its flavour and sweetness are very attractive to most people, at least for parts of their diets. It is labour-intensive and expensive to make honey, with fluctuations in specific gravity and production which result from the weather and from diseases among bees. Unfortunately, it is easy to extend limited honey supplies by extending it with glucose syrup. Although this adulteration is detectable, and illegal, it is also possible to provide bees with commercial sugar, from which they will make honey in place of nectar. This practice is used routinely to a small degree by bee-keepers at the end of the season, as a food for the bees, but it should not contribute to commercially available honey.

Glucose and fructose syrup

This is a sweet, syrupy mixture of glucose with other sugars and dextrins which is used extensively by the food industry. It is produced by the hydrolysis of starchy materials, such as maize, with dilute acids or by enzymes. The composition of glucose syrup (or corn syrup as it is known in North America) depends upon the extent to which the hydrolysis occurs (i.e. upon how far the amylose and amylopectin molecules in the starch are broken down). The degree of hydrolysis can be controlled to give a product which is largely glucose or a more viscous syrup containing substantial amounts of dextrins (i.e. partly hydrolysed amylose and amylopectin molecules). The more completely hydrolysed syrups, which contain a larger proportion of sugars, are sweeter than those containing substantial amounts of dextrins and they are widely used in the manufacture of sweet confectionery and cakes.

If fully hydrolysed glucose syrups are treated with the enzyme glucose isomerase up to half the glucose may be converted to fructose. The product is sweeter than glucose syrup because fructose is the sweetest of the sugars. It is claimed that, in addition to its greater sweetness, fructose has the effect of enhancing fruit flavours and 'high-fructose syrups' are widely used in soft drinks and jams.

SUCROSE, CANE SUGAR OR BEET SUGAR

Ordinary table sugar, whether produced from sugar cane (which can only be grown in tropical countries) or sugar beet (which can be grown in temperate zones) is almost pure sucrose. There is no difference between the sugar obtained from sugar beet and that obtained from sugar cane. Both provide only energy, in nutrition and brown sugar has no additional value. Sugar has been produced commercially from sugar beet for over 150 years. About 30 per cent of the total world production of sugar and 60 per cent of British sugar is produced from sugar beet. Sugar cane has been chewed by children in tropical countries for centuries, but it only became available to the rest of the world following the exploration of the sixteenth and seventeenth centuries. Its cultivation, particularly in the West Indies, had important economic and political impacts. It impacted eating habits (and tooth decay) from its happy conjunction with the arrival of tea, in adding new culinary possibilities to cakes and confectionery, and by providing a cheap source of fermentable material for beer-making. The soft-drink industry is more recent.

Production of raw sugar

Sugar cane is a type of giant grass which resembles bamboo and may grow to a height of 4 or 5 m with a diameter of 3–5 cm. The sugar, which amounts to about 15 per cent of the weight of the cane, is found in a soft fibre in the interior of the cane. From 3 to 8 tons of sugar are normally obtained from an acre of sugar cane. The sugar is extracted from the cane by crushing and spraying with water. The solution obtained contains about 13 per cent sugar and 3 per cent impurities, the remainder being water. This solution is purified and the clear solution obtained is concentrated by evaporation under reduced pressure until a mixture of sugar crystals and 'mother liquor' is obtained. The crystals are separated from the mother liquor by spinning the mixture very quickly in large drums. These drums have perforated sides through which the mother liquor, called molasses, is forced by centrifugal action, leaving the raw sugar behind. Molasses is used for the manufacture of rum and industrial alcohol.

The sugar content of sugar beet is similar to that of sugar cane, but only about 2 tons of sugar can be obtained from an acre of sugar beet. The sugar is extracted from the shredded beet by steeping in hot water; it diffuses through the cell walls into the water, leaving behind most of the non-sugar solids. Batteries of specially designed diffusers are used to ensure that the maximum amount of sugar is removed by the minimum quantity of water. The solution obtained contains about 14 per cent sugar and 4 per cent impurities, the remainder being water. It is treated to remove impurities and the clear solution obtained is concentrated by evaporation under reduced pressure to give sugar crystals and molasses which are separated by centrifuging as described for cane sugar. The raw sugar obtained is very similar to that produced from cane sugar but has a less attractive taste and smell, by virtue of the different impurities.

Sugar refining

Raw sugar, whether obtained from beet or cane, contains about 96 per cent sucrose. It consists essentially of sugar crystals coated with a layer of molasses. The first step in the refining process is to mix the raw sugar with sugar syrup to produce a stiff, semi-solid mixture of syrup and crystals. This is centrifuged and the syrup is forced out, leaving the sugar crystals within the centrifuge. The sugar crystals are then washed with water to remove the adhering syrup. A considerable amount of sugar is contained in the syrup and wash liquors from the centrifuge and this is recovered by evaporation of the water under reduced pressure.

The sugar crystals are next dissolved in water and treated with milk of lime (historically, crushed egg shells) and carbon dioxide to remove the bulk of the impurities. The remainder are removed by allowing the solution to percolate through a deep bed of charcoal which removes coloured impurities to produce a colourless liquid known as fine liquor.

All that remains to be done is to concentrate the fine liquor by evaporating the water, and crystallize the sucrose to produce uniform crystals of the correct size. The evaporation is carried out at reduced pressure in steam-heated 'vacuum pans', so that the water can be removed at a temperature much below the normal boiling point of the solution; this prevents any discoloration of the sugar.

The crystallization process produces a suspension of sugar crystals in syrup. Spinning in centrifugal machines removes most of the syrup, the remainder being removed by spraying with hot water and centrifuging. The syrup and washings contain about 40 per cent of the sugar originally present in the fine liquor and most of this is recovered by decolorizing and recrystallizing. This can be repeated several times. Eventually, however, the colour and quality of the sugar recovered from the syrup do not conform to the high standards required. When this happens, the syrup is used for the manufacture of golden syrup or is concentrated and crystallized to give a soft brown sugar.

Caster sugar is made in the same way as granulated sugar but the crystallization procedure is modified so that much smaller crystals are obtained. This is done by using a larger number of nuclei or by preventing the crystals from growing to granulated sugar size. Caster sugar is also obtained as a byproduct of the production of granulated sugar and it is separated from it by sieving the dry sugar. The particle size in icing sugar is even smaller than in caster sugar and it is made by pulverizing granulated sugar in special mills. Brown sugar is obtained by crystallizing the syrup obtained at the end of the refining process. The sugar obtained is slightly sticky because of the presence of a thin coating of mother liquor on each crystal. Genuine demerara sugar is a golden-brown, slightly moist sugar produced in this way in Demerara, Guyana. London demerara is a substitute made by coating white sugar crystals with molasses. Muscovado (or Barbados sugar) has a higher molasses content than demerara sugar and a 'treacly' flavour. Lump sugar is made by crystallizing the fine liquor (see above) in such a way that crystals of two different sizes are obtained: the larger crystals give the characteristic sparkle of lump sugar and the smaller ones bind the crystals together.

FOODSTUFFS MANUFACTURED FROM SUGAR

Sugar, as we have seen, occurs naturally in large amounts in fruits and in some specific plants but it is also present, sometimes in surprisingly large amounts, in many manufactured foods, where it has a variety of functions including taste and texture.

Sugar confectionery, chocolate and jam

The term 'sugar confectionery' is used to describe the large range of confectionery we commonly call 'sweets'. Boiled sweets, toffees and caramels, the filling used as centres for chocolates, marshmallow,

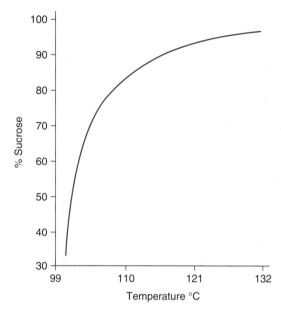

Figure 9.1 *The boiling points of sugar solutions*

nougat, pastilles and gums are all examples of sugar confectionery. This great variety of tooth-decay accelerators have one thing in common: they are all produced by controlled crystallization of sucrose from a supersaturated solution. The differences that exist between them depend upon water content, the extent to which crystallization of sucrose has occurred, and the presence of fat or milk, which enables emulsions to be formed, and flavouring agents.

When a concentrated solution of sucrose – a syrup – is heated, the temperature at which it will boil depends upon the amount of water present in the solution, as shown in Fig. 9.1. The water content of a sugar solution can be accurately determined from a knowledge of its boiling point. If boiling is allowed to continue, the concentration of the solution increases as water evaporates and the boiling point increases. Soft sweets, such as toffee, are cooked to a lower temperature than hard sweets such as butterscotch or boiled sweets. Sticky sweets stick to teeth and cause even more decay than boiled ones.

Boiled sweets

These are traditionally made by boiling sugar solutions with acidic substances to produce a certain amount of inversion. Boiling is continued until the temperature exceeds 150°C, by which time almost all the water has been driven off and, on cooling, the mass solidifies as a glass-like solid – the familiar boiled sweet. At the end of the cooling period only a small amount of water (a few per cent) is present. The glucose produced by the inversion process prevents the sucrose from crystallizing when the mass is cooled down. It is said to 'cut the grain'. Glucose itself does not crystallize easily from water and in a mixed solution of glucose and sucrose the glucose inhibits the crystallization of the sucrose. The final product is a supersaturated solution of sucrose, with smaller amounts of glucose and fructose, in a very small quantity of water. The amount of invert-sugar produced during the boiling must be carefully controlled because if too much is present the product will be prone to absorb water from the air and become sticky. This is because the fructose in the invert-sugar is hygroscopic. On the other hand, if too little invert sugar is produced it will be insufficient to prevent crystallization of the sucrose. About 10–15 per cent invert-sugar is required to give a non-sticky non-crystalline product.

Any acidic substance may be added to produce the inversion, and cream of tartar (potassium hydrogen tartrate) is commonly used. The amount of acid used depends upon several factors, including the hardness of the water, but it is quite small and, in the case of cream of tartar, is in the region of 0.15–0.25 per cent of the weight of sugar used. Boiled sweets are made commercially by heating a syrup of sucrose and glucose syrup which prevents crystallization of the sucrose in the same way as invert-sugar. The amount of glucose syrup used can amount to 30–40 per cent, but the product is not hygroscopic because it contains no fructose. Glucose syrup is less sweet than sucrose or invert-sugar and so the boiled sweets produced in this way are also less sweet. In addition, the dextrin in the glucose syrup is said to impart a certain toughness to the sweets and can sometimes cause cloudiness.

Fondant

This is the creamy material used for filling soft-centred chocolates and by biscuit and cake manufacturers for decorative purposes. It consists essentially of minute sugar crystals surrounded by saturated sugar syrup.

Fondant is made by boiling a sugar solution and adding glucose syrup or an inverting agent, as in the case of boiled sweets. No attempt is made to boil off all the water, however, and the mixture is only boiled to 115–120°C compared with 150–165°C in the case of boiled sweets. The syrupy solution obtained is cooled quickly to about 38°C by running onto a rotating water-cooled drum from which it falls into a beater. Here it is agitated violently to induce crystallization which occurs suddenly to produce a very large number of tiny crystals.

Fudge

This is simply fondant containing added milk solids, fat and chocolate solids which are suspended in the sugar syrup and give it added solidity.

Toffee

Fat, milk, sugar and glucose syrup are the main ingredients of toffee. It consists essentially of a dispersion of minute globules of fat in a supersaturated sugar solution. Various grades of sugar are used, depending upon the recipe, from refined granulated sugar to raw sugars and treacles, which contribute characteristic flavours to the product. As in the case of boiled sweets, sugars other than sucrose must be present to prevent graining. In home-made toffee, an acidic inverting agent such as vinegar or citric acid may be used to produce some invert-sugar from sucrose, but in commercial practice it is usual to employ glucose syrup to prevent graining.

The milk used makes an important contribution to the flavour and it is added as condensed milk, either full-cream or skimmed. The characteristic colour of toffee is largely due to caramelization of the milk solids during cooking. In addition, the casein of the milk acts as an emulsifying agent. Butter and various vegetable fats are used in the manufacture of toffee, and emulsifying agents, such as glyceryl monostearate or lecithin, may also be incorporated, if insufficient milk solids and butter are present, to aid in the dispersion of the fat and produce a stable emulsion.

In toffee manufacture, the ingredients are boiled together until the temperature reaches the required level. The temperature attained in the boiling process largely determines the consistency of the toffee produced because this depends, among other things, on the amount of water in the toffee. Very hard toffee such as butterscotch is heated to 146–154°C, which gives a water content of 3–5 per cent. Ordinary toffees and caramels are heated to 118–132°C when the mixture contains 6–12 per cent water.

Toffee and fudge are made from similar materials and they both contain about 10 per cent water. Why then are they so dissimilar in other respects? The short answer is that toffee, like boiled sweets, consists of sugar syrup surrounding other ingredients such as fat and milk whereas in fudge, as in fondant, part of the sugar is present in crystalline form. Toffee is in fact a thick, supersaturated syrup and not a solid at all, and this is why it has such a tough and chewy consistency.

There are innumerable varieties of toffees but in all of them there is a common background 'caramel taste'. This flavour is produced by caramelization or breakdown of some of the sugar molecules which occurs whenever carbohydrates are heated. During toffee-making a reaction also occurs between the heated sugars and the proteins present in the milk solids and this produces a brown colour. A browning reaction of this type (called the Maillard reaction or non-enzymic browning reaction) occurs whenever carbohydrates are heated with proteins (see p. 242).

Chocolate

The essential ingredients of chocolate are cocoa, cocoa-butter and sugar. The cocoa and cocoa-butter are both obtained from cocoa-beans which grow in pods on cacao trees in tropical countries. The pods are egg-shaped, about 20 cm long, and about 7–10 cm in diameter. Each pod contains 20 to 40 beans embedded in a soft, white, starchy pulp. The pods are split open and the beans, with adhering pulp, are scraped out and allowed to ferment for several days. A yeast fungus grows on the pulp and it liquefies owing to fermentation to alcohol. The liquid formed is allowed to drain away from the beans which during the process change in colour from their original light violet to dark brown. After drying in the sun the beans are ready for shipment to the cocoa manufacturers.

In the manufacture of cocoa and chocolate, the beans are first roasted in revolving drums and are then broken into small pieces by passing through special rollers. The husk is removed, leaving behind the small pieces of roasted bean which are known as nibs. This roasting process is of great importance

because it is at this stage that the characteristic chocolate flavour and aroma develop as a consequence of Maillard-type browning reactions occurring between carbohydrates and proteins present.

The nibs contain about 50 per cent of a fat known as cocoa butter and during the next operation, in which the nibs are finely ground in mills, the heat generated melts the cocoa butter to produce a viscous brown liquid as product. When the liquid, which is a dispersion of cocoa in cocoa butter is cooled, a brown solid known as cocoa mass is obtained. For the production of cocoa a proportion of the cocoa butter is squeezed out in powerful hydraulic presses. The residue, containing 20–30 per cent cocoa butter, is finely ground and sold as cocoa powder. It contains about 2 per cent theobromine and 0.1 per cent caffeine; these compounds are closely related alkaloids with properties similar to caffeine. The bitterness of cocoa and chocolate is a function of a range of antioxidant phenolic compounds also present. Milk proteins bind to the phenolic compounds, reducing bitterness and blocking the absorption from the gut.

Chocolate is made by mixing cocoa mass with sugar, cocoa butter and, for milk chocolate, dried milk or condensed milk. The mixing is carried out in melangeurs, in which massive rollers rotate in contact with a heated plate. The mixture then passes to a refining machine where it is pinched between rollers revolving at different speeds. To complete the process, the molten chocolate is then 'conched' for a period of up to 24 hours. In the conching process heavy rollers subject the chocolate to severe mechanical treatment and blend all the ingredients into a uniform velvety consistency.

Chocolate for coating purposes, such as is used in covering 'centres' to make individual chocolates or in covering biscuits, contains a larger proportion of cocoa butter than ordinary block chocolate. The purpose of this is to increase the fluidity of chocolate when warm. Chocolate-coated goods are made by passing the centre or biscuit to be coated through a curtain of molten chocolate in a machine called an enrober.

Conversion of liquid chocolate to the familiar solid chocolate bar is not simply a matter of pouring the chocolate into moulds and allowing it to cool. The fats present in cocoa butter can solidify in six different forms, or polymorphs, with different melting points. One of the polymorphs melts at 33.8°C and when only this form is present in solid chocolate it will be smooth and glossy and will easily melt in the mouth. To produce as much of this polymorph as possible chocolate is subjected to a special heat-treatment process called tempering. The molten chocolate is cooled until it just begins to solidify and then it is reheated to just below the melting point of the desirable polymorph. The chocolate is then stirred at this temperature, so that a high proportion of the fat will solidify in the preferred polymorphic form when the chocolate is finally moulded or used for coating.

If chocolate is incorrectly tempered, or if it is subjected to a series of temperature changes (e.g. if left in a shop window or a car) it may develop a white coating or 'bloom'. This may look like mould growth but it is in fact a harmless coating of fat crystals.

Molten chocolate is such a capricious substance that it is difficult to handle in the kitchen where precise temperature measurement and control is not easy. For this reason, chocolate-flavoured cake coating substitutes are available which contain vegetable fat in place of cocoa butter. Vegetable fat solidifies in only one form and hence the problems caused by the polymorphism of cocoa butter fats do not arise.

Chocolate is a nutritious food and a small bar (100 g) of milk chocolate provides about 9 g of protein and 220 mg of calcium – approximately one-sixth and one-third, respectively, of the reference nutrient intake (RNI) of these nutrients for a moderately active man. It would also supply about one-sixth of his energy requirements and 10–15 per cent of the RNI of iron, thiamin and riboflavin. The caffeine content of cocoa is similar to that of coffee. There has been recent interest in the high content of antioxidant phenolic compounds in chocolate. These compounds (mainly catechins and epicatechins) are extensively metabolized in the gut, but may have biological actions. Adding milk protein binds phenolics, masking the bitter taste of chocolate and blocking their absorption. The high sugar content of chocolate and its sticky texture leads to prolonged contact of teeth with sugar – especially if consumed between meals. Thus, chocolate has contributed considerably to dental caries and loss of teeth.

Jam

Jam is made by boiling fruit with sugar solutions and is essentially a gel or semi-solid mass containing pulped or whole fruit. A gel is really a very viscous solution, or dispersion, which possesses some of the attributes, such as elasticity, of a solid. The gel is formed from the sugar, the acids present in the fruit and the polysaccharide pectin (see p. 97).

Jam contains about 67 per cent dissolved sugar and this high concentration inhibits the growth of moulds and yeasts because the water activity (see p. 275) is too low (i.e. the osmotic content is too high) to permit their multiplication.

The quantity of pectin and acid in fruit for jam making is of great importance because gel formation only occurs when the concentrations of sugar and pectin and the pH of the mixture lie within certain limits. Some fruits, such as currants, damsons, gooseberries, lemons and bitter oranges, are rich in both acid and pectin and can easily be made into jam. Others, such as strawberries, blackberries, raspberries and cherries contain little pectin and some must be added before jam can be made successfully from them. A simple way of doing this is to add another fruit rich in pectin and acid, for example, apple or a concentrated pectin preparation (see p. 97). As the percentage of pectin in a jam increases so does the firmness of the gel produced on cooling. A satisfactory gel is obtained with about 1 per cent pectin, although for a given pH and sugar content the firmness of the gel is influenced by the 'quality' of the pectin as well as by the quantity present.

As we have already seen, pectin consists of large numbers of simpler molecules connected together to form a long thread-like molecule. The length of a pectin molecule depends upon its source. During gel formation the long molecules link loosely together to form a three-dimensional network which gives the gel its stability. If the pectin molecules are too short the gel may lack strength and be runny or soft.

Anyone who has tried to make jam at home knows that the jam obtained from ripe fruit is not as good as that from fruit which is almost ripe. This is because pectin will not form a satisfactory gel until the pH is lowered to about 3.5 and unripe fruit is usually more acidic than ripe fruit. To decrease the pH of a jam mixture an acidic fruit juice, such as lemon juice, may be added or a small amount of citric acid, malic acid or cream of tartar. A low pH during the cooking period may cause inversion of too much sucrose, and also hydrolyse the pectin to some extent. As both these changes are detrimental the pH adjustment is often carried out at the end of the cooking period.

When fruit is boiled with sugar, a certain amount of inversion occurs (see p. 91), and this is of the utmost importance because invert-sugar prevents the crystallization of the sugar in the jam when it is kept. Too much invert-sugar, however, is detrimental because it reduces the strength of the gel and may cause the jam to set to a honey-like mass on keeping.

Another reason why fruit used in jam making should not be over-ripe is that pectic substances, particularly protopectin, from which pectin is formed during jam making, are present in maximum amount just before the fruit is ripe. If jam factories could make jam only when supplies of fresh fruit were available they would be able to work for only a very short period each year. Moreover, the great amount of fruit harvested during these periods would be far too large to be made quickly into jam by the existing number of jam factories. To overcome this difficulty, large amounts of preserved fruits are used. The method of preserving the fruit is very simple; it is kept submerged in a weak solution of sulphur dioxide in water. Fruit can be preserved in this way either before or after cooking. In practice, strawberries, raspberries and blackberries are preserved raw, whereas plums, currants and gooseberries are usually preserved as a cooked pulp because sulphur dioxide tends to toughen the skins of the uncooked fruit. The fruit is bleached by the sulphur dioxide during the preserving but the colour returns when it is cooked. Almost all the sulphur dioxide is driven off during cooking and the finished jam must not contain more than 100 parts per million.

When jam is made at home, the fruit is first cooked until tender. Pectin is extracted during this process and the length of the cooking period depends upon the fruit being used. Cooking is complete when a sample of the fruit forms a coherent pectin clot when allowed to stand for a few minutes with several times its volume of methylated spirit. The clot should be strong enough to withstand pouring from one vessel to another without breaking. When a satisfactory pectin clot is obtained, the sugar should be added and the mixture boiled as rapidly as possible. The duration of the boiling period will depend on the fruit used and the size and shape of the pan; it varies from about 5 to about 20 minutes. A shallow pan, in which a large surface area of the jam is exposed for evaporation, is best because this permits rapid evaporation. The boiling period is usually complete when the temperature of the boiling mixtures reaches 104°C. The exact temperature at which boiling should be stopped depends upon the acidity and pectin content of the fruit, however, both of which influence the setting properties of the jam.

Jam making is carried out commercially in a much more scientific way than this. To begin with, the recipe is adjusted to give the correct amounts of sugar and pectin with the particular fruit being used and pH is also carefully controlled. Precooked pulp is often used and the boiling is usually carried out in open pans holding about 180 L of jam. The boiling time is very short and seldom exceeds 10 minutes. This short boiling time preserves the gel-forming properties of the pectin and also keeps the amount of invert-sugar formed to between 25 and 40 per cent. The time of boiling, and hence the amount of invert-sugar formed, can be controlled by altering the amount of water used. When the temperature reaches 104°C, the end of the boiling period is imminent. The boiling point is really an indication of the concentration of the solution being boiled, and this can be more accurately determined by measuring the refractive index with a refractometer. From a knowledge of the refractive index, the concentration of soluble solids in the jam can be calculated. To the soluble solids are added sugar and pectin together with sugars, acids and other solids extracted from the fruit. The soluble solid content varies from jam to jam but is usually about 70 per cent.

SUGARS IN THE DIET

As we have seen, sugars are soluble carbohydrates which are used by the body as a fuel for all its vital processes. Sugars naturally incorporated into the cellular structure of a food are referred to as intrinsic sugars. Those that do not form a natural part of the cell structure of a food but have been added to it (or are used on their own as a food) are known as extrinsic sugars. Thus, the sugars present in fruit are classed as intrinsic sugars, whereas honey and the sucrose added to food during cooking or at the table are classed as extrinsic sugars. The lactose in milk, although present naturally, is not intracellular and hence it is regarded as an extrinsic sugar. All other extrinsic sugars are classified as non-milk extrinsic sugars.

Sucrose is by far the most important dietary sugar but glucose, lactose and maltose may also be present in the diet to a minor extent. In Britain about 100 g of sugars are consumed by each adult every day (over half of this is non-milk extrinsic sugar) and this provides about 18 per cent of total food energy intake. Younger age groups obtain more of their energy from sugars – babies as much as 40 per cent and pre-school children about 25 per cent. These are average figures and, like all averages, should be treated with caution. The average figure is greatly exceeded by some individuals and not even approached by others. The variation in individual consumption is probably greater for sugars than for any other dietary item except alcohol. There are no obvious differences in consumption between rich and poor in Britain: the amount consumed increases with age up to about 16 years of age and then it tapers off. Males appear to be more sweet-toothed than females at all ages.

Why is so much sugar consumed? The main reason is probably the attraction that sweet-tasting foods have for many people – especially children. It has even been suggested that sugar can be mildly addictive. Regardless of how strong-willed one is, however, it is practically impossible to forgo all sugar because of its presence – often unsuspected – in a wide range of foods. In many cases, the reason for its presence is its sweetness, but it also has other properties which commend it to the food manufacturer.

1   In many cases, the sugar forms an indispensable part of the food. Sweets, jams and cakes, for example, could not exist in their traditional forms without sugar.

2   Sucrose has a high affinity for water and very concentrated solutions or syrups can easily be made. These syrupy solutions are smooth to the tongue and improve the 'mouth-feel' of semisolid foods.

3   Sucrose acts as a preservative when it is present in foods in high concentrations because it makes water unavailable to microorganisms. The sucrose present in jams and sweets, for example, acts in this way and helps to prevent spoilage through mould growth.

4   The texture of sugary solid foods may be varied from 'soft and pasty' through 'firm and chewy' to 'hard and crunchy' by adjusting the amount of sugar present and varying the cooking technique to control the water content.

5   Sucrose and other sugars play a part in making cooked food look more attractive by 'browning', either through caramelization of the sugar by heat or as a result of Maillard reactions (see p. 242) taking place between the sugar and amino acids present in the protein component of the food.

6   Sucrose can be employed with pectin and acid to form semisolid gels such as jam.

Not only can sugar do all these things, but it is also cheap – hence its presence in so many foods and its prominence in our diet.

Sugar and health

Suspicion has fallen on sugar as the causative agent of a number of diseases which are prevalent in developed countries where sugar consumption is high. Coronary heart disease, diabetes, gallstones, kidney stones, certain types of cancer and even behavioural abnormalities have all been speculatively linked to excessive sugar consumption. A great deal of research work has been carried out to see whether such links exist. The consensus of informed opinion is that there is no convincing evidence that sugar causes, or is a contributing cause of, any of these diseases. It is curious why so much suspicion about roles in such a wide range of disparate conditions has developed. It is reasonable to consider possible links between any nutrient and any disease, but evidence based solely on associations (e.g. countries with high rates of diabetes also have high sugar consumptions) cannot provide proof. Where proof has been sought, from experiments and more sophisticated cohort analyses, most of the proposed links between sugar and disease can be dismissed (including a direct link with diabetes).

Sugar and dental decay

It is now generally accepted that the eating of food containing extrinsic sugars is one of the main causes of tooth decay, or dental caries as it is more correctly called. Sucrose is the main offender because so much of it is eaten, but glucose, fructose and maltose are almost equally potent as tooth-rotting agents. Lactose does not cause dental caries. Some tooth decay may be caused by starchy foods because they are partly converted to glucose in the mouth by the action of salivary amylase. However, starch plays a much less important role than extrinsic sugars as a causative agent of dental caries.

Sugars themselves do not attack the teeth, but they are converted to acid by streptococcal bacteria in the mouth and the acids formed attack and erode the hard enamel surface of the teeth. This occurs rapidly after sugary food is eaten but the tooth surface has some ability to repair slight erosion and if enough time elapses between attacks no permanent harm is done. This repair process requires the essential mineral fluoride. If successive erosions occur too rapidly, however – through constantly eating sweets, for example – a cavity will form and the tooth will be permanently damaged. The frequency of ingestion and stickiness of food are as important in causing dental caries as the quantity of sugar eaten.

The bad effects of non-milk extrinsic sugars on dental health have been studied by a specialist panel of the committee which advised the government on the medical aspects of food policy (Committee on Medical Aspects of Food Policy, COMA). They made the following dietary recommendations:

1 Consumption of non-milk extrinsic sugars, especially sugary snacks, should be reduced. These sugars should be replaced by fresh fruit, vegetables and starchy foods.
2 Sugar should not be added to the bottle feeds of infants and young children. Sugared drinks should not be given in feeders where they may be in contact with teeth for long periods. Dummies or comforters should not be dipped in sugar or sugary drinks.
3 Elderly people who still have teeth should restrict the amount and frequency of consumption of non-milk extrinsic sugars because their teeth are more likely to decay owing to exposure of tooth roots and declining salivary flow.

Research has shown that fluoride helps to increase the resistance of tooth enamel to acid attack and fluoridation of drinking water and the use of fluoride-containing toothpaste are beneficial to dental health. For increasingly obscure reasons, powerful opposition to fluoridation of water has built up, related to spurious notions of evidence and of human rights. The evidence is that correcting fluoride-deficient water supplies to 1 ppm fluoride would enormously reduce dental caries, abolishing it completely for most people. The concept that this would contaminate a natural product (water) and remove a human right is specious, particularly since water supplies are already heavily treated for other reasons.

Sugar and obesity

It is widely believed that people become overweight or obese if they eat too much sugar or sweet food. Weight gain can only occur if the energy content of a person's diet exceeds his or her energy expenditure. Putting this in a more down to earth way we could say (what everyone knows) that if you eat too much you get fat. Excess energy derived from sugar is no different from that derived from other foodstuffs in this respect. Nevertheless, if an already adequate diet is 'topped up' by eating sweets, biscuits and cakes, the result is inevitable, and the sweet 'extras' usually get the blame even when their content of fat as per cent energy is as great as sugar. The sugar provided by soft carbonated drinks has become a major issue in recent years, especially for children. Most carbonated soft drinks contain 10 per cent sugar by weight. A 330 mL can thus contains 33 g sugar, or 124 kcal (528 kJ). Thus, two cans in a day would add about 16 per cent to the energy consumption of a child or 90 000 kcal/year, which would lead to about 10 kg fat deposition of weight gain per year. Apart from its energy content, sugar – whether white or brown – contributes absolutely nothing else to the diet. No harm would be done by excluding it completely if that were possible.

It is, of course, possible to become obese without consuming an excessive amount of sugar or, on the other hand, to remain slim while enjoying a sugar-rich diet. There is no reason to suppose that sugars, whether intrinsic or extrinsic, play a special role as a cause of obesity. Some studies have even shown the sugar consumption of overweight individuals to be lower than that of leaner people – possibly because sugars may have an appetite-suppressing effect. Nevertheless, it is obviously wise for obese people, and those likely to become obese, to limit their intake of extrinsic sugars as a contribution to a programme of calorie restriction.

Obesity is considered in more detail on pp. 29 and 260.

Lactose intolerance

The disaccharide lactose is present in mammalian (including human) milk. It is normally hydrolysed to its component monosaccharides in the small intestine by the enzyme lactase to form the monosaccharides glucose and galactose which are readily absorbed. About 95 per cent of Western Europeans secrete lactase throughout their life but about three-quarters of the population of Africa, India, Eastern Europe and the Middle and Far East do not and they develop lactose intolerance between the ages of 15 and 25 years, when lactase production ceases. They are unable to digest lactose, or are able to cope with only small amounts of it. The undigested lactose is converted to lactic acid by bacteria in the large intestine and this causes flatulence, discomfort and diarrhoea.

Most people who suffer from lactose intolerance are able to take small amounts of milk without too much of a problem. Most cheeses contain little lactose and hence they too can be digested without difficulty. The same is true of yoghurt – a frequent ingredient of Indian recipes – because the lactose which was originally present in the milk from which it was made will have been largely converted to lactic acid (see p. 79).

Man is the only animal to consume milk in any quantity after infancy and it may well be that lactose intolerance is the natural state of affairs. It is possible that an ability to digest lactose has persisted into adulthood only in those countries where milk has become a normal part of the adult diet.

CEREALS

The major part of the carbohydrate intake and about 30 per cent of the energy content of an average British diet is provided by foods of cereal origin. Cereals are cultivated grasses and the grain which we use as a food source is a seed which is really intended as a rich store of nutrients for the grass that would grow from it. The most important cereals are wheat, maize, rice, oats, rye and barley. Civilized societies in all parts of the world depend upon cereals for nourishment because they produce the maximum yield of food from a given area of ground. The cereal grains are obtained by threshing the harvested 'grass' to separate the grain from the chaff, which surrounds each grain, and the stalk, which supports the ear.

Cereals are major sources of carbohydrate but they also contain substantial amounts of protein (from about 6 per cent by weight in rice to about 12 per cent in oats and Canadian wheat), and because large quantities of cereal products are eaten, this may constitute quite a large proportion of the total protein intake. The proteins in cereals are low in the essential amino acid lysine. However, in balanced diets with the proteins from bread and also legumes, such as lentils, peas and beans, the balance of amino acids can be perfect. One of the proteins found in some cereals is gluten, which is important for bread making. Fats are also found in cereals (from about 1.5 per cent in wheat to about 5 per cent in oats); with the fats are some fat-soluble compounds including, importantly, vitamin E. Cereal grains contain substantial amounts of vitamins of the B group though, as will become evident, the quantity of these vitamins present in foods manufactured from cereals depends largely upon the degree to which the several parts of the grain have been separated in milling. The amount of moisture in cereal grains is quite small (from 7 per cent in oats to about 12 per cent in wheat) and this largely accounts for their good keeping qualities.

Wheat

Wheat is by far the most important cereal as far as people in the UK are concerned. It was first grown in the Middle East some 10 000 years ago, but in the course of centuries its cultivation has spread and varieties of wheat suitable for cultivation in zones as climatically different as the tropics and north European areas bordering on the Arctic Circle are now known. Some varieties of wheat, known as winter wheat, are sown in the autumn and harvested in the following August but spring wheat, which is sown and harvested in the same year, is grown in countries such as Canada where the winters are severe. Winter wheat, such as English wheat, usually contains less than 10 per cent protein and gives a 'weak' flour and a dough that bakes into small, close-textured loaves. Spring wheat (such as Canadian wheat) is richer in proteins (12–14 per cent) and because it has a hard and brittle grain it is described as a 'hard' wheat. Such wheat produces a 'strong' flour from which a strong elastic dough can be made. Strong flours give doughs which produce

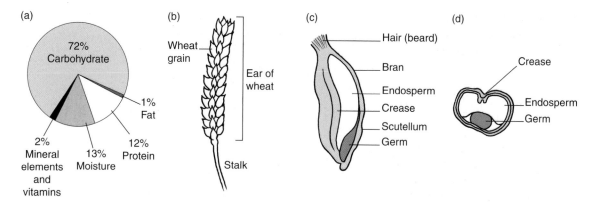

Figure 9.2 *(a) The composition of wheat. (b) An ear of wheat. (c) Longitudinal section of a wheat grain. (d) Transverse section of a wheat grain*

bold, well-risen loaves and they are very suitable for bread making. English flour and other similar 'weak' or 'soft' flours are more suitable for the manufacture of cakes and biscuits and for household use. Flour used for bread making in the UK is usually a blend of the two types.

Durum wheat, which is used for making macaroni and spaghetti, is a particularly hard wheat of high protein content.

The structure of a wheat grain

A grain of wheat is normally about 1 cm long and 0.5 cm broad. It is egg-shaped with a deep fissure or crease running along one side and a number of small hairs, called the beard, at one end (Fig. 9.2). The grain is enclosed in an outer covering called bran which consists of several distinct layers and constitutes about 15 per cent of the whole wheat. Bran contains a high proportion of B vitamins and about 50 per cent of the mineral elements present in the grain; it consists largely of cellulose which is indigestible by humans. The germ, which is situated at the base of the grain, is the actual seed or embryo and constitutes about 20 per cent of the wholegrain. It is rich in fats, protein, vitamins of the B group, vitamin E and iron. The combined fatty acids present in the fats are mainly essential fatty acids. A membranous tissue, called the scutellum, separates the germ and the endosperm; it is exceedingly rich in the vitamin thiamin and contains about 60 per cent of all the thiamin present in the grain. The endosperm is mainly starch and is intended as a reserve of food for the germ. It is by far the largest component and makes up

Table 9.2 Protein contents and yields from an English wheatflour[a]

Particle size range (mm)	Yield (%)	Protein content (%)
35–120	43	11.5
17–35	45	6.0
<17	12	15.6

[a] Parent flour = 9.5% protein content.

the major part of the wheat grain. The starch granules are embedded in a matrix of protein and the periphery of the endosperm is composed of a single layer of cells called the aleurone layer. This layer contains a higher proportion of proteins than the endosperm as a whole but, unfortunately, it is removed with the bran during the milling of the wheat.

So many varieties of wheat are grown and climatic and other conditions are so variable that it is not possible to give precise figures for the composition of wheat. The data given in Table 9.2 represent average values.

Flour milling

Wheat grains are almost always reduced to flour before being eaten and this operation is known as flour milling. Archaeological evidence shows that flour was made in hand mills in the Neolithic era. In later times, windmills or water mills were used in which the wheat was ground between two circular grooved stones, the upper of which revolved while the lower stone remained stationary. The wheat was

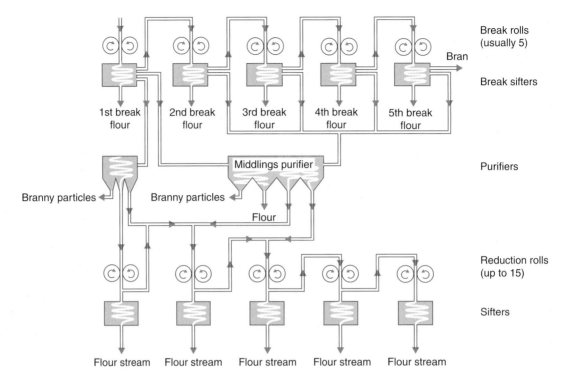

Figure 9.3 *Conversion of wheat to flour*

fed into the centre through a hole in the upper stone and was ground into flour during its passage to the periphery of the stones. In this process all the wheat grain was ground up so that the flour produced, called wholemeal flour, contained the germ, bran and scutellum, as well as the powdered endosperm. Wholemeal flour is dark in colour and bread produced from it may be rather coarse, depending upon the extent to which the bran particles have been reduced in size.

Modern milling processes differ greatly from the age-old method just described. The milling is carried out using steel rollers in place of revolving flat stones, and the germ, bran and scutellum are removed so that the flour produced consists essentially of powdered endosperm. The process is very complex but in essence it consists of separating the endosperm from the other constituents of the grain, then gradually reducing the size of the endosperm particles by passing them through a series of steel rollers as shown diagrammatically in Fig. 9.3. Before milling, different varieties of wheat may be blended together so that the flour obtained from the blend is best suited to the purpose for which it is intended.

After blending, the wheat is passed through a series of ingenious machines which remove stones, weed seeds and other extraneous materials, and may then be washed and brushed to remove adhering dirt.

Imported wheat is often too dry to be milled directly, and it must be 'conditioned' or brought to the optimum moisture content for milling. This can be done by storing the wheat in a moist condition for one or more days. The conditioning can be speeded up by passing the moist wheat through a machine known as a conditioner, in which is it heated to a temperature of 40–50°C for 30–90 minutes. Alternatively, the wheat may be exposed to live steam for a minute or so, followed by rapid cooling in cold water. During the conditioning process the distribution of moisture through the grain becomes more uniform, the bran becoming tougher and the endosperm more friable. This makes easier the separation of endosperm and germ from the bran in the milling operations which follow. English wheat often contains more water than is desirable, and when this is so it must be dried before milling.

The conversion of grain to flour begins with the operation known as breaking, in which the grain, or grist, is passed through four or five pairs of 'break rolls'. These rolls, which are made of steel, are finely corrugated and rotate at different speeds. The corrugations break the grain apart at the crease and scrape away the endosperm from the bran. After passing through the first break rolls the wheat is sieved through silk or fine wire gauze and separated into a small quantity of flour, termed 'first break flour', small particles of endosperm known as 'middlings' or 'semolina' and coarser particles of bran with adherent endosperm. The bran with its attached endosperm is passed onto the next set of break rolls. Each pair of break rolls is set closer together and has finer corrugations than the one before it and the branny residue from the final sifting is extremely thin with little or no attached endosperm.

The middlings produced at each set of break rolls are graded, or sized, by further sieving in machines known as purifiers. These consist of enclosed reciprocating sieves through which a current of air is blown. The blowing removes particles of endosperm, which are still attached to the bran, and these are treated in a separate part of the mill where the endosperm is scraped away from the bran by finely corrugated rolls similar to break rolls.

The graded semolina and middlings are converted to flour by a series of smooth rolls called reduction rolls. There are usually from 10 to 15 sets of reduction rolls and, as with the break rolls, the clearance between the rolls decreases from one set of rolls to the next. The reduction rolls crack the semolina particles and gradually produce smaller and smaller fragments without damaging the starch grains themselves. If the endosperm were simply crushed to a fine powder by being passed through a pair of rolls set very closely together the starch granules would be badly damaged and the resulting flour would be of very poor quality. The product from each set of reduction rolls is sieved to remove the flour, and the residue is divided into two parts; the finer of these two fractions progresses to one of the succeeding reduction rolls, and the less fine fraction is returned to one of the previous reduction rolls. The germ is not friable and so it is flattened rather than powdered by the reduction rolls, and is easily separated in the sifting operations.

The flour 'streams' obtained at each of the break rolls and reduction rolls differ markedly in composition. They may be mixed in various proportions to give flour suitable for special purposes, or they may all be combined to give what is known as a straight-run flour.

The milling technique described above can be modified to produce more or less flour from a given amount of wheat. The percentage of flour produced is termed the extraction rate of the flour. Wholemeal flour, which contains all the bran, germ, scutellum and endosperm of the wheat grain has an extraction rate of 100 per cent. In contrast, at an extraction rate of 70 per cent the flour produced is composed almost exclusively of crushed endosperm.

Because vitamins and minerals are lost from wheat during the milling of flour of low extraction rate, millers are required by law to add certain nutrients to all flour other than wholemeal flour of 100 per cent extraction rate. Sufficient iron, thiamin, niacin and purified chalk must be added to ensure that 100 g of the flour will contain not less than 1.65 mg of iron, 0.24 mg of thiamin, 1.60 mg of niacin and between 235 and 390 mg of calcium carbonate. The iron may be added as ferric ammonium citrate, ferrous sulphate or, rather surprisingly, as very finely divided metallic iron. Flour of any extraction rate may be produced provided that the above nutrients are present in the stated amounts.

Special flours

High- and low-protein flours The starch particles present in a sample of ordinary flour vary in size from below 5 μm to about 120 μm in diameter (1 μm = 10^{-6} m). The larger particles, of diameter greater than about 35 μm, consist of starch granules embedded in a protein matrix. Particles of sizes between 17 and 35 μm are, in the main, free starch granules and little protein matrix is present. Below about 17 μm the particles are mainly small starch granules, fragments of free protein and small particles of protein matrix with adherent fragments of starch. If flour is subjected to a further size-reducing process in an impact mill, many of the larger particles consisting of starch embedded in protein matrix can be broken down and more separate starch granules and protein fragments released. By separating the flour produced into three fractions it is possible to obtain two high-protein flours and one low-protein flour, as shown in Table 9.2.

Because the flour particles are so small it is not possible to separate the fractions by conventional sieving operations, but this can be done by using a piece of equipment known as an air classifier. In the classifier, flour particles in air are subjected to powerful centrifugal forces by being made to follow a spiral path at high speeds and at the same time, of course, each particle is experiencing frictional drag. The centrifugal force on each particle is proportional to its weight, whereas frictional resistance varies with particle size and not with weight. Because of this difference, the coarser particles migrate to the outside of the spiral path and finer particles accumulate in the centre. The fraction of largest particle size is noticeably coarser (because of the absence of fine particles) than normal flour and it has been used for biscuit making and for self-raising flour. The intermediate low-protein fraction is valuable as a high-ratio cake flour (see p. 63) because of its fine and even particle size.

Agglomerated flour   When ordinary flour is added to water, the particles float on the surface and tend to stick together to form lumps that are difficult to disperse. An 'instant' flour, which is easily wetted by water and can be dispersed in water without difficulty, is manufactured by allowing flour to fall through jets of steam. The outer surfaces of the flour particles are wetted and if they are then allowed to fall through cold jets of air the particles stick together, or agglomerate. The moisture content of the clusters is adjusted by passing the flour through heated chambers and oversized particles are reduced to a uniform particle size. As well as being easily dispersible in water, agglomerated flour, or instant flour, is free-flowing and dust-free because it consists of small clusters of flour particles above 100 μm in diameter. When agglomerated flour is added to water, the clusters are penetrated by water

as a result of capillary action and the wetted particles sink. Agglomerated flour is especially useful in soup and gravy powders or as a thickening agent, but it is likely to find many other applications in convenience foods.

Self-raising flour   When bread is made, it is aerated by carbon dioxide produced by fermentation (i.e. by the action of yeast on sugars present in the dough). Yeast can be successfully employed as a raising agent only with high-protein (i.e. 'strong') flours which give a strong elastic dough. Weak doughs, such as those used in pastry, are not fermented with yeast but a chemical raising agent (see p. 246) is used instead. Self-raising flour contains an acidic raising agent (e.g. monocalcium phosphate and sodium bicarbonate) incorporated into it in suitable amounts, so that carbon dioxide is formed during cooking and this aerates the dough.

Enzyme-inactivated flour   Enzyme-inactivated flour is discussed on p. 122.

Flour improvers

It was formerly the practice to store flour for several weeks after milling before it was used for bread making. During this period its bread-making characteristics improved, as a result of partial oxidation of the proteins which form gluten during dough making. Gluten obtained from 'aged' flour is stronger and more elastic than that obtained from freshly milled flour. The ageing period can be dispensed with if the flour is treated with a minute quantity of one of a number of oxidizing agents which are called flour improvers, and it is common practice for all flour except wholemeal flour to be treated in this way. The substances used as flour improvers, the proportions in which they may be used and their serial numbers (see p. 276), are listed in Table 9.3.

Table 9.3 Flour improvers

Serial number and name	Formula	Maximum permitted level (parts per million parts of flour) and restriction on use (if any)
925 Chlorine	Cl_2	2500 (for cakes only)
926 Chlorine dioxide (Dyox)	ClO_2	30
E220 Sulphur dioxide	SO_2	200 (for biscuits or pastry only)
E300 Ascorbic acid	$C_6H_8O_6$	200

Note: None of these compounds may be used with wholemeal flour.

The first four of the improvers listed increase the whiteness of the flour by bleaching the carotene and xanthophyll, which are always present and give the flour a slight yellow tinge; they are sometimes referred to as bleaching agents rather than flour improvers. Unlike the other flour improvers listed in Table 9.3, ascorbic acid is a reducing agent. The actual flour improver, however, is not ascorbic acid itself but dehydroascorbic acid. This is an oxidizing agent and it is formed in the bread mix by enzymic reduction of ascorbic acid.

The way in which improvers perform their functions is not fully understood, though many explanations have been put forward. It is likely, however, that the improvers produce some cross-linking between adjacent protein molecules by the formation of disulphide links (—S–S—) from neighbouring sulphydryl (—SH) groups, as shown in Fig. 9.4.

The sulphydryl groups belong to the amino acid cysteine which forms part of some protein molecules. The increase in molecular weight and molecular complexity produced by such a process of cross-linking produces a corresponding increase in the strength and elasticity of the gluten formed on treatment with water.

The enzymes of flour

Wheat flour contains α- and β-amylases which are capable of hydrolysing the amylose and amylopectin of starch. The hydrolysis does not occur to any significant extent in dry flour, but begins immediately a dough is made. β-Amylase attacks the damaged starch grains inevitably present as a result of milling and hydrolyses some of the amylose to maltose. It can also hydrolyse amylopectin and produce maltose by splitting off pairs of glucose units from the ends of the chains. With amylopectin only the 'free' ends of the chains can be attacked and hydrolysis ceases before the glucose unit which connects two chains together is reached. The links between the chains cannot be hydrolysed by β-amylase and a high molecular weight dextrin, which is not susceptible to further attack by β-amylase, is ultimately obtained. α-Amylase, which is present in flour made from sprouting wheat, attacks amylopectin in an entirely different way: it splits the links between chains to produce low molecular weight dextrins. These dextrins differ in structure, as well as in size, from those produced by β-amylase. They consist, like amylose, of strings of connected glucose units

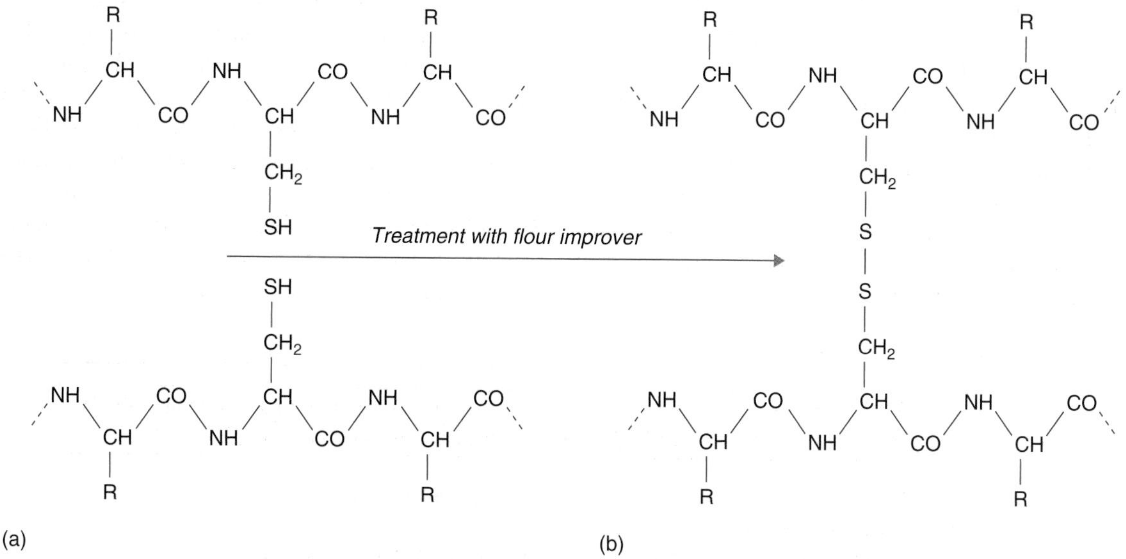

Figure 9.4 *Action of flour improvers. (a) Two protein molecules with adjacent sulphydryl groups. (b) One larger protein molecule formed by crosslinking*

whereas the dextrins produced by β-amylase are branched and three-dimensional like amylopectin.

The dextrins produced by α-amylase can be hydrolysed to maltose by β-amylase. Conversely, α-amylase can attack the dextrins produced by β-amylase to produce simpler dextrins which can be further hydrolysed to maltose by α-amylase. Clearly, by acting in conjunction, α- and β-amylase can produce a far greater quantity of maltose than either acting alone. The presence of too much α-amylase in flour can have a disastrous effect when it is made into bread: the low molecular weight dextrins it produces cause marked crumb-stickiness and may lead to collapse of the loaf. α-Amylase is active up to about 60°C and so its action may continue for some time after the bread has been put in the oven.

In practice, flour is not likely to contain excessive amounts of α-amylase because it is usually milled soon after being harvested. If the α-amylase content is too low, the amount of fermentable sugars in the dough may also be low and, in this case, insufficient carbon dioxide will be produced during bread making. Consequently, the bread obtained will be close-grained and lacking in volume. This can be prevented by adding α-amylase to the flour. Dough made from such flour rises strongly during fermentation and produces softer bread of greater volume.

A high α-amylase content may be undesirable in flour intended for use in gravies, thickening agents or powdered soups. If such a gravy or soup is kept hot, the α-amylase may break down the starch to such an extent that it is no longer able to act as a thickening agent. Enzyme-inactivated flour can be produced for special purposes such as this, and it is made by heating wheat with steam to 100°C. The wheat is subsequently dried and converted into flour in the usual way. Enzyme-inactivated flour is not suitable for bread making because the elastic properties of the gluten are destroyed by the steaming process.

Flour also contains peptidases (i.e. protein-splitting enzymes) and these also play a part in the 'ripening' of the dough. Peptidases also make available much α- and β-amylase which is combined with protein and would otherwise be unavailable. Lipases and lipoxidases also occur in flour and act upon the fats present. Lipases catalyse the hydrolysis of fats to glycerol and fatty acids and lipoxidases catalyse oxidation. Flour which has been stored for a long period may have a tallowy smell and flavour owing to the presence of oxidation products of fats. Phytase is another important enzyme present in flour. It splits phytic acid and phytates (see p. 127) and is active during the fermentation and early stages of baking.

Bread making

A type of bread, known as unleavened bread, can be made by mixing flour and water and then baking it. This is the forerunner of modern bread, but the product is hard and unattractive to most palates and the resemblance to bread, as we know it, is slight.

Bread is traditionally made from flour, water, salt and yeast. It has a honeycomb structure and may be regarded as a solid foam with a multitude of pockets of carbon dioxide distributed uniformly throughout its bulk. Sugars naturally present in flour, and the maltose made available by the action of amylases, are hydrolysed to glucose and this is fermented by zymase present in the yeast. Ethyl alcohol and carbon dioxide are formed and the latter aerates the dough.

$$(C_6H_{10}O_5)_n \xrightarrow[\text{flour}]{\text{amylases in}}$$
Starch
$$C_{12}H_{22}O_{11} \xrightarrow[\text{yeast}]{\text{maltase in}}$$
Maltose
$$C_6H_{12}O_6 \xrightarrow[\text{yeast}]{\text{zymase in}} C_2H_5OH + CO_2$$
Glucose   Ethyl alcohol

Most of the alcohol formed during fermentation is driven off during baking and many thousands of litres of alcohol enter the atmosphere daily from bakeries.

Small amounts of carboxylic acids are also produced during the fermentation period in addition to carbon dioxide and alcohol. The acids formed lower the pH of the dough and this affects the colloidal state of the gluten (see below) and assists in ripening the dough. The carbon dioxide retained by the dough also lowers its pH and so, in addition to its leavening function, it has a beneficial effect on the gluten structure. Some protein breakdown occurs during the fermentation period owing to the presence of proteolytic enzymes. During this period the yeast cells multiply and the yeast contributes substantially, together with the fermentation products, to the flavour of the loaf.

Two of the proteins present in flour – gliadin and glutenin – become hydrated and form an elastic complex called gluten when flour is kneaded with water. It is the presence of this elastic gluten which makes the manufacture of bread possible, because it forms an interconnected network which contains the carbon dioxide within the loaf and prevents its escape. The gluten is uniformly distributed throughout the dough and the carbon dioxide becomes trapped as small pockets of gas. As gas production continues, the gluten strands are stretched and it is thought that bonds between adjacent protein molecules are broken and reformed to produce an elastic, gas-retaining, three-dimensional network. A ripe dough (that is, one which is ready for baking) is springy and elastic; it can be fairly easily stretched out and shows a capacity to recover its former shape. An under-ripe dough is extensible (i.e. it can be stretched, but lacks elasticity). If fermentation is allowed to continue unhindered the dough becomes over-ripe and, as dough in this condition cannot be stretched far without breaking, its power to retain carbon dioxide is lost.

Salt is used in dough making and its most important function is to improve the flavour of the bread, which has a flat, insipid taste without it if the consumer's palate is accustomed to salty foods. The weight of salt added is about 1–2 per cent of the weight of flour used, although this figure varies slightly. It is possible to use less salt and bread manufacturers should be encouraged to gradually reduce the amount of salt in bread as it is a major source of sodium in the British diet. The palate soon adapts to low-salt foods. The amount of water needed to make a dough varies with the quality of the flour, but it is roughly half the weight of the flour used. Its temperature must be adjusted, so that the fermented dough has a temperature of 24–27°C. The quantity of yeast needed depends upon the time and temperature of fermentation but is usually about 0.3–1.0 per cent of the weight of the flour used. When bread is baked the carbon dioxide expands, the starch gelatinizes, and the gluten coagulates to produce a more or less rigid loaf. The changes which occur during baking are considered in more detail on p. 124.

Dough making

In the traditional method of bread making known as the long-fermentation process, the warm ingredients are thoroughly mixed to form a dough which is allowed to ferment in bulk. The dough is covered to prevent the formation of a skin and it is allowed to ferment for a period of 1 hour or longer, depending upon the quantity of yeast used and the temperature of the dough. Yeast functions best at a temperature of 26°C and the dough should preferably be kept at about this temperature. The dough is then thoroughly kneaded, or 'knocked back', to expel some of the carbon dioxide and tighten up the dough. This has the effect of bringing yeast cells into contact with a new environment and assists further fermentation. The dough is then covered again and allowed to ferment for a further period – usually about 2.5 hours – but, as before, this depends upon the amount of yeast used and the ambient temperature. At the end of this time, it is divided into pieces of the required weight which are shaped into balls.

A good deal of carbon dioxide is lost during the dividing and moulding process and the dough is given a further period of fermentation, referred to as first proof or intermediate proof, to allow more carbon dioxide to be formed. During this period the gluten fibres recover after the rather harsh treatment they have received during dividing and shaping. When the first proving period of 10–15 minutes is over, the dough is moulded to its final shape and, after placing in baking tins or on baking sheets, is given a final proof of about 45 minutes at a somewhat higher temperature (usually 32–35°C), during which it becomes fully inflated with carbon dioxide and assumes its final shape.

In a modern bakery, the mixing, knocking back, dividing and moulding to shape are carried out mechanically and the proving periods are often spent on conveyor belts which pass through temperature-controlled chambers. Because of the fairly long fermentation period, however, a considerable weight of dough is being dealt with at any one time in a large bakery and this has to be moved from place to place and, of course, it occupies considerable space. In modern bread-making methods, the fermentation period is replaced by a short period of intensive mixing (see below) and this overcomes one of the main drawbacks of the traditional bread-making process.

Most bread in the UK is now made by a short-fermentation process which is known as the Chorleywood bread process because it was developed by the Flour Milling and Baking Research Association

Table 9.4 Advantages of the Chorleywood bread process

Advantages	
Time	Less than 2 hours including baking – a saving of about 60 per cent
Premises	Dough-room areas are reduced by 75 per cent. Temperature and humidity control not required
Materials	Flour of low protein content may be used. Low fermentation losses
Product	Variability of product reduced. Bread has a lower staling rate

at Chorleywood in Hertfordshire, UK. In this method of bread making about twice as much yeast is used as in the traditional method and flour improvers are added to the bread mix. The long period of fermentation of the traditional method is replaced by a short period of high-speed mixing in the presence of about 75 ppm (based on weight of flour used) of ascorbic acid and other ingredients such as enzymes, emulsifiers and fats.

Dough made by the Chorleywood process is called mechanically developed dough. The ingredients for the dough are fed into a powerful mixing machine which is equipped with a meter to indicate how much energy is expended during the development period. The mixing and development are completed in as short a time as possible – usually about 5 minutes – and when the appropriate amount of energy has been expended the machine switches off. The mixing machine rapidly stretches the gluten and this replaces the stretching brought about more slowly by gas evolution in the long-fermentation process. It is believed that bonds between adjacent protein molecules are ruptured by the severe mechanical treatment and that this is followed by a rapid repositioning of the protein molecules. At this point, mixing must stop and bonds are rapidly reformed to give the required elastic network structure. If mixing is continued an inferior product is obtained.

When the mixing process has been completed the dough is divided into pieces of the correct weight for the loaves required and these are shaped into balls and given a first proof period of 6–10 minutes before being moulded to shape and being placed in baking tins. After a second proving period of about 50–60 minutes, the bread is ready for baking in the normal way.

Yeast is necessary in mechanically developed dough making, even though one of its jobs – the stretching and reorientation of gluten fibres – is done

mechanically. The yeast is still required for producing carbon dioxide, which aerates the bread in the usual way, and for flavouring.

Almost any flour can be used in the Chorleywood bread process and good bread can be obtained from weak flour. This means that English flour can be used, whereas for the normal bulk fermentation methods a stronger flour must be used. The reason for this is that some protein is lost during the long fermentation period; this does not occur to any extent with mechanically developed doughs.

Control of temperature is less important in the Chorleywood process than in long-fermentation methods and good results can be obtained throughout the range 27–32°C. Because of the large amount of energy expended during development of the dough, its temperature may increase by 11–24°C during the process.

The advantages of the Chorleywood bread process compared with the long-fermentation process are summarized in Table 9.4.

The special mixing machinery required for the Chorleywood process is usually found in large-scale bakeries, or 'plant bakeries' as they are known. Bakers who do not have the specialized equipment can considerably reduce the time taken for fermentation by using ordinary low-speed mixers and adding about 50 ppm (based on the weight of flour used) of the naturally occurring amino acid L-cysteine to the ascorbic acid used in the Chorleywood process. This process is called activated dough development.

Changes during baking

Bread is baked at a temperature of about 232°C for a period of 30–50 minutes, depending upon the type of bread and the size of the loaf. During baking, the dough first rises rapidly because the pockets of carbon dioxide in the loaf expand as the temperature increases. At first there may also be some slight increase in the activity of the yeast, resulting in increased production of gas, but this diminishes as the temperature increases, until at a temperature of about 54°C fermentation ceases. As the temperature increases, the water present causes the starch granules to swell and gelatinize, and during this period the starch probably abstracts some water from the gluten. Hot gluten is soft and devoid of its characteristic elasticity, and gelatinized starch now supports the structure of the loaf. The gluten begins to coagulate at about 74°C and the coagulation continues slowly to the end of the baking period. The temperature of the interior of the loaf never exceeds the boiling point of water, despite the high temperature of the oven. Water and much of the carbon dioxide and alcohol formed during the fermentation escape during baking. Considerable dextrin formation occurs at the outside of the loaf as a result of the action of heat and steam on the starch; the sugars formed are converted to caramel which imparts an attractive brown colour to the crust. Maillard reactions (see p. 242), which occur between the carbohydrates and proteins present, also contribute to the brown colour of the crust.

Bread quality

A loaf of bread has certain characteristics by which its quality is judged. The dough should have risen to produce an upstanding loaf, the interior of which should be uniform in porosity and firm and elastic to the touch. The crust should be golden-brown in colour and should be crisp and brittle rather than tough, to make cutting and chewing easier. Bread produced by the traditional long-fermentation process may be less consistent in quality than that produced from mechanically developed dough. A dough which has been insufficiently fermented will have a starch gel which is too stiff to permit expansion during baking and a small dense loaf will result. In an over-fermented dough, on the other hand, extensive starch breakdown will have occurred and the starch gel will be weak. The dough may be unable to stand the increased internal gas pressure which occurs during baking. Individual gas bubbles may coalesce to form large pockets and gas escape at the surface may prevent the loaf from rising properly. In addition, such a loaf may contain larger quantities of dextrins than are found in a properly fermented loaf, and as a result the interior of the loaf may be darker in colour.

Staling

When bread is kept and becomes stale, its crust becomes soft and leathery and loses its appealing flavour. At the same time the interior of the loaf loses flavour and becomes less elastic through crumb-staling.

Crust-staling is largely caused by the diffusion of water from the interior of the loaf. It occurs more rapidly with wrapped bread because the moisture is unable to escape.

Crumb-staling is not caused by drying out but by retrogradation (see p. 96) of amylopectin in the gelatinized starch which makes up the bulk of the loaf. This takes place as the bread ages and the amylopectin molecules become more regularly arranged. In fresh bread, the amylopectin molecules and the chains of glucose units of which they are built up are arranged in a completely haphazard and random manner in partially swollen starch granules. In stale bread, however, many amylopectin molecules may be arranged in a cluster and the chains of glucose units lie parallel to each other, almost as if they had been combed into position. The presence and absence of order in stale and fresh bread, respectively, has been confirmed by X-ray studies.

During the change from partially gelatinized starch to the more-or-less crystalline form, water is released and it is absorbed by the crust, which loses its crispness and becomes leathery. If the bread is left uncovered the crust will, in time, become hard again owing to diffusion of moisture into the air but the resulting dry crust bears little resemblance to a crisp, fresh crust.

Staling can be prevented by drying, because bread or breadcrumbs containing less than about 16 per cent moisture does not stale. Surprisingly, excess moisture can also prevent staling and wet bread remains fresh for long periods. Neither of these methods is of any practical importance, however. Temperature can play an important part and bread kept under controlled moisture conditions remains fresh above 60°C and below −10°C. At temperatures between these extremes bread becomes stale, with a maximum rate of staling at about 0°C. This has been put to practical use in the preservation

Table 9.5 Types of bread

Bread	
Wholemeal	Made from flour obtained by milling whole wheat grains including the bran and germ and no other cereal. May contain ascorbic acid if made by the Chorleywood bread process. Addition of L-cysteine or any of the flour improvers listed in Table 9.3 is prohibited. May contain any other permitted additional ingredients or additives (see white bread below)
Brown	Contains at least 0–6 per cent crude fibre (calculated on the dry matter) and flour other than wholemeal flour. May contain any other permitted additional ingredients or additives
Wheatgerm	Must at least 10 per cent processed wheatgerm (calculated on the dry matter). May contain any other permitted additional ingredients or additives
White	Defined by exception as bread which is not wholemeal, brown or wheatgerm. Contains flour made only from the endosperm, or central section of the grain. May contain a wide range of additional ingredients, including milk and milk products, liquid or dried eggs, wheatgerm, rice flour, oat grain (or oatmeal), soya bean flour (in limited quantities), salt, vinegar, oils and fats, malt extract, malt flour, sugars, wheat gluten, various seeds, wheat, malted wheat, rye or barley and, in limited quantities, starch. May contain one or more of 46 permitted additives
Softgrain	Made from white flour with additional grains of softene rye and wheat to increase the fibre content by 30% compared with conventional white bread
Granary	Brown bread made from special Granary flour (a trademark of the Hovis brand) which includes kibbled and whole grains
Soda	Contains sodium hydrogen carbonate (sodium bicarbonate, $NaHCO_3$) as an ingredient

of bread and sponge cakes (which normally stale in the same way as bread) by deep-freezing. Wrapped bread stays fresh longer than unwrapped (although crust staleness may develop more quickly) because of moisture retention, which prolongs the period for which the crumb remains soft.

Another method of delaying staling is the incorporation into bread of emulsifying agents, although it is not yet clear how these substances delay the onset of staling. The use of emulsifying agents in bread is controlled by the *Miscellaneous Food Additives Regulations* (1995) and only the substances specified in the regulations may be used as emulsifiers.

Types of bread

So many varieties of bread are made that it is sometimes difficult to be sure exactly what type of bread one is buying or eating. Certain types are listed in Table 9.5. Wholemeal and wheatgerm are prescribed by law in the Bread and Flour Regulations.

Bread as a food

Like all other foods of cereal origin, bread is eaten mainly as a cheap source of energy. It contains about 40–45 per cent available carbohydrate and has an energy value of 900–1000 kJ/100 g. Because considerable amounts of bread are eaten, its other constituents also contribute substantially to the daily intake of nutrients. It contains 8–9 per cent protein and significant amounts of minerals and vitamins.

The nutrients in wheat grains are not present in the same proportions in all parts of the grain, and so a change in the extraction rate (see p. 123) produces a change in the composition of the flour produced. In particular, unmodified flour (i.e. flour to which nutrients have not been added) of low extraction rate contains smaller amounts of the B vitamins (thiamin, riboflavin and niacin) and iron than flour of higher extraction rate. This is because these nutrients are mainly concentrated in the bran, germ and scutellum, all of which are removed in the production of low extraction rate flour. To compensate for the loss supplements, thiamin, niacin and iron are added to all flour produced in the UK other than wholemeal flour (see p. 119). Calcium carbonate (chalk) is also added to all non-wholemeal flour as a means of enhancing the calcium content of the diet. It is not added to wholemeal flour as calcium is naturally present in this flour. The composition of bread made from flour of different extraction rates is shown

Table 9.6 Composition of 100 g of bread

Nutrient	Extraction rate of flour used		
	White bread (72%)	Brown bread (85%)	Wholemeal bread (100%)
Protein	7.9 g	7.9 g	9.4 g
Fat	1.6 g	2.0 g	2.5 g
Sugars	3.4 g	3.4 g	2.8 g
Starch	43 g	39 g	39 g
NSP	1.9 g	3.5 g	5.0 g
Phytic acid	4 mg	202 mg	360 mg
Calcium	177 mg	186 mg	106 mg
Iron	1.6 mg	2.2 mg	2.4 mg
Thiamin	0.24 mg	0.22 mg	0.25 mg
Riboflavin	0.08 mg	0.07 mg	0.05 mg
Niacin	1.6 mg	2.8 mg	3.8 mg
Sodium	461 mg	443 mg	487 mg
Energy	931 kJ	882 kJ	922 kJ

NSP, non-starch polysaccharide.

in Table 9.6. Because bread is somewhat variable in composition, the figures given should not be regarded as constants, but rather as representative values.

The amount of bread eaten varies greatly between individuals but surveys show clearly that average consumption is decreasing. Purchases of bread were fractionally up in 2000, the first annual increase since 1994. Purchases of white bread rose by 2 per cent. Brown bread purchases continued to decline in 2000 and have fallen 40 per cent since 1990. Total bread consumption per head is greatest in households with low incomes and four or more children. Families in this category also eat the smallest proportion of wholemeal bread.

Surveys show that the average bread consumption in Britain is now only about 100 g per day – about three 'thickish' slices or four thin slices. This provides about 950 kJ or 227 kcal of energy, which is about one-tenth of the estimated energy requirement for a moderately active man. It also makes a substantial contribution to the iron, calcium, thiamin and protein content of the diet and provides about one-third of the NSP in the average British diet. Dietary recommendations for health encourage increased bread consumption, particularly wholemeal bread.

Although bread is an important source of protein, cereal protein contains only about 3 per cent

of the essential amino acid lysine (see Table 10.7, p. 144). This is not of great importance, however, because most people eat more protein than they need and it is unlikely that there will be an overall deficiency of lysine. In addition, bread is not normally eaten on its own and it is more than likely that the other foods eaten at the same time will compensate for the lysine shortfall. Many traditional diets have evolved over the centuries to include bread or pasta, complemented with legume foods (beans, peas, lentils) as characteristic pairings. How this came about is mysterious but the pairing allows the balance of amino acids to become nutritionally perfect, since legumes are higher in lysine, neatly complementing the deficiencies of cereals.

The calcium content of the notional daily average bread consumption of 100 g is about 106 mg for wholemeal bread and 170 mg for other bread. The reason for the big difference is, of course, the enrichment of non-wholemeal flour with calcium carbonate. Calcium in food may react with the phytic acid present in bread, especially wholemeal bread (see Table 9.6), to form insoluble calcium phytate. At one time it was believed that the body was unable to absorb calcium from calcium phytate. It is now known, however, that if phytic acid forms a regular part of the diet, the body is able to adapt to its presence and counteract its bad effect on calcium absorption. The effect of phytic acid on calcium absorption is also nullified to some extent by proteins present in the diet. The consensus of expert medical opinion is that phytic acid in bread made from high extraction rate flours does not prevent adequate absorption of calcium or other minerals.

All flour in Britain, except wholemeal flour, has iron added to it to compensate for that removed during milling. Despite this, wholemeal bread is considerably richer in iron than bread of lower extraction rate. It also contains more phytic acid and phytate but, just as with calcium, it is now believed that its presence has little or no effect on the absorption of iron from bread. Several studies have shown that iron, particularly the added iron, in metallic form is poorly absorbed from bread by the body and although about 10 per cent of the average iron intake is provided by bread and other flour products, most of it passes through the body unabsorbed. Thus, the difference in iron content between wholemeal bread and other types of bread is probably of little nutritional significance.

The high salt content of commercially made bread has become a major issue because sodium increases blood pressure. Stepped reductions from the current 1–2 per cent levels are planned.

Other wheat products

Biscuits

Biscuits are made from flour with the addition of other ingredients such as salt, fat, sugar and flavouring agents. Baking powder is sometimes added to make them rise a little and some biscuits, such as cream crackers, are leavened with yeast in much the same way as bread. The dough is rolled to a thin sheet, cut into appropriate shapes and quickly baked at a high temperature. The water content of biscuits is only about 3 per cent compared with about 39 per cent in bread. The energy value of sweet biscuits may be twice as high as that of bread because of their low water content and the extra sugar and fat they contain.

Pasta

Pasta is the collective name given to a number of wheatflour products which are cooked by boiling in water rather than baking. This custom was brought to Europe by Marco Polo from China, where he enjoyed noodles, and was adopted by the Italians as a national emblem. Macaroni, spaghetti, vermicelli and ravioli are all pastas, and there are many others. They are made from the endosperm of a particularly hard (i.e. protein-rich) variety of wheat known as durum wheat. Milling of durum wheat produces semolina, which consists of hard endosperm particles. Semolina is much grittier than normal wheatflour because the endosperm particles are considerably larger. Semolina and water can be made into a stiff dough from which the various pasta shapes – ribbons, tubes, spirals or sheets, to name but a few – are made.

When pasta is cooked in boiling water it absorbs up to three times its weight of water and becomes soft but, provided that it is not over-cooked, it does not disintegrate and form a paste as a normal flour dough would. Because of its high water content, large quantities of cooked pasta are required to provide a sustaining meal and this is why pasta is usually accompanied by other more nutritious foods such as cheese or a meat-rich sauce.

Other cereals

Oats, rye, barley, maize and rice are all important cereals (see Fig. 9.5) but their contributions to the British diet are much less than that of wheat.

Oats

Oats are richer in fats and mineral elements than other cereals and their protein content is also high. Flour made from oats is not suitable for making bread, however, because the proteins it contains do not form an elastic complex like the gluten of wheat when mixed with water. The soluble fibre content of oats helps to maintain lower cholesterol levels and thus is valuable in helping to prevent heart disease.

Oats are prepared for human consumption by cleaning, then drying and storing for a period before removing the closely adherent husk. The product, known as groats, can be ground to produce oatmeal or rolled into flakes after being partly cooked by steam. The rolling ruptures the cell walls and flattens the grains and this makes subsequent cooking easier.

Oatmeal contains roughly 11 per cent protein, 66 per cent carbohydrate, 9 per cent fat and 6.5 per cent non-starch polysaccharides: it has an energy value of

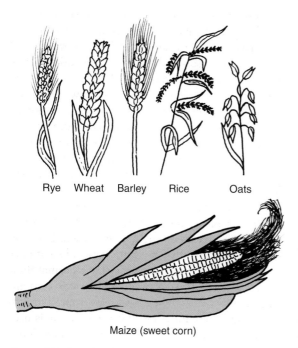

Rye   Wheat   Barley   Rice   Oats

Maize (sweet corn)

Figure 9.5 *Cereal grains*

about 1580 kJ/100 g. It must be remembered, however, that porridge made with water contains only about one-eighth of its weight from the oatmeal. Porridge can be made simply and with no mess in a microwave oven. It is valuable as a cheap, warming, nutritious, low-energy snack or meal replacement.

Rye

Rye can be grown in areas where the climate is too severe for wheat. The nutrients in rye are present in roughly the same amounts as in wheat. It is much less valued than wheat, however, because the proteins it contains do not give a strong gluten during dough making and, while large quantities of bread are made from rye flour, the product differs markedly from bread as we know it. Rye flour gives stodgy loaves which are unattractive to those accustomed to wheat bread. However, rye bread is still a staple article of diet in northern Europe. It may contain substantial proportions of wheatflour and this improves the appearance of the loaves obtained. Rye bread is not eaten to a large extent in Britain, but crisp rye biscuits (e.g. 'Ryvita') made from crushed whole rye grain are popular.

Barley

Barley is not eaten as a cereal in this country, but is grown extensively for the manufacture of malt for brewing and for animal fodder. Bread is never made from barley because its proteins do not form a gluten when mixed with water and an aerated loaf cannot be obtained. However barley is used in soups.

Maize

Maize is not widely used as a food for human consumption in Britain. In other countries, particularly America and South Africa, it forms an important part of the diet. It cannot be used for making bread because its proteins do not form a gluten. As a provider of energy, maize is as efficient as other cereals, but in other respects it is less desirable. Like all cereals its proteins are deficient in the essential amino acid lysine. Tryptophan, another essential amino acid, which can be converted by the body to the vitamin niacin, is also only present in small amounts. Maize contains niacin but it is bound to hemicellulose and is not available to the body when maize is eaten.

The deficiency disease pellagra is caused by a shortage of niacin and at one time it was a serious problem in parts of the world where maize was a staple food. It is still a serious health problem in parts of Africa and India, but because of improved standards of nutrition it is now rarely seen in Europe or USA.

A good deal of the maize crop is now used as cattle fodder or for conversion to glucose syrup or 'corn syrup'. It appears in the British diet mainly as cornflakes, which are toasted, malt-flavoured rolled maize. The nutritional deficiencies of maize are counteracted in cornflakes by means of lavish additions of iron, niacin, thiamin, riboflavin, vitamin B_6, vitamin B_{12}, vitamin D and folic acid. The amounts added are such that an average serving provides about one-quarter of the RNI of the added nutrients for a moderately active man (or one-third for a child).

Apart from cornflakes, maize is represented in British diets by sweetcorn and corn-on-the-cob, which are eaten as vegetables, and cornflour which is used in custard powder, blancmange powder and as a thickening agent (see p. 96). Cornflour consists of little but starch and is made by washing away the protein and fat from maize flour with dilute alkaline solutions. Worldwide, maize has supplemented indigenous crops and providing the major cereal source, being consumed in a wide variety of baked forms, as meal and porridge. Maize is a crop much of which has been genetically modified to make it more resistant to insect attack. However, there is controversy about its use and at the time of writing, genetically modified varieties are not grown in the UK for commercial production.

Rice

This is the main cereal of Eastern countries and one of the world's most important food crops. It is the poorest of all cereals in protein, fat and mineral elements and can hardly be called a nutritious food although, like all cereals, it is a cheap source of energy. Rice has an energy value of 1530 kJ/100 g and to provide over 10.5 MJ – the estimated average requirement (EAR) for energy of most men – about 700 g of rice would have to be eaten daily. This would weigh over 2 kg after cooking because of the large amount of water absorbed.

When rice grows the grains are surrounded by a loose, inedible outer husk which must be removed. The grain itself has a structure similar to that of a wheat grain. The starchy endosperm is surrounded by several layers of brownish bran which are removed, together with the germ, by a milling process. Unlike wheat, rice is not made into a flour and after milling the grains are polished to remove the aleurone layer, or silverskin, which surrounds the endosperm, and the membranous scutellum that separates the endosperm from the germ.

Many of the nutrients of whole rice are lost when the outer layers and germ are removed. The finished product, polished rice, contains about 85 per cent starch and 7 per cent protein. Some B-group vitamins remain in the endosperm but the amounts present are largely dissolved out and lost if rice is cooked in a large volume of boiling water. At one time many people who ate mainly boiled rice suffered from the deficiency disease beriberi which is caused by a lack of thiamin (see p. 207). This vitamin is required by the body to make use of carbohydrates in the diet and the amount required is related to the quantity of carbohydrate eaten. Thus, a diet which is rich in carbohydrates and low in thiamin is particularly likely to cause beriberi.

In India, rice is steeped in water after harvesting and it is then steamed and dried before milling. During this process, which amounts to parboiling, much of the vitamin content of the bran, germ and scutellum diffuses into the starchy endosperm and is retained there in the finished product. For this reason beriberi occurred less extensively in India than in other rice-eating parts of the world.

Beriberi is now a relatively uncommon disease, possibly owing to a general improvement in standards of nutrition. An understanding of the way in which it occurs and the availability of cheap synthetic thiamin have also been important factors in its eradication.

Key points

- Only plant-origin foods are rich in carbohydrates
  - Complex carbohydrates (polysaccharides including starch and NSP) mainly in cereal staples
  - Simple carbohydrates (mono and di-saccharides, i.e. sugars), naturally in sugar cane and fruits and in honey hydrolysed from starch from any plant food (especially beef)

Chapter summary

Starch is recommended to provide about half of all calories in a healthful balanced diet – from bread, cereals, rice, pasta, etc. Restricting sugar to about 10 per cent of calories is recommended, mainly to protect teeth and also to avoid weight gain in inactive subjects.

FURTHER READING

ADAM AC, RUBIO-TEXEIRA M, POLAINA J (2004). Lactose: the milk sugar from a biotechnological perspective. *Crit Rev Food Sci Nutr,* **44**(7–8): 553–557.

BELDEROK B (2000). Developments in bread-making processes. *Plant Foods Hum Nutr,* **55**(1): 1–86.

CHARALAMPOPOULOS D, WANG R, PANDIELLA SS, WEBB C (2002). Application of cereals and cereal components in functional foods: a review. *Int J Food Microbiol,* **79**(1–2): 131–141.

COMMITTEE ON MEDICAL ASPECTS OF FOOD AND NUTRITION POLICY (1994). *Nutritional Aspects of Cardiovascular Disease.* RHSS 46. London: HMSO.

FALCO MA (2001). The lifetime impact of sugar excess and nutrient depletion on oral health. *Gen Dent,* **49**(6): 591–595.

FOOD STANDARDS AGENCY (2002). *McCance and Widdowson's The Composition of Foods,* 6th edition. London: Royal Society of Chemistry, Food Standards Agency and Institute of Food Research.

JUKES TH (1986). Sugar and health. *World Rev Nutr Diet,* **48**: 137–194.

Websites

Wheat: www.wheatintolerance.co.uk/home.asp

Coeliac Association: www.coeliac.co.uk

Wheat Foods Council The Grain Nutrition Information Centre available at www.wheatfoods.org

Flour Advisory Board available at www.fabflour.co.uk

Bread Making tips available at www.aaoobfoods. com/breadmakingtips.htm

About Bread Making available at www.freerecipe.org/Old_Fashioned_Advice/About_Bread-Making/index.html

The Federation of Bakers fact sheets: How Bread is Made Factsheet no 7 http://www.bakersfederation.org.uk/resources/Fs7 per cent20- per cent20How per cent20bread per cent20is per cent20made.pdf

The Bread and Flour Regulations 1998 available at http://www.opsi.gov.uk/si/si1998/19980141.htm

The Miscellaneous Food Additives Regulations 1995 available at www.opsi.gov.uk/si/si1995/Uksi_19953187_en_2.htm

National Food Survey data can be found at http://statistics.defra.gov.uk/esg/publications/nfs/datasets/allfood.xls

Amino acids and proteins

Previous chapters have been concerned with fats and carbohydrates, substances containing almost exclusively the major elements carbon, hydrogen and oxygen, and it has been shown that these elements combined in the form of fats and carbohydrates are of fundamental importance in food science and nutrition. In addition to these major elements there is a fourth, namely nitrogen, which also plays a vital role in human life and which, when combined in the form of amino acids and proteins, constitutes a third group of 'macronutrient' compounds which are of basic importance in food and nutrition.

The way in which nitrogen is built up by stages into animal protein and then degraded in further stages back again into nitrogen is summed up in the nitrogen cycle (Fig. 10.1).

Elementary nitrogen occurs in almost limitless quantities in the atmosphere, while combined nitrogen is widely distributed in the soil as salts and, in the form of organic compounds, is found in all living matter. Combined nitrogen forms an essential part of the structure of the body, which requires a continuous supply of nitrogen in a suitable form. Unfortunately, the body is unable to synthesize its nitrogen compounds starting from elementary nitrogen; indeed, it is unable to perform such syntheses even when it is provided with a supply of inorganic nitrogen compounds. This means that humans must

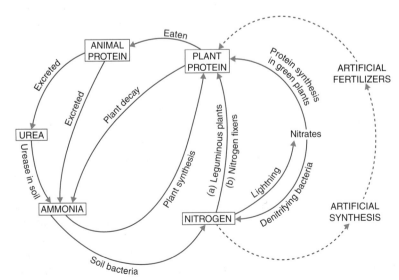

Figure 10.1 *The nitrogen cycle*

be supplied with nitrogen which has already been converted into a suitable organic form. This produces the paradoxical situation that although nitrogen is abundant in its elementary form, nitrogen compounds which can be utilized by humans are scarce. The explanation of this is to be found in the character of the element, which is noted for its inertness. This lack of reactivity makes it difficult to convert the element into its compounds, a process known as fixation.

Fixation of nitrogen into ammonia and subsequently into soluble ammonium salts is carried out commercially, but the amounts of fixed nitrogen thus produced are infinitesimal compared with the amounts required by living things. Fortunately, nitrogen fixation carried out with difficulty by chemists is performed with ease in nature, aided by microorganisms such as *Rhizobium*, which enable leguminous plants (e.g. peas and beans) to synthesize protein from nitrogen. Other green plants synthesize protein from nitrates present in the soil. Synthesis of protein is opposed by destructive processes which break down protein by stages into nitrogen, thus completing the cycle which is summarized in Fig. 10.1.

AMINO ACIDS

The structure of amino acids is relatively simple. Every amino acid contains an amino group —NH_2 and a carboxyl group —COOH. Amino acids of interest in nutrition have the amino and carboxyl groups attached to the same carbon atom, and to understand their structure it is easiest to start with acetic acid. If a hydrogen atom of acetic acid on the carbon next to the —COOH group is replaced by an —NH_2 group this forms the simplest possible amino acid, known as amino acetic acid or *glycine*.

CH_3COOH	CH_2NH_2COOH	$CHRNH_2COOH$
Acetic acid	Glycine	General formula

All amino acids encountered in food have a structure which can be expressed by the general formula $CHRNH_2COOH$, where the nature of R can vary considerably, as can be appreciated from Table 10.1 which gives the nature of R for the important amino acids obtained from food and body proteins.

The carbon atom to which the —NH_2 and —COOH groups are attached is known as the α-carbon and, except in the instance of glycine, this carbon atom has four *different* atoms or groups of atoms attached to it. Such structures may exist in two different spatial arrangements that are the mirror image of each other. In nature only one of these forms, the L-form, exists.

Classification of amino acids

More than 20 amino acids have been obtained from food and body proteins. They may be classified as being either neutral, basic or acidic, as shown in Table 10.1. Neutral amino acids are those, such as glycine, which contain one amino and one carboxyl group, basic amino acids contain one carboxyl but more than one basic group, while acidic amino acids contain one amino and two carboxyl groups. Three dietary amino acids contain sulphur as well as contain oxygen, hydrogen and nitrogen (cysteine, cystine and methionine).

Those amino acids marked with the letter 'E' in Table 10.1 are known as essential (or indispensable) amino acids, meaning either that they cannot be made by the body or that they cannot be made fast enough to meet the body's needs. Such amino acids must always be supplied by the diet. Eight amino acids are essential for adults and a further two – arginine and histidine – are essential for infants. During illness, the capacity for amino acid synthesis may be reduced so that other amino acids become 'essential'. For example, glycine may be required from the diet during 'conditioned essentiality' as a result of illness, especially in infancy.

Properties of amino acids

Amino acids are white crystalline substances that are soluble to some extent in water but which are mostly insoluble in organic solvents. The amino group, as its name suggests, is related to ammonia and like ammonia it has basic characteristics, while the carboxyl group is acidic. The combination of an amino group and a carboxyl group in the same molecule results in it being able to act as an acid or a base; such a substance is said to be amphoteric.

The formulae in Table 10.1 show the arrangement of covalent bonds in amino acids but they

Table 10.1 Structure of amino acids, $H_2NCHRCOOH$. Three amino acids, cysteine, cytine and methionine contain sulphur as well as C, H, O and N

Name	Abbreviation	R	Isoelectric point
Neutral			
Glycine	Gly	$H-$	6.0
Alanine	Ala	CH_3	6.0
Valine (E)	Val	$(CH_3)_2CH-$	6.0
Leucine (E)	Leu	$(CH_3)_2CHCH_2-$	6.0
Isoleucine (E)	Ile	$CH_3CH_2CH(CH_3)-$	6.0
Norleucine	Nor	$CH_3(CH_2)_3-$	6.1
Phenylalanine (E)	Phe	$C_6H_5CH_2-$	5.5
Tyrosine	Tyr	$C_6H_4(OH)CH_2-$	5.7
Serine	Ser	$HOCH_2-$	5.7
Threonine (E)	Thr	$CH_3CH(OH)-$	5.6
Cysteine	CySH	$HSCH_2-$	5.1
Cystine	CySSCy	$HOOCCH(NH_2)CH_2S_2CH_2-$	4.8
Methionine (E)	Met	$CH_3SCH_2CH_2-$	5.7
Tryptophan (E)	Trp	$-CH_2-$	5.9
Basic			
Ornithine	Orn	$H_2N(CH_2)_3-$	9.7
Arginine	Arg	$\underset{\text{NH}_2}{HN=CNH(CH_2)_3}-$	10.8
Lysine (E)	Lys	$H_2N(CH_2)_4-$	10.0
Histidine	His	$-CH_2-$	7.6
Acidic			
Aspartic acid	Asp	$HOOCCH_2-$	2.8
Glutamic acid	Glu	$HOOC(CH_2)_2-$	3.2

E, essential.

do not show the ionic character which amino acids display in solution. In solution amino acids may be more correctly represented as follows:

$$\overset{+}{N}H_3-CH-\overset{-}{COO}$$
$$|$$
$$R$$

This formula shows the ionic character of an amino acid and that it contains both a positive and a negative group. Amino acids are weak electrolytes and they ionize according to the pH of the system. We can represent this ionization as:

$$\overset{+}{N}H_3-CH-COOH \underset{\text{acid}}{\overset{+H^+}{\longleftarrow}} \overset{+}{N}H_3-CH-\overset{-}{COO} \underset{\text{alkali}}{\overset{-H^+}{\longrightarrow}} NH_2-CH-\overset{-}{COO}$$
$$|\qquad\qquad\qquad\qquad |\qquad\qquad\qquad\qquad |$$
$$R\qquad\qquad\qquad\qquad R\qquad\qquad\qquad\qquad R$$

Positive ion　　　　　　Zwitterion　　　　　　Negative ion

Thus, if acid is added to a neutral solution of an amino acid a positive ion is formed, whereas if alkali is added a negative ion is formed. Therefore an amino acid may be neutral, or positively or negatively charged according to the pH of the system.

When an amino acid is neutral, that is, when the positive and negative charges are equal, it is said to be at its isoelectric point and it is called a zwitterion or dipolar ion. Such zwitterions are effective buffers because of their capacity to combine with both acids and bases, thus preventing the change of pH that would otherwise occur. The buffering action of amino acids is very important, particularly in living cells where the cell can only function provided that the pH is maintained within a narrow range.

The isoelectric points of a number of amino acids are shown in Table 10.1. The isoelectric point is important because at this pH many properties have either a maximum or minimum value; for example, electrical conductivity, solubility and viscosity are all a minimum.

Importance of individual amino acids

Glycine is the simplest amino acid, normally synthesized in the body. During illness, in babies, this process may be insufficient to meet metabolic demands. Glycine is particularly abundant in fibrinogen, a protein involved in blood clotting and produced in increased amounts during illness. Arginine is a basic amino acid, formed in the liver and kidney and is involved in making urea in the liver. Lysine is an essential amino acid and, like arginine, basic in its reactions. It is used for producing carnitine in the body, a substance that transports fatty acids within cells. Cereals are deficient in lysine, but legumes are rich in it, and this is an important factor when planning diets that are adequate in protein (see p. 144).

Cysteine, cystine and methionine are all amino acids that contain sulphur and they constitute the main source of sulphur in the diet. They are found in cereals foods and in animal protein but little is present in legumes. The body can make cysteine from methionine, the latter being an essential amino acid. Cystine is one of the main amino acids of insulin, and is formed from cysteine in the body.

Glutamic acid is acidic in nature; it is not an essential amino acid though in the body it plays an important part in the metabolism of ammonia. It is of particular interest because its salt, monosodium glutamate, is used as a flavouring agent in food (see p. 302).

Glutamate occurs both in foods and in the body either free or as part of proteins. For example, proteins of foods such as milk, cheese and meat are rich in glutamate while some vegetables, notably mushrooms, tomatoes and peas, have high levels of free glutamate. The body contains glutamate both free and as part of the protein; about one-fifth of body protein is glutamate.

Histidine is a basic amino acid on account of the imidazole ring in its structure (shown in Table 10.1). The body's capacity to make it is limited so that during periods of rapid growth, as in infancy and childhood, additional amounts must be supplied by the diet. There is growing evidence that histidine remains essential into adult life. In the body, histidine is converted into histamine in a process called decarboxylation, in which amino acids are converted into related compounds called amines by the removal of the acid group. Histamine dilates blood capillaries and stimulates production of acid in the stomach.

Phenylalanine and tyrosine are neutral amino acids with a similar structure (see Table 10.1). The body cannot make phenylalanine for itself but can convert it into tyrosine, so that phenylalanine but not tyrosine is essential in the diet. They both contain a benzene ring in their structures, which enables them to provide the body with raw materials from which to make the hormones adrenaline and thyroxine.

Tryptophan occurs as part of the proteins casein (in milk) and fibrin (in blood). It is an essential amino acid in the synthesis of haemoglobin and plasma proteins. It is also of interest because the body can convert it into the vitamin niacin. However, only small amounts of niacin can be made in this way as it is not an efficient process, with 6 g tryptophan producing only 0.1 g niacin. Tryptophan is a component of the neurotransmitters serotonin and noradrenaline which signal satiety in the brain.

PEPTIDES

When two amino acid molecules combine, the acid group in one molecule reacts with the basic group in the other, with the elimination of water: a 'condensation' reaction.

$$\underset{\underset{R^1}{|}}{\overset{+}{N}H_3}CHCOO^- + \underset{\underset{R^1}{|}}{\overset{+}{N}H_3}\overset{\overset{R^2}{|}}{C}HCOO^- \longrightarrow \underset{\underset{R^1}{|}}{\overset{+}{N}H_3}CHCONH\overset{\overset{R^2}{|}}{C}HCOO^- + H_2O$$

The product formed is a dipeptide and contains the group —CONH—, which is the peptide linkage. Substances of relatively small molecular weight containing this group are called peptides.

A dipeptide still contains an amino and a carboxyl group and may react with another amino acid molecule to form a tripeptide. Theoretically, this procedure may be repeated again and again with the formation of polypeptides. In practice, amino acids do not react together in this way, but dipeptides, tripeptides and polypeptides may be synthesized indirectly.

A large number of peptides are known to act as hormones in the body. They are released in one cell, and transported in the extracellular space or blood to neighbouring or distant cells, where they are recognized by very specific receptors. When they combine with receptors, a signal in that cell is generated. Examples of peptide hormones are discussed in Chapter 2.

Peptide hormones are present in only minute amounts in the bloodstream, and in the specialized cells (endocrine cells) which make them. Even smaller changes in hormone concentrations have major effects on function, so for most functions the hormone concentrations are regulated by feedback systems to avoid erratic swings. There are also often sets of hormones with opposite actions (e.g. insulin promotes glucose uptake, glucagons and adrenaline promote its release), so changing one factor does not have profound metabolic effects. Many hormone actions interact with nutritional factors, and diet is involved in regulation of many endocrine systems. Appetite itself is regulated by several interacting peptide hormone systems.

PROTEINS

Protein molecules consist of chains of hundreds or even thousands of amino units joined together rather like beads on a string; they are the most complex substances known to man. This fact can be simply illustrated by comparing the molecular weights and formulae of proteins with those of other types of substance. A simple monosaccharide such as glucose has a molecular mass of 180 and a formula of $C_6H_{12}O_6$, whereas a simple protein has a molecular mass reckoned in thousands and a correspondingly complex formula. The protein lactoglobulin, for example, has a molecular mass of about 42 000 and a formula approximating to $C_{1864}H_{3012}O_{576}N_{468}S_{21}$. Large protein molecules are much bigger than this and have molecular masses of several millions.

Simple molecules can usually be classified readily as hydrophilic (water-soluble) or lipophilic. Large proteins have multiple hydrophilic and lipophilic sections, and they contribute to determining the three-dimensional shape of a protein. They do not exist as long chains, but as complicated folded forms, often suited to bridging through lipid (cell membrane) and aqueous regions. Their functions depend on what parts of the molecules are exposed in the three-dimensional shape, and this may involve rearrangement after binding with substrates, transmitters or peptide hormones.

Structure of proteins: primary and secondary structure

The way in which the complex structure of proteins has been worked out constitutes one of the major advances in biochemistry in recent years. The problem is one of awe-inspiring difficulty, but a notable step forward was made when, in 1951, Sanger determined the nature of the protein insulin. Insulin is a relatively small, simple protein built up from only 51 amino acid units (see Fig. 10.3), whereas large proteins may contain over 500 amino acid units. Persistent research enabled the structure of even complex proteins to be worked out, but knowing the conventions of the encoding genes allows scientists to work out the structure of any protein.

In addition to the elements carbon, hydrogen, oxygen and nitrogen, proteins often contain sulphur and sometimes phosphorus. On hydrolysis, proteins break down to polypeptides and eventually to amino acids, a single protein producing up to about 20 different amino acids. It is clear, therefore, that amino acids are the building units of which proteins are composed – but how are these units joined together to form a protein molecule? The answer is that they are joined together by peptide linkages. For example, although protein molecules contain few free amino or carboxyl groups, on hydrolysis about equal numbers of these groups are produced, as would be expected if peptide links are being broken.

Protein molecules are composed of large numbers of up to 20 different amino acids joined together by peptide linkages. X-ray analysis gives some indication of how the peptide chains are arranged in protein molecules. Such chains have a zigzag structure with the R-groups protruding alternately in opposite directions as shown in Fig. 10.2. The first major problem in working out protein structure is that of determining the sequence of amino acid units R_1, R_2, R_3 constituting the chain.

When it is considered that there are hundreds, and sometimes thousands, of amino acid units in a single protein molecule, and that there are over 20 different amino acids available to choose from, it is clear that the number of different protein molecules which can be constructed is almost limitless.

The determination of the sequence of amino acids in polypeptide chains reveals what is known as the primary protein structure, but this is only the beginning of the problem of working out the complete structure of a protein. In a protein molecule, polypeptide chains are linked together in a number of different ways giving rise to molecules of definite shape; this constitutes the secondary protein structure. Many of the R-groups in polypeptide chains contain reactive groups (see Table 10.1) which couple with reactive groups in adjacent chains so joining the chains together by crosslinking.

The most important R-group involved in crosslinking is that of cysteine which contains the SH-group. When two cysteine units in different polypeptide chains are adjacent, a disulphide bridge —S—S— may be formed between them by oxidation of the SH-groups, thus joining the chains together. Figure 10.3 shows how two such chains are joined together at two different points in insulin. It also shows how an internal disulphide bridge can be formed between cysteine units occurring in the same chain.

In addition to strong covalent cross-linking through disulphide bridges other weaker types of crosslink also play a part in protein structure. For example, when neighbouring R-groups in different polypeptide chains contain free NH_3^+ and COO^- groups the resulting electrostatic attraction holds the chains together,

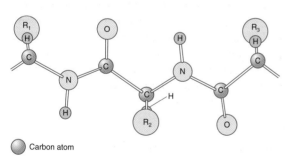

Carbon atom

Figure 10.2 *The zigzag structure of a polypeptide chain showing its three-dimensional structure*

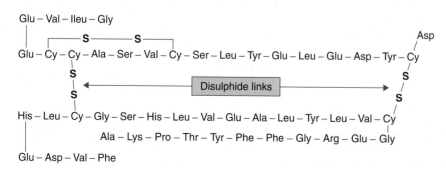

Figure 10.3 *The sequence of amino acids in insulin showing how two chains are joined by disulphide links*

although the strength of the attraction depends upon the pH of the system. Crosslinks are also created by salt formation between basic groups in one chain and acidic groups in another, and by ester formation between hydroxyl groups in one chain (e.g. threonine and serine) and groups such as phosphate in another. Crosslinks may also be produced by the formation of hydrogen bonds, although such links formed between hydrogen in one chain and, for example, oxygen in a neighbouring chain are much weaker than true chemical bonds. Figure 10.4 illustrates how such bonds are formed between adjacent polypeptide chains.

Classification of proteins: tertiary structure

Animal proteins can be classified according to their molecular shape as either fibrous or globular. Plant

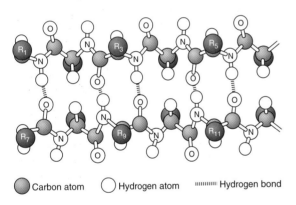

● Carbon atom   ○ Hydrogen atom   ⸏⸏⸏⸏⸏ Hydrogen bond

Figure 10.4 *Polypeptide chains joined by hydrogen bonds in a protein molecule*

proteins are more difficult to classify but, generally speaking, they can be divided into glutenins or prolamines. The nature of these different types is summarized in Table 10.2.

Fibrous proteins, which are simpler than globular proteins, are made up of individual zigzag polypeptide chains which are held together by crosslinks to form elongated or fibrous molecules with a fairly stable but elastic structure. They are characterized by being rather insoluble substances.

The fibrous proteins keratin and collagen have been much studied and will serve to illustrate typical features of this class of protein. Keratin is the main protein of hair. In its natural form, known as α-keratin, a hair or wool fibre consists of many polypeptide chains with the form of an α-helix (Fig. 10.5). These chains are held together by hydrogen bonds and by disulphide bridges provided by the sulphur-containing amino acid cystine. The chains are embedded in an insoluble protein matrix. When α-keratin is subjected to moist heat and stretching, the hydrogen bonds break, the α-helix structure disintegrates and a permanently stretched, inelastic form, known as β-keratin is formed. This is the basis of the 'permanent' waving of hair.

Collagen is the most abundant protein in the body. It occurs mainly in skin, cartilage and bone and is the body's major structural protein. The main amino acids in collagen are glycine, proline and hydroxyproline, and these prevent the formation of an α-helix structure. Instead, the polypeptide chains wrap round each other in threes to form a triple helix (Fig. 10.6), which has a rope-like structure. The strands of the 'rope' are held together by hydrogen bonds and the

Table 10.2 Simple classification of proteins

Type	Solubility/function	Examples/source
Animal		
Fibrous	*Insoluble, elastic proteins forming structural part of tissues*	*Keratin (hair); collagen (connective tissue); elastin (tendons, arteries); myosin (muscle)*
Globular	*Relatively soluble. Part of fluids of all body cells. Many food proteins*	*Enzymes; protein hormones; albumins, globulins (blood); casein (milk); albumin (egg white)*
Plant		
Glutelins	*Insoluble in neutral solutions. Soluble in acids and alkalis*	*Glutenin (wheat); hordenin (barley); oryzenin (rice)*
Prolamines	*Insoluble in water. Soluble in alcohol*	*Gliadin (wheat); Zein (maize)*

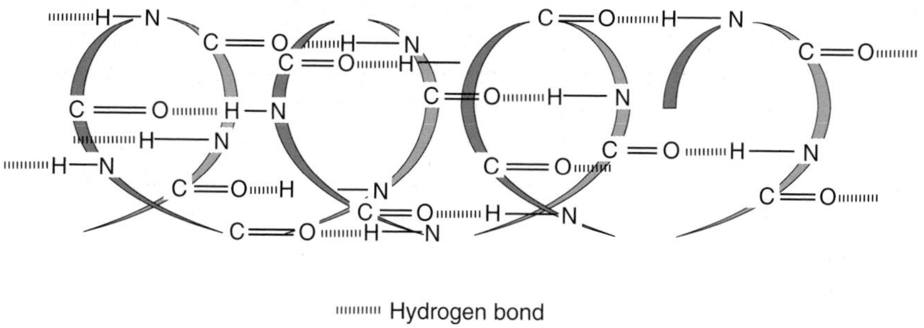

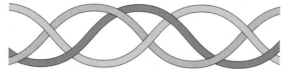

Figure 10.5 *α-helix showing how the links in the coil may be held together by hydrogen bonds*

|||||||| Hydrogen bond

Figure 10.6 *Collagen, showing its triple helix structure*

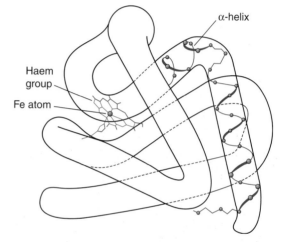

Figure 10.7 *An impression of a molecule of myoglobin showing the helical nature of a section of the chain and the way in which the chain is folded (after R. E. Dickerson)*

whole structure has great tensile strength as well as being insoluble in water.

Globular proteins are more complex than fibrous proteins because the α-helix chain is folded in various ways to form molecules with an irregular but bulky shape. The particular way in which folding takes place depends upon the points in adjacent coils at which disulphide and other crosslinks are formed. One of the complexities of determining the structure of globular proteins is that there is no general pattern of folding and so the exact nature of folding – called the tertiary structure – needs to be determined for each protein individually. Figure 10.7 gives an impression of how the α-helix is folded in the myoglobin molecule, about three-quarters of the chain being in the form of an α-helix. It can be seen that the structure is complex and non-symmetrical, although the overall shape is approximately spherical. Globular proteins are very important in the body as they include all proteins found within body cells and many food proteins.

The structure of plant proteins is less well understood than those of animals, but they can conveniently be divided into two categories. Glutelins are characterized by their insolubility in neutral solutions and their solubility in acids and alkalis. Prolamines, on the other hand, are insoluble in water but soluble in alcohol. Examples of both classes are shown in Table 10.2. It is worth re-emphasizing the importance of the presence of both glutenin and gliadin in wheat.

In combination these constitute gluten, the significance of which in bread making was discussed on p. 123.

Simple and conjugated proteins

The proteins encountered so far consist entirely of combined amino acids. They are distinguished from conjugated proteins whose molecules contain combined amino acids and also a non-protein component, called a prosthetic group. The main types of conjugated protein are summarized in Table 10.3.

Genes contain the nucleic acids ribonucleic acid (RNA) and deoxyribonucleic acid (DNA). These are of particular interest and importance because they play an essential part in the synthesis of all body proteins, including enzymes. Almost all human cells

Table 10.3 Classification of conjugated proteins

Type	Prosthetic group	Examples
Nucleoproteins	Nucleic acid	DNA combined with protamines
		RNA combined with ribosomes
Lipoproteins	Lipid	Distinguished by density e.g. LDL (low density); see Table 6.10
Chromoproteins	Coloured group containing a metal	Haemoglobin (blood)
Glycoproteins	Carbohydrate	Some enzymes and hormones
		Mucins (egg white)
Phosphoproteins	Phosphate	Casein (milk)

contain nucleoproteins in which nucleic acids are bound to different proteins; RNA occurs mostly outside the nucleus while DNA occurs inside. The DNA carries the genetic code which determines the nature of the proteins that must be made to maintain hereditary character. It passes this information to RNA which controls the synthesis of these proteins. Neither DNA nor RNA need to be supplied by the diet as the body can make all it requires. Nevertheless, certain foods do contain them, particularly fish roe, liver and kidneys.

With the arrival of post-genomic technology, the detailed structure and chemistry of even the biggest and most complex proteins can be ascertained with certainty, and interest is focused on mutations that give rise to polymorphisms of protein structures. Very small errors in the amino acid sequences of proteins can have profound effects on function, and such polymorphisms underpin many diseases.

Properties of proteins

Proteins normally exist in complex environments which contribute to their physical and functional properties. Isolated proteins lose most of these properties and change in tertiary structure. Some have been obtained in crystalline form. The solubility of proteins in different solvents may show wide variations, especially in water, salt solutions and alcohol, and this diversity is used to classify them. Although we talk about the solubility of proteins they do not give true solutions but, because of their relatively large size, they form colloidal dispersions or sols. The colloidal character of proteins is important in many foods as we have already seen in connection with the

colloidal food systems, such as milk, butter and ice cream, discussed in Chapters 6 and 7. Colloidal proteins, such as in milk, can bind a range of smaller molecules, including bitter tannins, so improving palatability.

The properties of proteins are similar in many ways to those of the amino acids from which they are constructed. For example, they contain free amino and carboxyl groups at the ends of the polypeptide chains, and as these carry a positive and negative charge, proteins form zwitterions; consequently, they are amphoteric and they act as buffers. The net charge on protein molecules varies with pH and is zero at the isoelectric point. The isoelectric point is important in considering the behaviour of food proteins because at this pH many properties are either a maximum or minimum; some values are shown in Table 10.4.

The properties of fibrous proteins are distinct from those of globular proteins. The former are relatively insoluble, being resistant to acids and alkalis, and they are unaffected by moderate heating, whereas the latter are soluble and are affected by acids, alkalis and heating. Globular proteins are very sensitive to chemical and physical conditions on account of the weak crosslinks that hold the folded α-helix chains in position. A small change of pH or a small rise in temperature is sufficient to disrupt such crosslinks and cause the chains to unfold, a process that is known as denaturation. When proteins are denatured their properties are completely altered; biological activity is destroyed, solubility decreased and viscosity increased. Moreover, the change is irreversible.

Denaturation may be brought about by controlling pH and occurs most readily at the isoelectric point, when proteins are least stable. For example, casein,

Table 10.4 Molecular mass and isoelectric points of some food proteins

Protein	Source	Molecular mass	Isoelectric point
Casein	Milk	34 000	4.6
β-Lactoglobulin	Milk	35 000	5.1
Ovalbumin	Eggs	44 000	4.6
Gliadin	Wheat	27 000	6.5
Gluten	Wheat	39 000	7.0
Gelatin	Bones	Variable	4.9
Myosin	Meat	850 000	5.4

which is the main protein of milk, has an isoelectric point of 4.6, and this explains why, when milk turns sour and the pH drops, it is quick to curdle. It also explains why milk is coagulated or clotted in the stomach so easily by rennin, for the pH is low and not far removed from the isoelectric point of casein. The denaturation of milk proteins is discussed in more detail on p. 78.

Many proteins are denatured by heat. For example, if egg white is heated, coagulation begins at about 60°C when the protein ovalbumin starts to separate out as a solid. As the temperature is raised, coagulation continues until the whole mass is completely solid. It is clear that coagulation occurs in the cooking of protein foods. For example, the proteins in lean meat coagulate on heating. Coagulation starts at about 60°C, as with albumin, and if cooking temperatures are kept somewhat below 100°C, coagulation is slow and the coagulated protein is not too hard. In this state, protein is most digestible. However, if a temperature of 100°C or over is used, as in boiling and basting, coagulation is more rapid and the denatured protein forms a rather hard, solid mass.

Partial coagulation of proteins may be brought about by beating them into a foam. For example, when egg white is beaten the foam that is formed is stabilized by the partial coagulation of the ovalbumin. Ovalbumin constitutes over half the protein content of egg white but foam formation is dependent on other proteins, such as globulins, which are better at lowering surface tension. If such a foam is heated, it becomes rigid because of further coagulation of the ovalbumin and conalbumin. Such foaming occurs most readily at the isoelectric point when the ovalbumin is least stable, and it may be promoted by addition of an acidic substance which lowers the pH to a value near the isoelectric point. Proteins are

precipitated out of solution by certain salts such as ammonium sulphate, sodium chloride, mercuric chloride and lead acetate. Thus, the presence of mineral salts affects the denaturation of proteins by heat treatment. The fact that lead acetate precipitates with ovalbumin in egg white explains why white of egg is used traditionally to treat cases of lead poisoning, since by reaction with egg white a soluble lead salt is rapidly converted into an insoluble compound that is not assimilated. However, this is rather theoretical and no longer used as a treatment, since lead poisoning usually occurs over long periods of time, in a slow, cumulative way.

Tests for proteins

In order to detect the presence of nitrogen (and sulphur) in a substance, Lassaigne's test may be used. The substance to be tested is heated with sodium, which reacts with nitrogen and sulphur forming sodium cyanide and sodium sulphide, respectively. Sulphide ions give a purple colour on addition of sodium nitroprusside solution and cyanide ions give a blue precipitate or colour with a mixture of ferrous and ferric ions.

Lassaigne's test detects the presence of nitrogen in a substance, but further tests are required to determine whether the compound containing nitrogen is a protein. Proteins may be detected by means of colour tests. For example, in the Biuret test proteins give a characteristic purple colour when they are heated in the presence of strong alkali and copper sulphate solution. A similar colour is given by any substance containing more than one —CONH— grouping, so that the test is not specific for proteins but is positive for all polypeptides.

Most proteins give a positive result in the Xanthoproteic reaction in which the suspected protein is heated with concentrated nitric acid. In the presence of protein the solution turns yellow and, on the addition of alkali, orange. Millon's reaction may be used to detect proteins which on hydrolysis yield tyrosine. The only common protein which does not give a positive result in this test is gelatin. The substance is warmed with Millon's reagent (which contains mercurous and mercuric nitrates in nitric acid) and if a protein is present a white precipitate turning red is obtained. The conventional laboratory method to measure the amount of protein is Lowry's method, which involves a dye, Coomassie blue, which develops in the presence of protein.

Gels and gelatin

Gels are remarkable colloidal systems in which large volumes of liquid are immobilized by small amounts of solid material, the liquid constituting the dispersion medium and the solid the disperse phase. Gels are of considerable importance in food preparation on account of the rigidity that such systems possess. For example, gels formed by polysaccharides, such as pectin gels in jam and starch gels in cooked starchy foods, have been discussed in Chapter 9. Proteins also form gels and the gel formed by gelatin is of particular importance in food preparation.

Gelatin is made from the protein collagen, which occurs widely in the skin, hair and bone of animals. The molecules of collagen are made up of three chains which are intertwined to form a triple helix and held in position by covalent crosslinks and other weaker links (see Fig. 10.6). When collagen is treated with hot water and acid or alkali all the weak crosslinks and, according to the harshness of the treatment, a proportion of the covalent crosslinks, are broken down. The resulting product, commercial gelatine, is soluble in water and contains a range of protein molecules and about 12 per cent water and 1 per cent mineral salts. It is produced both in granular form and in thin sheets, the former being the more common.

When cold water is added to gelatin it swells owing to the absorption of water. This is because the different protein molecules that constitute gelatin are in the form of zigzag polypeptide chains that are weakly linked together to form a three-dimensional network. Water becomes entangled and immobilized in this network in much the same way as water is held by a sponge. Additional water is bound to the gelatin by hydrogen bonding. If hydrated gelatin is heated with water above 35°C it liquefies and forms a sol. On cooling, the sol 'sets' and becomes solid, a process which is known as gelation. As little as 1 per cent gelatin is sufficient to produce such a gel. The gel formed is semi-rigid, although it loses its rigidity on heating or shaking; the solution thus formed is not coagulated by heat.

The setting powers of gelatin are utilized in the preparation of food. Commercial table jellies are made from syrups of glucose and sucrose. Gelatin is added to the hot syrup and, after it has dissolved, acid (usually citric), flavouring and colouring are added and the mixture is cooled until it sets. Gelatin is also responsible for the setting of stews and of broth prepared by boiling bones. If a gelatin sol is cooled until it is viscous but not firmly set, it can be beaten into a foam. A foam is most easily formed at the isoelectric point of gelatin (see Table 10.4), when the gelatin particles adhere to each other most strongly. During beating, air is incorporated into the mixture and because the gelatin at this stage has a certain elasticity it is able to stretch and surround the air bubbles without breaking. Whipped cream and flavouring may be added to such foams in making gelatin desserts.

Gelatin is also used as a stabilizing agent for emulsions, and its use in this connection was discussed with reference to ice cream on p. 60.

Protein quality

The quality of protein in food is usually judged by the number and amounts of essential amino acids it contains and the degree to which it is digested and absorbed by the body. Foods with the highest quality protein are those which provide all the essential amino acids in the proportions needed by humans (Table 10.5). This approach, based on 'goodness of fit', tends to assume a fixed need for each amino acid. In life, these needs do vary with growth, age, activity and health. Thus the need for specific amino acids varies, and there is of course a need for non-essential amino acids.

Table 10.5 Essential amino acid content of high-quality animal proteins (mg/g protein)

Amino acid	Eggs	Milk	Beef	Suggested pattern for adults[a]
Histidine	22	27	34	16
Isoleucine	54	47	48	13
Leucine	86	95	81	19
Lysine	70	78	89	16
Methionine and cysteine	57	33	40	17
Phenylalanine and tyrosine	93	102	80	19
Threonine	47	44	46	11
Tryptophan	17	14	12	9
Valine	66	64	50	5

[a]FAO/WHO report 1985, assuming a safe level of protein intake for adults of 0.7 g/kg body weight. Reprinted with permission.

Protein quality: biological evaluation

The biological value (BV) of a protein food is usually measured by feeding the protein under test to young rats as the only source of nitrogen and at a level below that required for maintaining nitrogen balance (see p. 145).

The biological value is calculated by measuring the nitrogen intake and the amounts of nitrogen lost in the urine and the faeces. The nitrogen lost in urine measures the nitrogen that has been absorbed and used by the body, while the nitrogen lost in the faeces measures the nitrogen that has not been absorbed.

$$BV = \frac{\text{Nitrogen intake} - (\text{Nitrogen lost in urine + faeces})}{\text{Nitrogen intake} - \text{Nitrogen lost in faeces}} \times 100$$

$$= \frac{\text{Retained nitrogen}}{\text{Absorbed nitrogen}} \times 100$$

The BV is defined as the percentage of absorbed protein that is retained in the body (i.e. that which is converted into body protein).

The BV value of a protein takes no account of the digestibility of the protein, and if this is taken into account we measure the net protein utilization (NPU). The NPU is defined as the percentage of protein eaten that is retained in the body.

$$NPU = \frac{\text{Retained nitrogen}}{\text{Nitrogen intake}} \times 100$$

$$= BV \times \text{digestibility}$$

As most proteins have a digestibility exceeding 90 per cent (see Table 10.8), BV and NPU values do not differ greatly, as is demonstrated by Table 10.6. As biological evaluation of protein quality is usually done on rats there is no guarantee that the results for BV and NPU values are accurate for humans. In practice, it is believed that the results are reasonably reliable, although they tend to underestimate protein quality for humans, especially adults. The NPU value of a good mixed diet is about 70.

Protein quality: chemical evaluation

The protein quality of a food can be evaluated in chemical terms by measuring its amino acid content and comparing it with that of a reference protein. Whole-egg protein is usually taken as the reference protein and given a score of 100. Chemical score values are found to match up fairly well with biological values, as shown in Table 10.6.

Limiting amino acids

An inspection of Table 10.5 shows that eggs, milk and beef provide high-quality proteins because they contain all the essential amino acids and in sufficient amounts to meet the needs of an adult. However, in other foods one or more amino acids may be present in amounts that are below human requirements. The amino acid which is furthest below the human requirement is known as the limiting amino acid. The limiting amino acid in a variety of foods is shown in Table 10.7.

Table 10.6 Protein quality of some foods comparing biological value (BV), net protein utilization (NPU) and chemical values

Food	BV	NPU	Chemical score
Whole egg	98	94	100
Milk	77	71	95
Soya flour	70	65	74
Wheat	49	48	53
Maize	36	31	49
Rice	67	63	67
Gelatin	0	0	0

Table 10.7 Limiting amino acids in animal and plant foods

Animal source	Limiting amino acid	Plant source	Limiting amino acid
Milk	None	Wheat	Lysine
Eggs	None	Maize	Tryptophan
Beef	None	Legumes	Methionine
Cheese	Methionine	Soya	Methionine
Gelatin	Tryptophan	Nuts	Methionine

Complementary proteins

The evaluation of protein quality in an individual food is of little practical value, given that we all eat mixtures of foods with a variety of protein profiles. Where the proteins provided by a particular food are relatively deficient in an essential amino acid, the disadvantage may be overcome simply by eating more of the protein in question. However, in some circumstances, such as in times of food shortage or with infants, this may not be possible.

Normal diets contain a mixture of proteins and the fact that any one protein is of high or low biological value is of no great significance. The important dietary requirement is that the total protein intake should supply all the essential amino acids in suitable proportions for our needs. Thus, although a certain protein may be of low quality because it lacks a particular amino acid, provided that it is eaten on the same day, or preferably as part of the same meal, as a second protein that lacks a different essential amino acid, the mixture is of high biological value. Such proteins are said to complement each other. This principle is illustrated by a mixture of gelatin and bread. The limiting amino acid of wheat is lysine, whereas that of gelatin is tryptophan. As gelatin is relatively rich in lysine the two complement each other. Examples of other complementary proteins are fish and rice and maize and beans, pasta and lentils or beans.

Provided that a diet contains a mixture of different proteins, it is unlikely to be deficient in any essential amino acid. Even vegetarian diets of underdeveloped countries, usually fulfil adult requirements for essential amino acids. It is only in the case of children, with their relatively greater need for specific amino acids at particular stages, that such diets lack sufficient essential amino acids. In absolute terms, the total protein requirement of infants is very low. Human milk provides only about 6 per cent of energy as protein, which is evidently adequate. The general conclusion reached is that provided diets contain a variety of protein sources the total mixture will have high biological value. Only where 70 per cent or more of dietary proteins comes from one staple food, which is very low in protein (such as cassava or plantains) need there be concern that protein quality will fall below an acceptable level.

Digestibility and assimilation of proteins: nitrogen balance

Digestibility of protein is usually measured as the assimilation or retention of nitrogen in the body.

Table 10.8 Relative digestibility of different foods

Food	Digestibility
Reference: egg, milk, cheese, meat, fish	*100*
Wheat, refined	*101*
Peanut butter	*100*
Peas, mature	*93*
Rice, polished	*93*
Oatmeal	*90*
Wheat, whole	*90*
Maize	*89*
Beans	*82*

Source: FAO/WHO, 1985. Reprinted with permission.

In a normal, weight-stable adult, there is a state of 'nitrogen balance'. What goes in equals what comes out (in urine and stools) because there is no capacity to store nitrogen and proteins. Negative nitrogen balance indicates inadequate intake to match losses, and only occurs during illness or weight loss unless the diet is extremely low in protein, using very bizarre foods. Positive nitrogen balance occurs during growth (including pregnancy) and recovery from illness. Nitrogen balance cannot be influenced by dietary intake except if the diet is truly deficient in protein and essential amino acids.

As most nitrogen leaves the body in urine, assessing nitrogen balance and protein digestibility depends heavily on having an accurate, complete urine collection. In practice, this is very difficult, so nitrogen losses are commonly underestimated (suggesting positive nitrogen balance).

The digestibility of specific amino acids or protein can be studied using isotope-labelled compounds. Radioactive isotopes are of course to be avoided in humans. As it is now believed that few diets provide insufficient amounts of essential amino acids, more attention needs to be given to digestibility, especially of diets in developing countries.

It is evident from Table 10.8 that while animal proteins are highly digestible, plant proteins may have a much lower rate of digestibility. This factor needs to be taken into account when considering protein requirements (see below). The digestibility of protein in foods or diets is related to their content of dietary fibre which increases excretion of nitrogen in faeces and hence reduces the apparent digestibility.

Protein requirement and DRVs

In considering how much protein should be supplied to the body in the diet, account must be taken of its nature; consequently, it is much more difficult to estimate the optimum dietary intake of protein than that of carbohydrate or fat. Whereas a certain amount of protein of high nutritional value may satisfy the body's protein requirements, a much larger amount of low-quality protein will be needed. It is, therefore, only possible to calculate the minimum protein intake necessary for health on the assumption that this amount of protein furnishes the body with the minimum of essential amino acids that it requires.

Protein requirement for an individual is defined as the lowest level of dietary protein intake that will balance the losses of nitrogen from the body in persons maintaining energy balance at modest levels of physical activity. In children and pregnant or lactating women, the protein requirement is taken to include the needs associated with the deposition of tissues or the secretion of milk at rates consistent with good health.

In practical terms, protein requirement is measured when a person is in neutral nitrogen balance (i.e. when the nitrogen intake from diet is equal to the nitrogen output in the urine, faeces and skin, see above). The requirement is simply the minimum amount of protein needed to maintain nitrogen balance. In seeking to measure such a protein requirement two reference points have been established, namely those of a young child and those of a young male adult. For other groups, estimates have been made based on the reference points. The dietary reference values for protein are given in Table 10.9 and are based on the values in the World Health Organization (WHO) report of 1985 which are derived from the amounts of high-quality egg or milk protein required for nitrogen equilibrium as measured in nitrogen balance studies.

Table 10.9 shows that the RNI for men aged 19–50 years is 55.5 g/day, and 45.0 g/day for women of the same age. On this basis, protein intake needs to provide less than 10 per cent of total dietary energy, which was the recommendation of earlier British Standards. Most people eat much more in practice. The most recent dietary survey indicates, that in practice, if the estimated average requirements of other energy-providing nutrients are met, protein

Table 10.9 Dietary reference values for protein

Age	Weight (kg)	Estimated average requirement (g/day)	Reference nutrient intake (g/day)
0–3 months	5.9	–	12.5
4–6 months	7.7	10.6	12.7
7–9 months	8.8	11.0	13.7
10–12 months	9.7	11.2	14.9
1–3 years	12.5	11.7	14.5
4–6 years	17.8	14.8	19.7
7–10 years	28.3	22.8	28.3
Males			
11–14 years	43.0	33.8	42.1
15–18 years	64.5	46.1	55.2
19–50 years	74.0	44.4	55.5
50+ years	71.0	42.6	53.3
Females			
11–14 years	43.8	33.1	41.2
15–18 years	55.5	37.1	45.4
19–50 years	60.0	36.0	45.0
50+ years	62.0	37.2	46.5
Pregnancy			+6
Lactation			
0–6 months			+11
6+ months			+8

The reference nutrient intake (RNI) values applicable to pregnant and lactating women are to be added to the adult requirement through all stages of pregnancy and lactation.
Henderson *et al.* (2003). Crown copyright material is reproduced with the permission of the Controller of HMSO and the Queen's Printer for Scotland.

provides about 17 per cent of the energy intake in the diet of the average British adult.

Human adaptability

Although a great deal of effort has gone into establishing minimum protein requirements, it is known that adults can adapt to a wide range of protein intake. The reason why humans can adapt so well to different intakes of protein depends upon the action of the liver, which has the ability to transform amino acids into urea, which can then be excreted from the body. When protein intake is high, the enzyme argininosuccinase is active and is responsible for the formation of urea with consequent loss of protein from the body in urine. When protein intake is low, enzymes responsible for using amino acids for protein synthesis are active, so that in these conditions little protein is lost from the body.

It is worth noting that the body's adaptability with regard to protein intake is in sharp contrast to its adaptability with regard to energy intake. In the latter instance, the energy requirement is exactly determined by energy expenditure. If the intake exceeds or falls below energy output the body is unable to adapt and responds by storing energy in the form of fat or wasting away, respectively.

The body does not contain stores of protein as such. All the body's protein is incorporated into its cells and functioning organs. If protein intake falls below the requirement for balance, or in starvation, or during illness with high protein breakdown and loss, the shortfall for essential organs must be made up by recycling proteins from less-critical tissues. Thus, commonly, the skin thins, hair stops growing and underused muscles waste rapidly during illness or starvation. These processes are under endocrine control and the process is reversed in the recovery phase. Extra dietary protein is not usually needed, since we normally eat more than the minimum needed in health. Furthermore, recent research suggests that we are able to reclaim some of the nitrogen excreted as amino acids into the bowel after protein metabolism, through the activity of colonic bacteria which can convert it back to amino acids. The idea that protein assimilation can be increased or that muscle growth can be increased by eating more protein (in health or disease) is erroneous.

High protein intake

Is a high intake of protein desirable or harmful? In attempting to answer this question the health of groups of people with both high and low levels of protein intake has been studied. The warriors of the Masai tribe of Central Africa, for example, appear to be healthy and of good physique and have a high-protein intake of up to 300 g/day. In contrast, many people in developing countries have a low protein intake of around 45 g/day, and provided that their diet is adequate in other respects, they too are healthy.

These findings confirm that the body can adapt to a wide range of protein intake values. However, there is some evidence that a high protein intake may be harmful and may contribute to demineralization of bone and to a deterioration of kidney function in patients with kidney disease. Consequently, the Committee on Medical Aspects of Food Policy (COMA) Panel on Dietary Reference Values (COMA, 1991) concludes that it is prudent for adults to avoid protein intakes of more than twice the RNI, i.e. 1.5 g protein per kilogram per day.

The notion that people with high energy needs, such as athletes, benefit from a high protein diet is without foundation. Protein intake for athletes, like that for the general public, should not exceed twice the RNI. They need more energy (calories) and that is best provided by more carbohydrates.

Paradoxically high-protein diets have been marketed for treating obesity. Excess protein is metabolised much like carbohydrate, but can blunt appetite and ultimately nauseate. For short-term

use they can be as good as high carbohydrate diets, but they are harder to tolerate, and expensive.

Protein in malnutrition

We have already established that adults rarely suffer from protein deficiency even when they have to subsist on poor diets consisting mainly of vegetables. However, protein deficiency does occur among children in underdeveloped countries. Alternatively, children in such countries may simply lack sufficient food; that is they may exist on diets that are lacking in both energy and protein (and other nutrients). Between these two extremes of lack of protein and lack of food lie a variety of diets which are lacking in varying combinations of protein and energy (and other nutrients). The whole range of such diets gives rise to what has become known as protein-energy malnutrition (PEM).

Protein-energy malnutrition constitutes the greatest health problem in underdeveloped countries today. In such countries, PEM is a major cause of death and as many as half the children do not reach the age of 5 years.

Protein deficiency in children presents as the disease known as kwashiorkor, which arises when, after a period of breast feeding, children are weaned onto a diet in which the staple food is either cassava or green bananas (matoke) and therefore low in protein. If total food supply dwindles, and particularly if there is infection such as gastroenteritis or measles, at this age the body swells with oedema because the main protein in the blood (albumin) is very low. Patches of pigmentation develop in both hair and skin; it also produces apathy and reduces immunity to other infections. It is also associated with other deficiency diseases such as pellagra caused by deficiency of niacin.

Lack of food in older children produces starvation, a condition which is known as marasmus. While it is caused by lack of food, it is also made worse by susceptibility to repeated infections caused by poor hygiene. Marasmus produces shrunken, dehydrated children with wasted muscles; it is often accompanied by diarrhoea. If blood protein falls, then oedema (kwashiorkor) can develop.

Protein-energy malnutrition is the result of poverty and ignorance. Tradition also plays a part, resulting in the father of a family being given any meat or other protein food which is available, the rest of the family having to make do with what other food remains.

Proteins in the body

Digestion

During digestion proteins are broken down into amino acids. Their degradation is brought about progressively by peptidases, as explained in Chapter 2. Peptidases are hydrolysing enzymes which operate by catalysing the hydrolysis of the peptide links in the protein molecule, so breaking down the protein into smaller units.

In the stomach, the gastric glands secrete pepsinogen which, at the low pH of the gastric juice, becomes activated forming the enzyme pepsin. The action of pepsin is extremely specific; it catalyses the hydrolysis of only those peptide links that are joined to particular groupings. Moreover, it is an endopeptidase and acts only on inner peptide links of polypeptide chains. Figure 10.8 shows part

of a protein molecule, and the only point at which pepsin could act is indicated. As a result of the action of pepsin, proteins are broken down into smaller peptone units. The enzyme rennin is also present in the gastric juice and brings about the coagulation of the casein of milk.

In the small intestine, endopeptidases such as trypsin and chymotrypsin continue the hydrolysis of proteins and complete their breakdown into peptones. The action of these enzymes is just as specific as that of pepsin, each enzyme attacking only a certain type of link. The points at which they could attack a typical protein fragment are illustrated in Fig. 10.8. Peptones are further broken down by a group of exopeptidases, called erepsin, which are present in the intestinal juice. These enzymes catalyse the hydrolysis of peptones into dipeptides which are broken down into amino acids by a series of dipeptidases. Proteins are thus completely hydrolysed to amino acids before passing from the small intestine into the blood. The amino acids are, however, rapidly removed from the blood by all the cells of the body, but particularly by the liver.

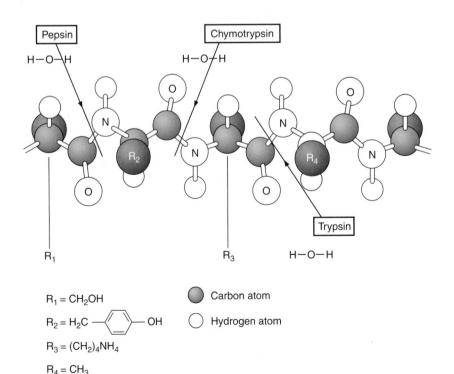

Figure 10.8 *Hydrolysis of a protein fragment*

Enzymes

The supreme importance of enzymes in the body and their protein nature have already been emphasized in Chapter 2. Now that the structure of proteins has been considered, it is possible to gain a clearer insight into the nature and mechanism of enzyme activity. It must be admitted, however, that despite the success of current research we still have a great deal to learn about the way enzymes act, although this is hardly surprising considering the complexity of tertiary (three-dimensional) protein structure. Moreover, the results of recent research show that few generalizations may be made in this field and that each enzyme needs to be investigated individually.

Enzymes are globular proteins which, as we have already seen, are the most complex proteins known and consist of folded α-helix chains, the method of folding being irregular and dependent on the nature of the crosslinks formed between adjacent helical coils. Such structures are very sensitive to both chemical and physical conditions on account of the ease with which the crosslinks are broken. This explains why enzymes are so sensitive to changes of temperature and pH. Moreover, the zwitterion structure of enzymes enables them to resist changes of pH in living systems by acting as buffers.

The lock and key theory of enzyme action was outlined in Chapter 2 and this theory has the merit of extreme simplicity. Modern developments have confirmed the essential correctness of this theory but have shown that the details are a good deal more complicated. It appears that the lock should be regarded as being flexible and that a substrate must not only fit the enzyme lock exactly, but that it must also induce a change in the enzyme structure, thus causing a reorientation of the enzyme groups involved in catalysis. Thus, the specificity of an enzyme is due not only to a good fit between lock and key, but also to the ability of the key to bring about certain structural changes in the lock.

The structures of the enzymes lysozyme, ribonuclease and carboxypeptidase are known and show that these molecules are folded in such a way as to contain a jaw-like groove into which substrate molecules fit. In the case of carboxypeptidase it has further been shown that the substrate protein brings about structural changes in the enzyme molecule which are essential to its catalytic activity. Not all enzyme molecules possess jaw-like grooves, however, and in such cases (e.g. chymotrypsin) some other mechanism must operate.

As already mentioned in Chapter 2, certain substances promote enzyme activity and three main types have been identified, namely coenzymes, cofactors (or activators) and prosthetic groups. Coenzymes are large organic molecules such as several members of the B-group of vitamins. The coenzyme is not firmly bound to the enzyme, but may become attached to it during enzyme activity only to be released later so that, like the enzyme itself, it may be reused.

Cofactors are usually ions, either metallic or nonmetallic, which become temporarily attached to an enzyme during enzyme activity but which are later released. The action of chloride ions as a cofactor for the enzyme salivary amylase has already been mentioned (p. 16).

Prosthetic groups are non-protein groups which are permanently bound to enzymes to form conjugated proteins (see Table 10.3). The enzyme catalase present in vegetables (see p. 279) is an example in which the prosthetic group contains a ferrous ion known as haem. The haem group is the key functional element of haemoglobin, the red-coloured protein in blood whose main function is to transport oxygen safely around the body.

Metabolism

The present picture of protein metabolism is quite different from earlier theories which assumed that the proteins of living tissues were stable and only required replacement after a long period of service. It is now known that far from being stable, body proteins are in a constant state of flux and are continually being degraded and resynthesized in a manner similar to fat molecules. On one hand there are the complete body proteins, and on the other a reservoir of amino acids derived partly from food and partly from degraded body proteins. During life the proteins and amino acids are in dynamic equilibrium with each other and there are also episodic demands for specific protein produced (e.g. fibrinogen from the liver during illness or injury). Fibrinogen is very rich in the amino acid glycine, and its increased production can have short-term knock-on effects for protein turnover elsewhere. Such an equilibrium involves the continual hydrolysis of the peptide links of protein molecules and the continual resynthesis of proteins from amino acids.

The synthesis of proteins takes place throughout all the cells and tissues of the body. The amino acids that are required for this synthesis are taken from the liver, both essential and non-essential amino acids being involved. If non-essential amino acids are not available from the pool of amino acids in the liver they may be made in body cells by a process of transamination in which an amino group is transferred to a substance that does not contain nitrogen, thereby converting it into an amino acid. This process is controlled by enzymes known as transaminases and by the coenzyme pyridoxal-5-phosphate (PLP) derived from vitamin B_6. Such syntheses are extremely rapid, the amino acids being correctly assembled into proteins through the action of DNA and RNA.

removed from the amino acid as ammonia. The ammonia formed in deamination is poisonous and is rapidly converted into urea, which is then excreted by the kidneys in urine. Some is excreted into the bowel, where it is utilized by colonic bacteria.

Deamination, which requires the presence of the B vitamins nicotinic acid and riboflavin in the form of dinucleotides, results in the formation of an organic acid which may be either glucogenic or ketogenic. Glucogenic acids are broken down into glucose while ketogenic acids are converted into fatty acids. Both these substances may be broken down to produce energy, as described previously, illustrating how carbohydrates, fats and deaminated amino acids all follow closely related metabolic pathways. If energy is not required by the body the non-nitrogenous residues of deamination are converted into fat.

Protein as a source of energy

Although the primary specific function of food proteins is the provision of amino acids for the production and maintenance of body proteins (including enzymes), they are ultimately broken down to urea with the liberation of energy. The secondary role of proteins is, therefore, as a supplementary energy source. In practice, in a stable adult all dietary protein is ultimately metabolized to produce energy, and it functions very like carbohydrates in this way.

The first step in the breakdown of amino acids is normally deamination, in which the amino group is

Key points

- Proteins (structural and enzymes) are made from a chain of amino acids, which contain nitrogen
- Protein in foods are hydrolysed to amino acids in the process of enzymatic digestion in the gut
- All human adult proteins can be made from eight 'essential' amino acids, required from the diet. In infancy and illness others may be required. They are supplied by foods of animal origin or by combinations of cereal and legume foods

Chapter summary

Proteins occur in all cells, so virtually all foods. They provide function in metabolism, change and movement. In foods, the huge variety of proteins contribute to structure, consistency and taste and to the consequences of cooking. Enzymes in raw foods may promote decay which causes spoiling.

FURTHER READING

CHARLEY H, WEAVER C (1998). *Foods: a Scientific Approach*. 3rd edn. Merill: Prentice Hall.

COMA (1991). Report on dietary reference values. www.nutrition-matters.co.uk/misc/1991 COMAreport.htm

DEPARTMENT OF HEALTH (1991). *Dietary Reference Values for Food Energy and Nutrients for the United Kingdom*. London: HMSO.

FAO (1990). *Report of the Joint FAO/WHO Expert Consultation on Protein Quality Evaluation*. Rome: FAO.

HENDERSON L, GREGORY J, IRVING K, (2003). *The National Diet and Nutrition Survey: Adults Aged 19 to 64 Years, Energy, Protein, Carbohydrate, Fat and Alcohol Intake*, Volume 2. London: The Stationery Office.

WHO (1985). Energy and protein requirements. Report of a joint FAO/WHO/UNU expert consultation, technical report series no. 724. Geneva: WHO.

11

Protein-rich foods

There is no such thing as a pure protein food (i.e. one which contains 100 per cent protein). As can be appreciated from Table 11.1, even those foods that are highest in protein do not contain more than 45 per cent by weight, and even this value is exceptionally high. Because these foods vary widely in water content and in portion size the nutritional values are rather different. So some 'protein-rich' foods contribute little to nutrition.

The normal requirement for dietary protein is about 8 per cent of dietary energy, assuming a normal variety of foods which provide a balance of essential amino acids. Human breast milk contains only about 6 per cent energy as protein, but with a perfect amino acid profile that exactly matches the metabolic demand for growth and maintenance of a healthy, growing baby. Most nutritionally adequate diets provide 10–15 per cent of the energy in the form of protein and this allows for some redundancy if the 'goodness of fit' of amino acid profile is not perfect. Thus, Table 11.2 makes it easy to assess whether foods are poor, adequate or good as protein sources in relation to their energy content.

Some foods which are valuable as sources of protein, such as milk and cheese, have already been considered in Chapter 7. In this chapter other foods particularly valued as sources of protein, namely meat, fish, soya and eggs, will be described.

MEAT

Lean meat is the flesh or muscular tissue of animals. Its composition is different from that of the internal organs, such as kidneys and liver, which are referred to collectively as offal. The composition of flesh of different animals shows considerable variation and the composition of even a single type of meat, such as beef, varies according to breed, type of feeding and the part of the animal from which the meat has come.

Muscle tissue consists of about three-quarters water and one-quarter protein together with a variable amount of fat, 1 per cent mineral elements and some vitamins. It is the variation in fat content which is the main factor in nutritional difference in different meats. Structurally, the tissue is composed of microscopic fibres, each of which is made up of cells. The main constituent of the cells is water in which the proteins and other nutrients are either dissolved or suspended. Numbers of fibres are held together by connective tissues to form a bundle. A quantity of such bundles is enveloped by a tough sheath of connective tissue which forms a tendon joining the muscle to the bone structure (Fig. 11.1).

The cells of the muscle fibres contain a number of proteins, the most important being myosin (7 per cent) and actin (2.5 per cent). Myosin is a relatively large elastic protein which can exist in

Table 11.1 The protein content of some animal and plant foods

	Protein (%)	Average portion (g)	Protein per average portion (g)
Animal foods			
Cheese, Cheddar	25	40	10
Bacon, lean	20	46	14
Beef, lean	20	140	44
Cod	17	120	26
Herring	17	119	24
Eggs	12	50	6
Beef, fat	8	50	8
Milk	3	100	3
Cheese, cream	3	30	1
Butter	<1	10	0
Plant foods			
Soya flour, low fat	45	30	14
Soya flour, full fat	37	30	11
Peanuts	24	13	3
Bread, wholemeal	9	36	3
Bread, white	8	36	3
Lentils (cooked)	8	40	3
Rice	7	180	5
Peas, fresh	6	70	5
Baked beans	5	135	6
Potatoes, old	2	175	3
Sweet potato (cooked)	1	130	1
Cabbage (cooked)	1	95	1
Bananas	1	100	1
Apples	<1	100	1
Cassava (cooked)	<1	100	1

Table 11.2 Protein content of foods expressed in terms of their contribution to the energy provided by each food

Value of food as protein source	Per cent of total energy from protein
Poor	
Cassava	3
Sweet potatoes, plantains	4
Adequate	
Potatoes	8
Rice	8
Wheat flour	13
Good	
Peanuts	19
Milk	22
Lentils	31
Beans and peas	26
Beef, lean	38
Soya beans	45
Eggs	33
Cabbage	50
Chicken	67

stretched and unstretched forms and which is classified as a fibrous protein (Table 10.2, p. 138). Actin has two forms; a small globular form of molecular weight about 70 000 and a fibrous form in which a series of globular units are arranged in a double chain. The cells also contain ATP (adenosine triphosphate) which, as we saw in Chapter 8, provides the energy used when muscle fibres contract. After death, ATP is broken down and in its absence myosin and actin combine to form rigid chains of actomyosin. In this state, known as rigor mortis, meat is rigid and tough and it is therefore not consumed until, after a period of storage known as conditioning, the stiffness has diminished and tenderness and flavour have improved.

The changes that occur during conditioning are complex, as might be expected from the protein nature of meat; moreover, they are affected by a number of variables of which temperature, pH and length of storage are all important. Although the

(a)

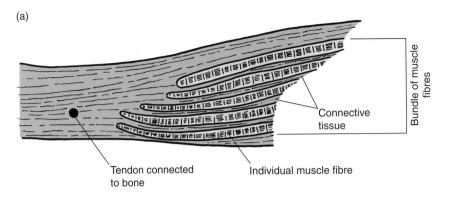

Bundle of muscle fibres

Connective tissue

Tendon connected to bone

Individual muscle fibre

(b)

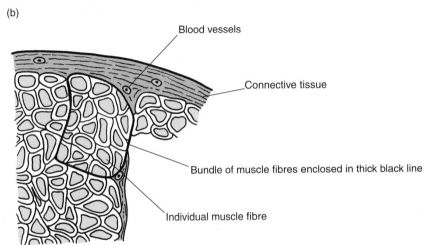

Blood vessels

Connective tissue

Bundle of muscle fibres enclosed in thick black line

Individual muscle fibre

Figure 11.1 *Meat. Diagrams of muscle showing fibres and connective tissue: (a) longitudinal section; (b) transverse section*

changes that constitute conditioning are complicated and still not completely understood it is a very important process resulting in the conversion of the muscular tissue of animals into the 'meat' of our diet.

After an animal's death the glycogen present in its muscular tissue is broken down by stages to lactic acid with a consequent fall in pH. The final pH is usually about 5.5, which is close to the isoelectric point of the main muscle proteins (the isoelectric point of myosin is 5.4). As we have already noted, proteins are least stable and most readily denatured at the isoelectric point, and during conditioning proteins of muscular tissue are denatured, although the proteins of connective tissue are not. Denaturation is followed by some breakdown of denatured proteins resulting in the formation of peptides and amino acids and an increase in tenderness. A further important change results from the fact that the solubility of proteins is a minimum at the isoelectric

point and hence during conditioning some water is lost from meat.

During conditioning the colour of meat changes from reddish to brown and this is associated with the conversion of the main muscle pigment myoglobin into metmyoglobin. The myoglobin molecule consists of a protein part, consisting of folded chains of α-helices, as shown in Fig. 10.7, together with a non-protein coloured haem group containing an iron atom in the ferrous state. During conditioning myoglobin is denatured and oxidized, ferrous iron being converted into ferric iron, and the resulting metmyoglobin is brown in colour.

The connective tissue of meat which surrounds the bundles of muscle fibres is mainly collagen, while the walls of the muscle fibres are mainly elastin. Both these proteins are classified as fibrous proteins (see Table 10.2), collagen containing inelastic polypeptide chains joined by cross-links and elastin having an unstretched α-helix form. Collagen and elastin, being

Table 11.3 Percentage of different types of fatty acids in meat and poultry fat

	Saturated	Monounsaturated	Polyunsaturated
Beef	44	50	4
Lamb	52	40	5
Pork	43	47	8
Chicken	35	48	16

Table 11.4 Composition of 100 g edible portions (raw weight) of meat and poultry

	Beef		Lamb		Pork		
	Lean	Fat	Lean	Fat	Lean	Fat	Chicken
Energy (kJ)	517	2625	679	2762	512	2259	508
Protein (g)	20.0	9	21.0	6	22.0	10.00	21.0
Fat (g)	5.0	67	9.0	72	4.0	56.00	4.0
Calcium (mg)	7.0	10	7.0	7	7.0	9.00	10.0
Iron (mg)	2.0	1	2.0	1	1.0	0.40	1.0
Niacin (mg)	5.0	–	6.0	–	7.0	2.00	8.0
Riboflavin (mg)	0.2	–	0.3	–	0.3	0.13	0.2

Dash indicates values that are difficult to obtain; small amounts may be present.

insoluble and tough, are difficult to digest. However, when meat is cooked in the presence of moisture the collagen is converted into gelatin, which is soluble in water. This makes the digestion of connective tissue much easier, and enables the digestive juices to come into intimate contact with the myosin of the muscle fibres. The greater the age of the animal and the more active its life, the greater is the amount of connective tissue and the thickness of the walls of the fibres. Thus, meat of old animals is more difficult to digest than that of young ones and muscular tissue of active animals is more difficult to digest than that of inactive ones.

Embedded in the connective tissue is a variable amount of invisible fat. There is also a much larger amount of visible fat which is stored in the fat depots of the animal's body. Such fat is mainly found under the skin, interleaved between bunches of muscle fibres and around internal organs; it is not a part of lean meat but is apparent in the marbling of fatty meat as well as lying between muscle and skin.

The fat of meat is of some nutritional interest because it is predominantly saturated in character, as is evident from Table 11.3. Chicken fat is notable in having a greater proportion of polyunsaturated fatty acid (PUFA) than other types of meat fat. Reflecting awareness of the role of saturated fat in cardiovascular disease, and also in obesity, consumers are increasingly showing a preference for lean meat and for types of meat or meat products low in saturated fatty acids and high in PUFA. Although red meats contain higher amounts of fat than other protein-rich foods, moderate amounts of quality meat can be eaten even in slimming diets. The real menace is high-fat processed meat products.

Apart from protein and fat, meat contains small quantities of mineral elements and vitamins, but is notable for its lack of carbohydrate, in which respect it resembles eggs. Meat is a good source of iron in the most available form (haem), although the amount present is small except in certain organs, such as kidney and liver, which are relatively rich sources. Meat is a good source of zinc, but a poor source of calcium. Meat is a useful source of the B group of vitamins, notably niacin. The amount of thiamin in meat is not large except in the case of pork, which contains about 0.6 mg/100 g of meat. Riboflavin occurs in useful quantities, especially in internal organs such as the kidneys. Lean meat contains very little vitamin A, and practically no vitamin D or ascorbic acid. Table 11.4 summarizes the differences in nutrient content between beef, lamb, pork and chicken and highlights the considerable differences in the nutrient content of lean and fat meat.

The flavour of meat is one of its main attractions and is partly due to the presence of a variety of substances known as meat extractives that are soluble in water. These include some produced during muscular activity in the living animal, such as lactic acid and some derived from ATP, and substances that are the result of protein metabolism, such as amino acids (e.g. glutamic acid) and urea. Meat extractives aid digestion by stimulating the secretion of saliva and gastric juice. The fat content of meat also contributes to its flavour, texture and mouth-feel.

Although much is known about the flavour of meat it is a complex matter and is incompletely understood.

Cooking of meat

The main reasons for cooking meat are as follows:

1. To improve its texture by making it tender and digestible.
2. To improve its flavour, especially by the development and retention of extractives.
3. To improve its colour by making it more pleasing to the eye and palate.
4. To improve its safety by destroying bacteria.

Tenderness

As already mentioned, tenderness of meat depends on the age of the animal, the amount of activity in its life and correct conditioning after slaughter. Muscle tissue which has been involved in much activity develops longer and thicker muscle fibres and more connective tissue to hold them together than tissue that has been rarely used. This explains why, in the same animal, the neck and the leg will always be tougher than fillet or rump.

In addition to improving the tenderness of meat by cooking, it can be made more tender in a number of other ways.

The most effective way of tenderizing meat is to inject an animal with a proteolytic enzyme before slaughter. This reduces the time required for conditioning by 1–2 days. Care must be taken not to over-tenderize the meat or an unpleasant flavour and mushy texture are produced. Proteolytic enzymes may also be added to meat after slaughter to help break down muscle fibre and connective tissue. Juice from the papaya fruit, for example, contains the proteolytic enzyme papain, and may be added to meat before cooking. Its enzyme activity is most effective at low cooking temperatures. The enzymes bromelin, obtained from pineapples and ficin, obtained from figs, may also be used to tenderize meat.

Meat, particularly in the form of thin sections such as steaks, can be made more tender by mechanical breakdown of muscle fibre and connective tissue brought about by pounding with a heavy object such as a mallet.

If salt is added to meat it increases the capacity of meat proteins to hold water when the meat is cooked and this promotes tenderness. A nutritionally preferable approach is to seal the meat with initial high-temperature frying, while the interior cooks less and more gradually.

Meat may be marinated, that is, soaked in an acid solution of wine, vinegar and spices for several days before cooking. The meat may then be cooked in the marinade to improve flavour and tenderness.

Hanging allows the action of endogenous and bacterial enzymes to increase tenderness and impart a rich flavour.

Chemical and physical changes

The tenderness of meat considered in the previous section can be further improved by cooking and, as we have already mentioned, this is one of the principal reasons for cooking meat. Cooking improves tenderness by increasing the denaturing of muscle protein initiated during conditioning and by converting collagen to gelatin, this latter process being assisted by water.

Cooking brings about chemical changes including the breakdown of nucleoproteins and similar substances which result in producing the desirable flavour of cooked meat. Cooking also changes the colour of meat. A cut meat surface is bright red in colour because the reddish-coloured myoglobin is oxidized in air to oxymyoglobin. When meat is allowed to stand, myoglobin is converted into brown-coloured metmyoglobin. Cooking produces an attractive brown coloration, partly owing to metmyoglobin and also to non-enzymic browning.

Cooking also produces a number of structural and physical changes in meat. Protein is coagulated and this reduces its hydration, resulting in water, together with water-soluble substances dissolved in the water, being lost from the meat. The consequence of this loss of water is that meat shrinks during cooking. Fat is melted during cooking and if very high temperatures are used some fat may become charred.

The way in which tenderness, flavour and colour are affected by cooking, and the way in which individual nutrients are affected, depends upon whether dry or moist heat methods of cooking are employed; also on the cooking time and the quality of the meat being cooked.

Dry heat methods

Dry heat methods of cooking meat include roasting and grilling. As the temperature rises to 60°C some proteins start to coagulate. If the temperature remains low, coagulation is slow and the protein will be in its most digestible form. Conversely, if high temperatures are used, coagulation is more complete and the protein becomes harder and tougher. Heat alone does not increase tenderness very much because, apart from coagulation, the tough elastin remains unchanged and conversion of collagen into soluble form is slow. Thus, dry heating methods are best used for cooking meat that contains little connective tissue.

At high temperatures some protein may be rendered unavailable by reaction with carbohydrate (non-enzymic browning), as described in Chapter 16. One of the amino acids liable to be rendered unavailable in non-enzymic browning is lysine and the loss of this amino acid, which occurs during the cooking of meat, has been studied under a variety of conditions. For example, it has been found that beef cooked for 3 hours loses one-fifth of its lysine at a cooking temperature of 120°C, but that when the temperature is raised by 40°C, the amount lost increases to one-half.

At a temperature a little above 60°C meat starts to shrink because of the contraction of the proteins of the connective tissue. Shrinkage results in some of the 'juice' in the meat being squeezed out, and the higher the cooking temperature the greater is the shrinkage and loss of juice. In roasting, for example, shrinkage causes the weight of meat to decrease by about one-third. The juice is mainly water but it also contains mineral salts, extractives and small amounts of water-soluble vitamins.

During roasting in open containers, water reaching the surface of the meat rapidly evaporates, leaving behind the non-volatile material. This causes the brown outer layer of the meat to have a good flavour but also to be dry. Occasional basting of the meat with hot fat can prevent dryness. In closed containers and at lower temperatures the rate of evaporation is much slower and the juice drips from the surface of the meat, so reducing its flavour. However, where such methods are used the juice is usually collected and eaten with the meat as gravy.

Fat near the surface of the meat melts during cooking and most of it passes into the cooking vessel, although a small portion of melted fat penetrates the lean meat. The greater the cooking temperature the greater is the loss into the cooking vessel and if too high a temperature is used some meat may become charred as in barbecuing.

Some B vitamins are lost when meat is heated. On average about 20 per cent of B vitamins are lost when meat is roasted, fried or grilled.

Moist heat methods

Moist heat methods of cooking meat include boiling, stewing, simmering and braising. The particular advantage of these methods relates to the relatively low temperature of the cooking medium. In stewing and simmering (and particularly when using slow cookers) the conduction of heat through the muscle tissue to the centre of the meat is a slow process and thus the denaturation of protein to the toughening and shrinking stage is delayed and tenderness is at a maximum.

Tenderness is also improved by the action of water and heat because these bring about the conversion of collagen to soluble gelatin, so allowing the muscle fibres to separate from each other. The other protein of connective tissues, elastin, remains unchanged, so that parts of an animal containing a high proportion of this protein, such as the neck, never become tender no matter how long cooking is prolonged.

Moist heat methods of cooking involve inevitable loss of water-soluble substances by leaching into the water used for cooking. In such methods the surface of the meat is in contact with the cooking water.

Table 11.5 The legal minimum meat content of meat products

Food	Meat (%)	Comment
Sausages		
Pork	*42*	
Other	*30–32*	
Burgers	*62–67*	
Economy burger	*41–50*	*Percentage depends on type of meat used*
Hamburgers	*67*	*Pig meat only*
Luncheon meat	*67*	
Corned beef	*120[a]*	*Must contain only corned beef*
Chopped meat	*70–75*	
Meat pie, pudding	*12.5*	*Refers to total weight of pie before cooking*
Scotch pies	*10*	*Refers to total weight of pie before cooking*
Sausage rolls, pasties	*6*	*Refers to uncooked products*

[a]On a fresh weight basis as it loses water during processing.

When protein shrinks, juice is forced to the surface of the meat and soluble matter dissolves in the water. Thus, mineral salts, extractives and thiamin are lost from the meat, which in consequence has less flavour and less nutritional value than if it had been cooked by a dry heat method. However, as such meat is normally eaten with the liquor in which it has been cooked this is not important from a nutritional point of view.

Meat products

A number of meat products are made by processing those parts of an animal that cannot be sold as carcass meat. Such parts include meat scraps recovered mechanically after most lean meat has been removed by hand, and offal. Now that carcases are carefully trimmed of visible fat, to attract health-conscious customers, a lot of fat is sold in unvisible form in cheap (and even expensive) processed meat products. Most processed meat products are made from minced or ground meat which may be compacted or moulded and to which other ingredients, such as fillers, fat, preservatives and other additives including salt and monosodium glutamate (MSG) may be added. However, a recent European Union (EU) directive has changed the definition of meat such that it no longer includes this mechanically recovered meat or parts such as skin or gristle or any parts of the animal that are not skeletal muscle.

The main types of processed meat products are sausages, which may be fresh, cooked or dry and other meat products such as burgers, pies, pasties, rolls and balls. The composition in terms of meat content is now controlled by the EU directive and defined in the Meat Products Regulations (2003 in England, 2004 in Scotland and Northern Ireland). Table 11.5 gives the minimum legal requirement of lean meat for a number of such products, the importance of which is growing with the increase in 'fast food' catering.

The legislation of meat products has come under close scrutiny recently, both for reasons of nutrition and food safety.

Sausages

Fresh sausages are made from some raw meat, large amounts of fat, a filler (rusk, bread, flour), water and seasoning. The mixture is filled into a casing and the product must be cooked, usually by frying or grilling, before it is eaten. Cooked sausages use similar ingredients to fresh sausages except that the fillers (binders) used may be corn flour (liver sausage), rice flour (polony) or oatmeal (black pudding). Additional ingredients give a special character to certain products such as black pudding, in which fresh pigs' blood (defibrinated to prevent clotting) is a main ingredient. These products are cooked before sale though some, such as black pudding and frankfurters, are heated through before eating.

Dried sausages are similar to the fresh variety, except that the meat is cured either before processing or early in the process, and they are dried under controlled conditions. German salami is a typical example of a dried sausage. It is made from lean beef and pork with pork fat which are finely minced, cured, mixed with garlic and other seasoning, moistened with Rhine wine, dried in air for 2 weeks and cold smoked.

French charcuterie includes many traditional varieties of diced sausages. They are very high in fat but eaten in small amounts so without detriment to health.

Other types

Many other different types of meat product are made, some being produced from meat trimmings left over from carcass meat (e.g. burgers), while others are made from offal (e.g. brawn, haggis). Beefburgers, the staple item of so many fast food outlets, are made from minced beef trimmings, pork fat, cooked chopped onions, breadcrumbs (or rusks) and seasoning. They are moulded into shape and fried or grilled before serving. Haggis, the source of innumerable jokes, is made from sheep's lungs, liver, heart and spleen coarsely chopped and mixed with oatmeal, suet stock, spices and seasoning, which are put into a sheep's stomach (or nowadays a synthetic equivalent) before being boiled and eaten with neeps and tatties (mashed swedes and potatoes).

Many processed meat products are prone to spoil and should therefore be stored with care after manufacture. They have been the cause of many cases of food poisoning and, for this reason, they may be preserved using a permitted preservative. Sausages and burgers, for example, may be preserved with sulphite (but it destroys the vitamin thiamin) and cured and pickled meats with nitrite.

FISH

The flesh of fish is composed of bundles of short fibres called myomeres, which are held together by thin layers of connective tissue composed of collagen. Thus, the protein of fish differs from that of meat in having less connective tissue and no elastin. The absence of tough elastin, and the conversion of collagen into gelatin which occurs during cooking, make the protein of cooked fish easily digestible. Fish contains rather more water than meat.

Fish may be divided into two classes: white fish, such as haddock, cod, whiting and plaice, which contain very little fat (usually less than 2 per cent), and 'oil-rich' or 'fatty' fish such as herring, trout and salmon, which usually contain 10–25 per cent fat.

The flesh of most white fish contains no fat, as fat in these fish is concentrated in the liver, which is often removed and used as a source of vitamins (e.g. cod-liver oil). A few white fish (e.g. halibut) contain small amounts of 'invisible fat' dispersed in the flesh. Fatty fish contain a considerable amount of invisible fat which is of particular interest because it is rich in n−3 PUFA. The actual amount varies, being highest just before spawning.

The fat content of farmed fish (trout, salmon, sea bass, etc.) is often much higher than in wild fish, and its fatty acid profile lower in n−3 PUFAs. Fish are of value mainly as a rich source of protein, the amount and quality of protein in fish being similar to that in lean meat (Table 11.6). Fish contain no carbohydrate but are a good source of phosphorus, though not of calcium unless the bones are eaten. They are not usually a good source of iron, although sardines are an exception. Sea fish are a valuable source of iodine. Fatty fish are valuable sources of the fat-soluble vitamins A and D, fish-liver oils being exceptionally good sources of these vitamins. They also contain useful amounts of the B group of vitamins. White fish do not contain useful amounts of vitamins A and D, and usually contain less of the B vitamins than oil-rich fish.

Unlike meat, fish deteriorate rapidly after death because the lack of connective tissue makes the muscle protein more vulnerable to spoilage. Such rapid deterioration and the fact that fish are often caught far from land, has led to most fish being salted or frozen at sea immediately after they have been caught. Consumption of fresh fish has rapidly declined in recent years in Britain, while consumption of frozen fish and frozen fish products, such as fish fingers, has increased. In nutritional terms, frozen is as good as fresh.

The varieties of fish consumed have also changed in recent years. In the UK, cod, together with haddock, halibut and plaice, have traditionally been the most popular fish. However, restricted fishing in the areas where these fish are found has led to their replacement by others, such as mackerel, coley and whiting.

Table 11.6 Nutrient composition of 100 g fish (raw weight)

	Cod	Haddock	Plaice	Herring	Mackerel	Salmon
Energy value (kJ)	337	345	336	791	914	750
Protein (g)	18.3	19.0	16.7	17.8	18.7	20.2
% Energy from protein	92.3	93.6	84.5	38.3	34.8	45.8
Total fat (g)	0.7	0.6	1.4	13.2[a]	16.1[a]	11.0
% Energy from fat	7.7	6.4	15.4	61.7	65.2	54.3
PUFA (g)	0.4	0.3	0.3	2.7	3.3	3.1
Calcium (mg)	9	14	45	60	11	21
Iron (mg)	0.1	0.1	0.3	1.2	0.8	0.4
Vitamin A (µg)	2	0	0	45[b]	45[b]	13
Thiamin (µg)	0.04	0.04	0.2	0.01	0.14	0.23
Vitamin D (µg)	0	0	0	19.0	8.2	5.9

PUFA, polyunsaturated fatty acid.
[a]Value varies through the year being highest in July–October.
[b]Expressed as retinol equivalents.

Fish farming is also a developing industry, both salmon and rainbow trout being produced inland, sea bass and halibut in seawater, in this way in Britain.

Cooking of fish

When fish is cooked, the changes that take place are similar to those that occur during the cooking of meat. As there is less connective tissue in fish than in meat, and no elastin, cooking is not required to make the fish tender but only to render it as palatable and digestible as possible. Raw fish is eaten widely throughout the world – best very fresh and sliced thin. Fish should be cooked as little and as gently as possible as fish proteins coagulate quickly and easily. If fish is overcooked the flesh becomes rubbery and dry.

There are less extractives in fish than in meat, and fish should therefore be cooked in such a way that as much flavour as possible is preserved. During cooking, proteins coagulate, collagen is converted into gelatin and some shrinkage occurs. Shrinkage, however, is less than with meat because of the smaller amount of connective tissue. Shrinkage causes water and soluble matter to be squeezed out of the fish and in moist heat methods of cooking, water, extractives and soluble mineral salts are lost. In boiling, for example, over one-third of the extractives and soluble salts are lost, so that fish cooked in this way is rather tasteless. Dry heat cooking, on the other hand, causes rapid evaporation of water from the surface of the fish

while the non-volatile soluble matter remains behind. Thus, fish cooked in this way has much more flavour than fish which has been boiled or steamed. Fatty fish, such as herring or trout, are best cooked by a dry heat method such as grilling or baking since their high fat content keeps them moist.

Both white and fatty fish may be cooked by frying, and this is particularly effective if the fish are coated in batter before frying because the batter helps to retain the structure of the flesh, even if relatively long cooking times are used. Heavily battered fish in British fish and chip shops is grossly overcooked, necessitating the heavy batter which absorbs large amounts of old cooking fat. Less cooking and much less batter would improve flavour and health consequently.

Microwave cooking is particularly suited to fish and minimizes cooking smells. Microwave cooking fish is a quick and simple cooking method, although seasoning is essential to enhance the flavour. It is also important to adhere to the recommended standing time, usually about 2–3 minutes, to allow the fish to cook through as foods will keep cooking after the microwave is off.

Fish products

Apart from being preserved by freezing, canning and smoking, fish is also converted into a number of convenience products, such as fish fingers, fish cakes

Table 11.7 The fish content of fish products

Food	Fish content (%)
Fish cakes	35
Fish pastes and spreads	70
Potted fish	95
Potted fish and butter	96 (fish and butter)
Fish paste with one other main ingredient	80

Table 11.8 The nutrient content of eggs per 100 g

Nutrient	Nutrient content per 100 g
Energy (kJ)	612
Protein (g)	12.3
Fat, total (g)	10.9
Fat, saturated (g)	3.4
Fat, polyunsaturated (g)	1.2
Carbohydrate (g)	0
Water (g)	75
Cholesterol (mg)	450
Calcium (mg)	52
Iron (mg)	2
Sodium (mg)	140
Vitamin A (μg)	140
Thiamin (mg)	0.09
Riboflavin (mg)	0.47
Niacin (mg)	3.68
Vitamin C (mg)	0
Vitamin D (μg)	1.75
Vitamin E (mg)	1.6

and fish spreads. Fish fingers, for example, are made from blocks of frozen filleted white fish which are cut into fingers, dipped into a batter and breadcrumbs and refrozen.

The fish content of some typical fish products is shown in Table 11.7. Fish fingers usually contain 50–70 per cent fish, while fish cakes (which also contain potato, herbs and seasoning) contain at least 35 per cent fish.

A variety of additives is used in preparing fish products. Permitted additives include colour (yellow in smoked fillet, brown in kippers), flavours and emulsifiers. Antioxidants and preservatives, while not being added to the finished product, may be present in the ingredients used. Frozen, fried fish, for example, contains antioxidant present in the oil used for frying. Other additives that are not controlled by law may also be used. For example, both smoke solutions and polyphosphates may be added as these prevent the loss of water which takes place during traditional curing processes.

EGGS

The hen's egg, which is the only variety to be discussed here, is a most interesting food because it is designed to accommodate a living organism. It contains a sufficient store of nutrients to supply a developing chick embryo with all that it needs during its early stages of growth. It is, therefore, a complete food for a growing chick embryo, and although it is not a complete food for humans, it is, nevertheless, a valuable one. The nutrient content of eggs is shown in Table 11.8.

The egg consists of three main parts – the shell, the white and the yolk – and these are shown in Fig. 11.2. The outer shell forms a hard protective layer composed

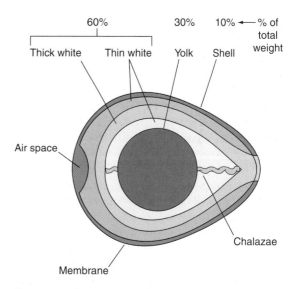

Figure 11.2 *The structure of a hen's egg*

mainly of calcium carbonate and, as it is porous, it allows a developing embryo to obtain a supply of oxygen. The colour of the shell may vary from white to brown although, contrary to popular opinion, this gives no indication as to the quality of the contents of the egg. Egg shell is also a calcium store for the growing chick. It is gradually absorbed as the chick uses calcium for bones etc., so the shell becomes thinner, allowing easier exit at hatching time.

Inside the shell is a viscous colourless liquid called egg white which, in a fresh egg, is divided into regions of thick and thin white and which accounts for about 60 per cent of the total egg weight. It is a dilute aqueous sol, being about one-eighth protein and seven-eighths water. The main protein is ovalbumin, though smaller quantities of several others are present, including mucin, which accounts for the viscosity of the liquid. Also present are small quantities of dissolved salts and the vitamin riboflavin.

In the centre of the egg is the yolk, which is a thick yellow or orange oil-in-water emulsion stabilized by lecithin. It is suspended in the white, being held in position by the chalazae, and it is a rich source of nutrients, being much more concentrated than egg white. It is roughly one-third fat, one-half water and one-sixth protein; it also contains a supply of mineral elements and vitamins.

The only type of nutrient not present in an egg is carbohydrate. Its presence might be expected, because it would provide a ready source of energy for the growing chick. However, the size of the egg is limited and fat, which weight for weight has more than twice the energy value of carbohydrate, forms the sole source of energy. The fat of eggs is concentrated in the yolk, which is also a rich source of cholesterol.

The proteins of eggs, particularly those of egg white, have been intensively studied. Nine proteins have been identified in egg white and the nature and properties of the principal ones are summarized in Table 11.9. In addition to those mentioned in the table, two globular proteins, identified as G_2 and G_3 and a small amount of a protein called avidin are present. Avidin is of some nutritional importance as it combines with the vitamin biotin, rendering it unavailable to the body. However, avidin is inactivated during cooking, so that all the biotin of cooked eggs is available. The presence of the protein conalbumin in egg white prevents the absorption of the iron in eggs.

The main proteins of egg yolk are the phosphoproteins lipovitellin and lipovitellenin which comprise about 30 per cent of the total egg yolk solids. The phosphorus content of these proteins is in the form of phosphoric acid esterified with the hydroxyl groups of hydroxy amino acids. They also contain a lipid part as their names suggest, and this is mainly lecithin.

The proteins of an egg are of high nutritional value and because of the quantity present – about 12 per cent of the edible part – eggs must be considered as a valuable protein food. Moreover, the properties of egg proteins, particularly the ease with which they coagulate, cause eggs to be used in many methods of food preparation.

The nutritional value of an egg may be summed up by saying that it supplies the diet with valuable amounts of iron, phosphorus and protein of high nutritional value and useful amounts of fat, vitamin A and calcium. It also supplies some vitamin D, riboflavin, thiamin and biotin.

Egg shell provides calcium, magnesium and phosphate in ideal form for the growing chick, and possibly for women concerned about osteoporosis, but is seldom eaten. Instead, it is often used to clear visible contaminants from drinks such as wine.

Eggs in cooking

When eggs are heated, the proteins are coagulated. Overcooking can produce excessive coagulation of protein and a consequent rubbery texture, particularly

Table 11.9 The principal proteins of egg white

	Ovalbumin	Conalbumin	Lysozyme	Ovomucin	Ovomucoid
Per cent of total protein	70	9	3	2	13
Type	Albumin	Albumin	Globular	Conjugated	Conjugated
Molecular weight	44 000	74 000	15 000	8 000 000	28 000
Non-protein part	Phosphate carbohydrate	None	None	Carbohydrate	Carbohydrate
Isoelectric point	4.6–4.8	5.6–6.0	11.5–11.0		3.9–4.5
Coagulated by heat	Yes	Yes	No	No	No

of the egg white. The rate at which egg proteins coagulate depends upon conditions such as pH, salt concentration and temperature. Egg white coagulates readily into a white solid on heating and at its normal pH of around 9, coagulation starts at about 60°C. At higher temperatures the rate of coagulation increases until eventually it is nearly instantaneous. Egg yolk coagulates less readily than the white and does not coagulate appreciably below 70°C. As coagulation proceeds, the viscosity of the yolk increases until eventually it becomes solid.

Cooked eggs form an easily digestible food and, provided that they are not overcooked, there is little loss in the nutritional value of the protein. There is, however, some loss of B vitamins on cooking and typical losses are shown in Table 11.10. It is evident that losses are more severe when eggs are baked than when they are scrambled or made into omelettes. Folate is more readily destroyed than other vitamins when eggs are cooked.

Eggs, as we have already noted, have many uses in food preparation. This versatility is mainly due to the properties of egg protein. Eggs may be used as thickening agents, in which the coagulation of the egg proteins is used to thicken sauces, custards, soups and lemon cheese. Eggs are also used as binding agents when the coagulation of egg proteins gives cohesion to a mixture containing dry ingredients, as in rissoles and croquettes. Eggs are used as coatings, as when a mixture of eggs and breadcrumbs is used to coat fish before it is fried. The coagulation of the egg during frying forms a strong coating which holds the fish structure together. Beaten egg is used as a protective covering for fried food because, on heating, the egg white hardens quickly; this has the additional benefit of preventing the food being penetrated by the oil during frying.

Table 11.10 Typical percentage loss of vitamins when eggs are cooked

Vitamin	Scrambled	Omelette	Baked dishes
Thiamin	5	5	15
Riboflavin	20	20	15
Niacin	5	5	5
Pyridoxine	15	15	25
Folate	30	30	50
Pantothenic acid	15	15	25

Egg white, as we saw in the previous chapter, has the ability to entrap air and form foams. Foam foundation is brought about by beating the egg white and is promoted by the addition of acid, which lowers the pH to a value near the isoelectric point of ovalbumin. Heating causes further coagulation of ovalbumin and produces a solid foam as when making meringues. Whole eggs, when beaten, also entrap air and are able to lighten the texture of baked goods such as sponge cakes. They also act as emulsifiers and assist the formation of a stable emulsion from a creamed mixture of fat and sugar during cake making. Egg yolks are used to emulsify oil and vinegar in making mayonnaise.

Whole eggs can be used to improve texture and enrich flavour especially when making baked goods such as cakes. The yolks also contribute a rich yellow colour. The fat of the yolk also exerts a shortening effect (see p. 64) in the making of biscuits, shortbread and cakes.

The versatility of eggs in cooking is enhanced by the fact that the white and yolk may be used either separately or together. The making of meringues illustrates the use of egg white while the making of the filling for a lemon meringue pie illustrates the use of egg yolk, which is mixed with cornflour and lemon. The exotic-sounding and delicious desert Zabaglione is made by the careful blending together and subsequent very gentle heating of egg yolk, caster sugar and Marsala wine. The gentle thickening produced by the slow coagulation of the egg yolk contributes the particular smooth, delicate, creamy texture of this dish.

Whole eggs are used to make egg custard when a mixture of beaten eggs (strained to remove the chalazae) sugar and milk are heated together. The rate and duration of heating can be adjusted to produce either a viscous stirred custard, produced by partial coagulation of the egg proteins, or a solid baked form, produced by more complete coagulation. Slow and even coagulation is essential in making both products if a successful texture is to be achieved. Rapid heating can easily cause curdling.

SOYA

As long as 5000 years ago, soya beans were cultivated in China and used as food. It was not until 1804, however, that soya beans arrived in the USA, and even then it came about by accident, when they were carried as ballast aboard a ship from China. When these beans were cultivated, it was for curiosity without any thought of their potential as a food.

It was not until the First World War that the value of soya beans as a source of oil was recognized and not until the Second World War that shortage of animal protein focused attention on the potential of soya beans as a possible alternative. Currently, large quantities of soya beans are grown, the USA being the largest producer with Brazil and China as the other two major producers.

Soya beans grow in pods on bushy plants which are able to fix nitrogen (Fig. 11.3), and in warm temperate climates where they grow best they reach maturity in about 4 months. Like peas and lentils they are legumes; all have similar nutrient contents.

As Table 11.11 demonstrates, soya beans have a high food value and they are a valuable source of protein of high biological value. They are also a rich source of oil which may be extracted from the beans. The oil is rich in PUFA, particularly linoleic acid which accounts for about half the fatty acid content. Soya beans are also a useful source of iron, calcium and some B vitamins.

In China, soya beans have an amazing variety of uses. They are used as a vegetable and in salads and the seeds are used to produce soya sprouts. The dried bean is roasted and used as a coffee substitute (which is caffeine-free) and fermented beans form the basis of soya sauces. The bean, or flour derived from it, is used to make a form of 'milk' which has about the same protein content as cows' milk and can be used in a similar way. The milk is used to make a form of cheese or curd known as tofu.

Soya beans are often converted into a form of flour which is made by removing the outer seed coat, crushing the beans between rollers to convert them into flakes which are then ground into flour. Soya bean flour is a high-protein flour and may be added to wheat flour as a protein supplement. It is an important ingredient in many baby foods and in slimming and 'health' food products. It cannot be used alone for making bread because it is lacking in starch and gluten and its fat content is too high. However, it may be added in small amounts to wheat flour where it helps to improve colour (the enzymes in soya flour help to bleach the yellowish pigments of wheat flour), improves texture and keeping qualities and imparts an attractive nutty flavour to the baked loaf.

Genetic modification

Soya, like other legumes is a rich source of phyto-oestrogens – compounds which bind to receptors and act like weak oestrogen. It has been proposed that, if eaten in large amounts this effect may reduce risks of osteoporosis and heart disease and may reduce symptoms of the menopause, but evidence is largely lacking.

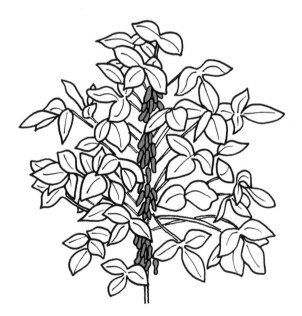

Figure 11.3 *The soya bean plant*

Table 11.11 The nutrient content of 100 g soya beans and soya flour

	Cooked beans	Flour	Low-fat flour
Energy value (kJ)	648	1871	1488
Protein (g)	13.1	36.8	45.3
Total fat (g)	6.8	23.5	7.2
Polyunsaturated fat (g)	3.8	13.3	4.2
Carbohydrate (g)	9	23.5	28.2
Calcium (mg)	87	210	240
Iron (mg)	3.2	6.9	9.1
Thiamin (mg)	0.4	0.75	0.90
Riboflavin (mg)	0.1	0.31	0.36

There has been some controversy recently regarding the use of genetically modified (GM) soya. Soya has been genetically modified so that it is not destroyed by certain weedkillers. Soya is used as an ingredient in 60 per cent of processed foods. The USA is one of the major sources of soya and do not separate GM soya from conventionally grown product. It has therefore been difficult for UK manufacturers to respond to consumer pressure to produce products that are GM-free. Recent European legislation has required manufacturers to declare the content of GM ingredients New rules for GM labelling come into force in April 2004 which cover all EU member states. In the EU, if a food contains or consists of genetically modified organisms (GMOs) or contains ingredients produced from GMOs this must be indicated on the label. Any GM food products which are sold loose must have information displayed next to the product indicating that it is GM. The GM Food and Feed Regulation (EC) (see Further reading section) details rules that cover all GM food and animal feed, regardless of the presence of any GM material in the final product. For example, products such as flour, oils and glucose syrups will have to be labelled as GM if they are from a GM source.

NOVEL PROTEIN-RICH FOODS

For over 20 years, from the 1940s to the 1960s, great significance was attached to a perceived world shortage of protein and consequently to ways of replacing expensive animal protein, which was in short supply, with new forms of protein foods derived from plants. It is now appreciated that the world food problem is one of a lack of food rather than a lack of protein and that most mixed diets provide an adequate supply of protein. The original impetus to develop concentrated protein-rich foods, known as 'novel protein foods', has therefore diminished. Nevertheless, animal protein remains expensive and the conversion of plant foodstuffs into animal protein in the bodies of cattle and other animals is an extremely inefficient and extravagant use of the world's food resources. It is still appropriate, therefore, to consider novel protein-rich foods derived from non-animal sources.

Novel protein foods are of two types:

1 Those produced by processing plant foods.
2 Those produced from sources not previously used as food, including (a) plants and (b) microorganisms.

'Soya protein'

The most widely used novel protein foods are those derived from soya beans, the proteins of which, unlike most vegetable proteins, are of high biological value. Such products are often made to simulate meat and are intended as a cheaper alternative to it. 'Soya protein' is badly named. It is not pure protein. A comparison of the amino acid pattern of soya beans with beef (Table 11.12) shows that the

Table 11.12 Essential amino acid content of novel proteins (mg/g protein) compared with beef

Amino acid	Beef	Soya	Grass	Yeast	Fungi	Bacteria
Isoleucine	53	62	93	45	43	43
Leucine	82	79	130	70	55	68
Lysine	87	53	72	70	51	59
Methionine (+ cystine)	38	16	21	18	10	24
Phenylalanine (+ tyrosine)	75	49	93	44	39	34
Threonine	43	37	67	49	25	46
Tryptophan	12	11	21	14	21	9
Valine	55	53	103	54	60	56

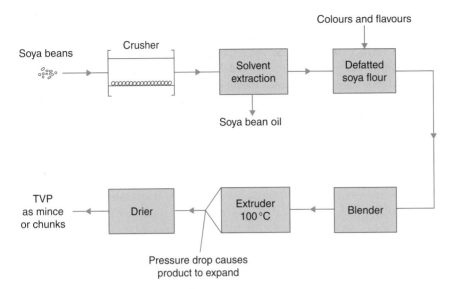

Figure 11.4 *How extruded textured vegetable protein (TVP) is made from soya beans*

former is low in methionine, which is the limiting amino acid, but otherwise they are broadly comparable. Soya bean products are made from soya flour and the conversion of soya flour into products having a meat-like texture is now carried out on a large scale (Fig. 11.4). The simplest way of doing this is to convert the flour into a dough, heat under pressure above 100°C and extrude through a nozzle into atmospheric or reduced pressure. The sudden drop in pressure causes the material to expand and achieve the desired texture. The material is cut into pieces and dried. It can either be used in its natural form or flavours and colours may be added to the dough so that the final product, known as textured vegetable protein (TVP), has a somewhat meaty colour and texture. It is used mainly as a meat extender and is available as chunks or granules for addition to meat products such as mince, stews and pies.

Another type of product, known as spun vegetable protein is made by extracting the protein from soya flour, dissolving it in alkali and forcing the resulting solution through the tiny holes of a spinneret to give many fine threads of spun material. The threads of precipitated protein are stretched and twisted into bunches of fibres having a meat-like texture, to which additives such as colour, flavour, fat and protein binders may be added. The final product may be frozen or, more usually, dried.

Spun products have a more fibrous texture than textured ones, but are more expensive to produce.

Vegetable proteins are regularly used in schools, hospitals and canteens, usually as a meat extender to replace part of the meat in traditional dishes. It is recommended that in the UK not more than 10 per cent of meat should be replaced by vegetable protein, although in the USA the limit is 30 per cent. Vegetable proteins are also being used as components of simulated meat products such as stews, curries and burger and burger-style dried mixes.

Other sources of novel protein foods

Large amounts of plant materials are grown as a source of vegetable oils. In addition to soya beans, groundnuts, cotton seed and other seeds are used; after the oil has been extracted a protein-rich residue remains. Concentrated protein can be extracted not only from such oil seeds but also from grass and other indigestible, but often abundant, vegetable material, and from fish. At present, such processes are only carried out on a small scale.

One product that has proved popular in the UK is Quorn, a protein-rich meat substitute produced from a fungus. The main ingredient in all Quorn products is mycoprotein, which is protein from a member of the fungi family. This ingredient provides the taste and texture to the meat-free products. Quorn offers chilled and frozen products. Its range includes mince, pieces, fillets, burgers and sausages, some of which have been approved by the Vegetarian Society. Quorn also offers a range of pre-packed chilled sliced meat alternatives and ready meals which include lasagne and enchiladas. It has been said that mycoprotein has beneficial effects on appetite control and maintaining healthy blood cholesterol levels but well designed, conclusive research is lacking.

Key points

- Interest in protein-rich foods arose largely from historical misunderstandings over 'protein-energy malnutrition'. It is now recognized that protein is required only as 8–10 per cent of dietary energy, protein deficiency almost never exists
- Very high protein intakes (over 25 per cent of dietary energy) have no known medical or health value. They tend to nauseate so promote weight loss, and can overload and damage the kidneys

Chapter summary

Several classes of foods are high in protein. These include animal products (meat, meat products, fish, eggs, cheese) which are rich in the essential amino acids but also tend to be high in saturated fatty acids, and protein-rich plant foods, e.g. pulses and legumes, which are also valuably rich in carbohydrate and dietary fibres but lack some essential amino acids, which must be provided by grain and cereal foods. Some novel protein-rich foods made from bacteria, fungi and legumes (e.g. 'soya protein' - which is not just protein) may hold attractions for some vegetarians but claims for any health value are generally overstated.

FURTHER READING

ADVISORY COMMITTEE ON NOVEL FOODS AND PROCESSES (1991). *Guidelines on the Assessment of Novel Foods and Processes*. London: HMSO.

BRITISH NUTRITION FOUNDATION (1993). *Nutritional Aspects of Fish*. BNF Briefing Paper No. 10. London: BNF.

FOOD STANDARDS AGENCY (2003). *Labelling and Composition of Meat Products – Guidance Notes*. http://www.food.gov.uk/multimedia/pdfs/meatguidance.pdf

HOLLAND B. *et al.* (1993). *Third Supplement to McCance and Widdowson's The Composition of Foods*, 5th edn: *Fish and Fish Products*. Cambridge: Royal Society of Chemistry.

Cooking seafood: http://www.seafish.org/plate/buying.asp?p=gc179

http://www.foodstandards.gov.uk/gmfoods/gm_labelling

http://www.scottish-haggis.com (Haggis, the McKean Family of Haggis)

http://www.microwavecooking.com

http://www.marlow-foods.ch/

http://www.quorn.co.uk/index.php

http://www.food.gov.uk/multimedia/pdfs/meatguidance.pdf

GM FOOD AND FEEDING REGULATION (EC) – www.food.gov.uk/multimedia/pdfs/reg18292003.pdf

ROSE J (1998). What is Haggis? Available online at www.freep.com/fun/food/ghaggis21.htm

12

Water and beverages

Under heaven nothing is more soft and yielding
than water. Yet for attacking the solid and
strong, nothing is better

(Lao Tsu, Tao Te Ching 78, 600 BC)

Water, water, see the water flow
Glancing dancing see the water flow
O, wizard of changes, water, water, water
Dark or silvery mother of life
Water, water, holy mystery, heaven's daughter

God made a song when the world was new
Water's laughter sings it is true
O, wizard of changes, teach me the lesson of flowing

*(The Hangman's Beautiful Daughter,
Incredible String Band, 1968)*

WATER

Without water there could be no life; water is essential to the life of every living thing from the simplest plant and single cell organism to the most complex living system known – the human body. Moreover, while living things may exist for a considerable time without the other essential nutrients, they soon die without water. Living things contain a surprising amount of water: never less than 60 per cent of their total weight and sometimes as much as 95 per cent. About two-thirds of the body is water and all the organs, tissues and fluids of the body contain water as an essential constituent. Only a few parts of the body, such as bones, teeth and hair contain little water.

Water is continually being lost from the body, partly in the urine, partly from the surface of the body as sweat and partly as water vapour in the gases expelled in respiration. Some water is also lost in the faeces. If the body is to function successfully the water that is lost must be replaced, to maintain balance between intake and output. The main source of water for the body is food and drink, although some is produced when nutrients are oxidized to produce energy. For example, when glucose is oxidized it breaks down to form carbon dioxide and water. A kilogram of glucose produces just over half a litre of water on oxidation. The balance between input and output for a person living a sedentary life in a temperate climate and having a diet which provides 8.8 MJ per day is shown in Table 12.1.

Water is unlike the other essential nutrients, in that most of it does not undergo chemical change within the body. Whereas proteins, for example, are broken down into amino acids during digestion, most water passes through the body unchanged. The functions performed by water mainly result from physical action and depend upon its ability to transport nutrients through the body, to dissolve substances or hold them in colloidal suspension and, above all, to remain liquid over a wide range of temperatures. This latter property enables water to provide a liquid medium in which the thousands of reactions necessary to life can occur. Physical activity increases the losses from lungs and skin to maintain body temperatures. In hot climates, skin loss is greater. These are compensated by increased drinking.

Table 12.1 Approximate water balance in the body of an average adult in a temperate climate

Source	Water intake (mL/day)	Source	Water loss (mL/day)
Food	*1000*	*Urine*	*1000*
Drink	*1000*	*Lungs*	*300*
Metabolism		*Skin*	*920*
(oxidation) of nutrients	*280*	*Faeces*	*60*
Total:	*2280*	*Total:*	*2280*

Although most of the water in the body is involved in physical changes, some is involved with chemical changes. Some chemical changes, such as the enzymic and hydrolytic breakdown of nutrients during digestion, involve the uptake of water, whereas others, such as the oxidation of absorbed nutrients to provide the body with energy, release water.

The earth is unusual in having a lot of water, and in having an average surface temperature at which water is liquid. Water therefore provided a remarkably stable environment over millions of years, in which life was able to develop. Even when water freezes, it has the unusual physical property of having a density lower than when liquid. Thus, ice gathers at the surface, and provides effective insulation such that even quite small ponds retain liquid during severe winters. This allowed fragile and complicated organisms to evolve: most animal cells are destroyed by freezing.

One of the basic principles of all living things is the need to maintain the 'milieu interieur'. That is, to maintain constant concentrations inside the body of all the chemicals which allow cells to function. Life developed initially in water and needed physiological structures and processes to keep excess water out, which would otherwise dilute the composition of the body. As a very broad generalization, the body starts to malfunction if there is a 5 per cent excess of water, vital organs may be critically damaged and both physical and mental functions are seriously affected by 10 per cent dilution.

When life emerged onto dry land, the opposite problem, dehydration, became a possibility. It is also possible to lose water in strong salt solutions, by osmotic effects, so physiological processes were already in place. As another generalization, organ functions, physical and mental performance are adversely affected by 2–5 per cent loss of water, and critically affected by 10 per cent dehydration.

Water forms a very large proportion of our bodies, around 60–80 per cent by weight. The proportion depends on how much fat we carry: fat contains no water. The absolute amount of water is rather difficult to measure exactly and not critical. What is more important is fluctuation in water content, and that is easily measured over the short term by changes in body weight. Other parts, like fat, take long periods to change. The body works optimally, in terms of function and performance over a very narrow range.

We are constantly losing water, in urine, in sweat, and as vapour in our breath. The amount of water being lost varies considerably under the influence of environmental conditions, activity, factors in food and drink, drug effects, etc. It is therefore necessary to drink at different rates in order to match the losses from the body, and this gives rise to the concept of 'fluid balance'.

Under usual climatic conditions, and without physical activity, the minimal 'insensible' fluid losses from sweat and in breath is about 500 mL water daily. Another 200–300 mL or so is lost from the bowel in stools, and it is necessary to pass at least 750 mL to keep the kidneys functioning and remove toxic waste products of metabolism. So, for health, in round terms we need to consume a minimum of about 1500–2000 mL water daily, in drinks and in foods. The absolute minimum varies between individuals, mainly according to size, and we cannot establish that minimum for any individual.

This minimum water consumption necessary to achieve 'fluid balance' varies with physical size. Larger people have a greater skin area so produce more sweat, and also have higher metabolic rates, so they require more oxygen (as well as food calories) and thus need to breathe more, and more water evaporates in the breath. Therefore, larger people need to drink more, and that is particularly marked during physical activity.

In hot temperatures, causing more rapid water evaporation from skin and lungs, and at high levels of physical activity, it is possible for healthy people to lose water at up to 1.5 L/hour. So the maximum water requirement to avoid dehydration might occasionally be towards 20 L/day. However, it would be dangerous to drink this amount under normal conditions, because it would exceed the maximum capacity of the kidneys to excrete excess water, leading to 'water intoxication'.

Dehydration

It is certainly a general truth that many people would feel better if they drank more water, and that many common day-to-day symptoms are aggravated by not drinking enough. Central heating commonly contributes to mild dehydration and a lot of avoidable headaches. However, like many principles in biology, it is possible to overdo it.

As a land-species, the relationship with water is always critical, and the balance vulnerable which accompany mild dehydration. Dehydration can mean death, not just the headaches, tiredness and loss of performance, so we have sophisticated systems to conserve and retain water. In the primordial soup we lived and breathed water, but water-living species still had to develop protective mechanisms to avoid getting washed out. The skin serves to keep the inside in and the outside out, but originally its main function, complemented by kidneys, was to stop us becoming diluted in an aqueous environment.

Water overload – 'Water intoxication'

It is possible for a healthy person to drink too much water, too fast, for the kidneys to remove. The nervous system is the first to suffer, producing a variety of serious consequences – confusion, unsteadiness, fits and coma. A healthy person has to drink a lot to develop 'water intoxication', but it can occur more easily in infants or children. Prolonged swimming is

said to cause continued excessive water ingestion by small children, and water intoxication can occur. It can even develop in dogs after swimming in water for several hours. There was a scare when diabetic children developed epileptic seizures. Initially, the artificial sweeteners in sugar-free drinks were blamed, but the answer ultimately seemed to be the sheer volume consumed (2–3 L at a time). Large volumes of beer might just do it in adults, or any drink which exceeds the limit of the kidneys to excrete excess water – about 1–2 L per hour. Water intoxication has also been reported in fanatical marathon runners who drink water excessively for fear of dehydration. Electrolyte-containing sports drinks are better. Before water intoxication causes fits, earlier signs include restlessness, confusion, vomiting and unsteadiness. These are all signs of 'cerebral oedema' – excess water in the brain. Visible accumulation of fluid (as 'oedema') usually swelling of the legs, is not marked, but sensation in the fingers and feet can be altered.

Water intoxication can also develop in a gradual way, without gross excess drinking, in a condition called syndrome of inappropriate antidiuretic hormone (SIADH). The hormone ADH (antidiuretic hormone or vasopressin) is produced in the pituitary gland (at the base of the brain) and it is one of the main defence systems against dehydration. Normally the kidneys produce lots of dilute urine, getting rid of excess water and waste products. If dehydrated by 1 or 2 per cent, muscle function and brain function start to suffer. Effects of dehydration are marked with 5 per cent dehydration, and 10 per cent loss of body water can be fatal. Long before that, changes in the chemical concentrations of blood and tissue are detected by sensors in the body. Nerve messages link to the pituitary gland, which releases ADH. The role of ADH is to reduce water loss from the kidneys (i.e. making the urine more concentrated). It also constricts blood vessels around the body, temporarily reducing the volume of blood needed to carry oxygen and nutrients round. It is this constriction of arteries in the brain that causes the characteristic headache of minor dehydration – cured by drinking more water.

In SIADH, the hormone ADH is released, inappropriately, when there is no dehydration. The kidneys therefore retain extra water, and this produces both the headache normally associated with ADH in dehydration and also the confusion, tiredness and ultimately seizures of water intoxication. Luckily the syndrome is quite rare – at least in a severe form – although a range of diseases, chest infections, extreme physical exertion, surgical stress, head injuries, certain drugs and cancers can cause it. The diagnosis is made by finding the urine to be concentrated (an antidiuretic effect) when blood chemistry shows dilution. As a response to physical stress or illness, it presumably had some survival value if access to water was temporarily problematic. It usually passes in time, and it is easily resolved by fluid restriction, but its effects can be debilitating when caused by chronic or progressive conditions.

If the pituitary gland fails to produce ADH, the kidneys will fail to concentrate urine, and a condition called diabetes insipidus develops. Huge volumes of dilute urine are produced and a great thirst develops to keep up with it. Dehydration, with headaches, fatigue, etc., is more likely. Diabetes insipidus (unrelated to the more common diabetes mellitus) is treated with a synthetic form of ADH, called DDAVP.

A little understood psychiatric condition, polydipsia (drinking up to 20 L a day), is relatively common in psychotic disorders and produces water intoxication whose symptoms must in some way be counterbalanced by pleasure from drinking.

Humans do a pretty fair job at maintaining a stable, physiological 'milieu interieur' over a range of water intakes. We need more to drink in centrally heated environments, or if physically active, on long air flights because of excess losses from lungs and skin. We need more if we take diuretics, either as prescribed drugs or as the 'social diuretics', alcohol and caffeine.

The structure of water and ice

A water molecule contains two atoms of hydrogen linked to one atom of oxygen, the bond angle being about 105° as shown in Fig. 12.1a. The electronegativity of oxygen, that is its attraction for electrons, is greater than that of hydrogen. This results in unequal charge distribution over the molecule, the oxygen atom carrying a partial negative charge ($\delta-$), balanced by partial positive charges ($\delta+$) on the hydrogen atoms. Such molecules are said to be polar and they attract each other; in water, hydrogen bonds are formed between adjacent polar molecules as

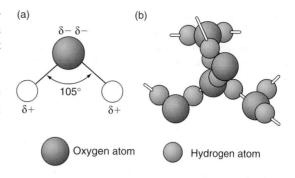

Figure 12.1 (a) A water molecule showing its polar character and bond angle. (b) Hydrogen bonding in water gives rise to its tetrahedral structures

shown in Fig. 12.1b. It will be noted that, because of the shape of water molecules, such intermolecular attraction results in water molecules grouping together to form tetrahedral structures in which each water molecule is linked to four others.

Hydrogen bonds are weak electrostatic links which are easily broken, and in water such bonds are constantly being formed, broken and reformed. If water is heated, the thermal energy of the molecules is increased, and their resulting increased motion favours the breaking, rather than the formation, of hydrogen bonds. In water vapour no hydrogen bonds are present and the water molecules exist as single units. Conversely, if liquid water is cooled the loss of thermal energy and the resulting decreased motion of the water molecules favours the formation of hydrogen bonds. In ice, hydrogen bonding is so extensive that all the water molecules are linked together by hydrogen bonds so forming a rigid and regular structure. The tetrahedral structure of groups of water molecules is preserved, but the tetrahedra are further linked together to form layers of hexagonal rings which are joined to give a very open structure. The open structure of ice compared with that of water explains why ice has a larger specific volume and lower density than water. Under different conditions, hydrogen bonds form during freezing, leading to an almost infinite number of patterns in snowflakes.

The physical characteristics of water

Water is the commonest of all liquids and perhaps for this reason it is often considered to be unremarkable.

Because it is ubiquitous its presence, like that of air, is taken for granted. Yet, it is fortunate that water is so readily available for, in reality, it is a most remarkable liquid, having properties that make it uniquely suited to the endless purposes for which it is used or needed, including the support of life itself.

Water is a colourless, odourless and tasteless liquid which, under normal atmospheric conditions, boils at 100°C and freezes at 0°C. These facts are well known and are readily accepted. Yet, in view of its low molecular mass, it is surprising that water is a liquid at all. The reason is that, because of hydrogen bonding, individual molecules group together forming unstable units with an effective 'molecular mass' that is much higher than that of a single molecule.

Although water boils at 100°C at normal atmospheric pressure, its boiling point decreases or increases as the pressure is lowered or raised. At the top of Mount Everest, for example, its boiling point is about 72°C, whereas in a pressure cooker working at maximum pressure ($1.05\,kg/cm^2$), it boils at 120°C. The temperature at which water boils is also affected by the presence of dissolved substances. These increase the boiling point by an amount that is proportional to their molecular concentration. Thus, in jam making, when fruit is cooked in water containing dissolved sugar, the boiling point is greater than 100°C. If boiling is continued, the concentration of the solution increases and, consequently, the boiling point rises. Indeed, as mentioned on p. 113, the end of the boiling period can be judged from the boiling point, a knowledge of which enables the composition of the mixture to be determined.

The freezing point of water is lowered by the presence of dissolved solids, the lowering being proportional to the molecular concentration of dissolved material. Thus, water in plant tissues and foods does not freeze until below 0°C. This fact must be taken into account when preserving foods by cold storage, where temperatures of −18°C are normally used to ensure that the water in the food is frozen. When water freezes, its volume increases because of an increase in hydrogen bonding and the formation of a hexagonal structure which is very open. This causes ice to float on water, thereby conserving the heat of the water beneath; this has important consequences in nature as it enables aquatic plant and animal life to continue beneath ice surfaces. Other noteworthy effects of ice formation are the bursting of plant tissues, which occurs when the plant sap freezes, and the breakdown of the tissues of frozen food, which occurs if large ice crystals are allowed to form.

The specific heat capacity and the specific latent heat of vaporization of water are high compared with their values for other liquids. If liquids where there is no hydrogen bonding are heated, all the thermal energy supplied increases the kinetic energy of the molecules and hence the temperature. In water, however, some of the thermal energy is used in breaking hydrogen bonds and therefore more heat energy must be supplied to obtain a given temperature rise than in liquids containing no hydrogen bonds. This is important in the body because the high specific heat capacity of water allows it to act as a heat reservoir, so preventing its temperature from rising quickly when heat is absorbed.

The specific latent heat of vaporization of water is high for a similar reason, namely that energy is required to break hydrogen bonds, making necessary a greater supply of heat to vaporize a given mass of water than would be needed for the same mass of a non-hydrogen bonded liquid. The high specific latent heat value of 2300 kJ/kg means that 2300 kJ are required to vaporize a kilogram of water at a given temperature. Thus, when sweat evaporates from the surface of the body a relatively large amount of heat is absorbed from the skin, which is thereby kept cool.

Snow and ice will readily vaporize directly, without needing to go through a liquid phase. Deep-frozen food must be kept in sealed containers to prevent spoiling by desiccation. The process of freeze-drying uses this principle to remove water by using low temperature and low pressure, for example to produce powdered coffee and tea.

Water as a solvent

Water has unique solvent properties that enable it to dissolve a very large number of substances. It is sometimes called an ionizing or polar solvent because it will dissolve electrovalent substances such as acids and salts and, importantly, carbon dioxide. It will also dissolve some covalent compounds (e.g. sugar, urea and oxygen), though others (e.g. fat) do not dissolve in water to an appreciable degree. The importance of the solvent action of water cannot be emphasized too strongly; it enables water to dissolve a large number of substances that are essential to plant and animal life. These dissolved substances can then be transported through the organism to areas where they are needed. In the absence of water, or some other solvent, they could not be utilized by living things.

The explanation for the excellent solvent properties of water is to be found in the nature of the molecule itself: to be more specific it depends upon the polar character of the water molecule. To understand this, consider the way in which a typical salt, such as sodium chloride, forms a solution in water. Sodium chloride exists in the form of ions; in it, sodium exists as a positively charged particle or ion and chlorine exists as a negatively charged ion.

A crystal of sodium chloride contains many millions of sodium ions and an equal number of chloride ions. The ions are arranged in a three-dimensional geometrical pattern known as a space lattice, as shown in Fig. 12.2a. This represents about one five-million-million millionth part of a 1 mm cube of sodium chloride. It shows clearly the geometry of the space lattice but suffers from the defect that the sodium and chloride ions appear to be widely separated, whereas in fact they are closely packed. In Fig. 12.2b a portion of the lattice has been enlarged

and is shown in a more realistic way. In the interior of a sodium chloride crystal each sodium ion is surrounded by six equidistant chloride ions and, similarly, each chloride ion is surrounded by six equidistant sodium ions.

A sodium ion is not associated with a particular chloride ion and, in this sense it is wrong to think of a sodium chloride molecule. However, it is convenient and customary to speak of the sodium chloride molecule, and its formula is written NaCl and not Na^+Cl^-. The lines in the diagram do not, of course, represent bonds between the ions, but merely indicate the geometrical properties of the space lattice.

When sodium chloride dissolves in water, this orderly space lattice breaks down and the ions are separated from each other and become free to move. This process of separating the ions is difficult to achieve because it requires a large amount of energy. Water is able to effect this because it hydrates the ions, and the energy liberated in hydration is sufficiently great to compensate for the energy required to separate them. In other words, the overall process of dissolving a salt in water, that is, separating and hydrating the ions, requires little if any energy, and therefore occurs readily. The result is that ions never exist free in solution; they are always

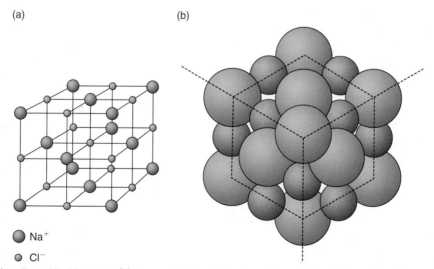

(a)   (b)

● Na$^+$

○ Cl$^-$

Figure 12.2 *A sodium chloride lattice. (a) Representation of about one five-million-million millionth part of a 1 mm cube of sodium chloride. It shows clearly the geometry of the space lattice but suffers from the defect that the sodium and chloride ions appear to be widely separated whereas in fact they are closely packed. (b) A portion of the lattice has been enlarged and is shown in a more realistic way. In the interior of a sodium chloride crystal each sodium ion is surrounded by six equidistant chloride ions and, similarly, each chloride ion is surrounded by six equidistant sodium ions*

hydrated, in which form they are firmly bound to surrounding water molecules.

Water is also a good solvent for substances which, although they are not ionic, contain polar groups and which are able to form hydrogen bonds and other weak electrostatic links with water molecules. Thus, low molecular mass alcohols, for example, ethanol (C_2H_5OH), which contain polar hydroxyl groups, are readily soluble in water, although as molecular mass increases and the proportion of non-polar hydrocarbon chain increases, solubility decreases. Molecules which contain a number of hydroxyl groups, such as simple sugars, are very readily soluble in water because the greater number of polar groups that they contain increases attraction between them and water. The ability of water to dissolve covalent substances, provided that they contain a reasonable proportion of polar groups, is very important in the body. It means that after food has been broken down during digestion into relatively small polar molecules, such as simple sugars and amino acids, it is dissolved by the body fluids, which are mainly water, and transported through the body in solution.

Water supplies

There is no such thing as pure natural water. Rain water, which is the purest form of natural water, contains small amounts of dissolved gases, such as oxygen, carbon dioxide and, owing to industrial pollution, it may also contain dissolved oxides of sulphur and nitrogen (when it is known as 'acid rain'). It also contains small quantities of dust. Other types of natural water, such as spring and river water, in addition to the impurities of rain water, contain dissolved salts and in the latter case further impurities from vegetation and drainage. Water is not important as a supplier of salts, except for fluoride, only about 1 ppm is needed to preserve teeth against decay, but 3–4 ppm may be enough to discolour teeth (fluorosis).

An adequate supply of clean, wholesome water is one of the essentials of modern life and water for domestic consumption must be carefully treated before use, so that it is not injurious to health. A considerable proportion of the water supply in Britain is obtained from reservoirs which receive their water from moorland catchment areas. The water which is withdrawn from such reservoirs is treated in a number of ways before being supplied to the consumer. The essential stages are settlement, filtration and sterilization. Some water used for drinking is also treated by fluoridation, as described on p. 195. Water which has been treated in these ways is wholesome and suitable for human consumption, although for industrial purposes it may also require to be softened. Since 1985 the quality of water supplies has had to comply with European Union (EU) regulations which lay down strict requirements for the bacteriological and chemical quality of water supplies.

Water which needs to be softened is said to be hard because it does not easily give a lather with soap. The hardness of water results from the presence of certain mineral salts – chiefly the sulphates and bicarbonates of calcium and magnesium – and because of this hard water makes good drinking water. For industrial purposes, however, hard water is unsatisfactory because the mineral salts tend to precipitate out and form insoluble deposits in boilers, water pipes and other equipment. Consequently, water required for industrial purposes is often treated before use by removing the calcium and magnesium ions by a process of ion-exchange in which these ions are exchanged for sodium ions.

Sterilization

Natural water always contains organic matter and dissolved oxygen and is therefore a natural breeding ground for bacteria. Typhoid fever, cholera and jaundice are caused by the infection of water supplies, and in order that bacteria causing these and other diseases may be eliminated, water which is to be used for human consumption is usually sterilized before use.

Water is normally sterilized by adding 0.5 ppm of chlorine; this small concentration is sufficient to kill all bacteria but not to impart a taste to the water. Water which is to be used for canning or bottling may be sterilized by adding 1 or 2 ppm of ozone. This treatment is more expensive than chlorination but has the advantage that ozone breaks down into oxygen, which has no taste.

Mineral waters

Mineral waters come from natural springs and sales of bottled mineral water are increasing in the UK. Natural mineral water originates in an underground water table or deposit and emerges from a spring tapped at one or more natural or bore exits. The sale and composition of such water is legally prescribed and as such is distinguished from spring water and bottled water. Mineral water contains certain mineral salts such as sodium chloride, sodium carbonate and sodium bicarbonate as well as similar salts of calcium and magnesium. A few mineral waters also contain iron salts or hydrogen sulphide, the latter being responsible for the unpleasant 'bad egg' smell of certain mineral waters. The total of dissolved mineral salts may be as low as 0.1 g/L and is rarely more than 3.5 g/L. Ordinary tap water may come from the same origin, and may be chemically identical. Mineral waters from limestone regions are rarely naturally aerated with carbon dioxide. More commonly they are artificially aerated with synthetic carbon dioxide.

Mineral waters, especially the better known, such as Evian, Perrier, Vals or Vichy waters, have for many years been considered to have special health-giving properties and to be less likely to cause illness than tap water because they are free from bacteria. However, these special claims are quite unfounded and, as already explained, tap water in most developed countries is quite safe and of high quality.

The use of mineral waters allows people to drink water that has a pleasant, sharp taste and that is without the unpleasant taste of chlorine sometimes noticeable in tap water. They may also be preferred by people who object to drinking water that has been treated in various ways. Curiously, some large soft-drink manufacturers are now marketing ordinary tap water which has been reprocessed and deionized. Some consumers assume that these bottled waters are the same as mineral waters and buy them at inflated prices.

NON-ALCOHOLIC BEVERAGES

Although water is essential to humans, drinking tap water has become an unpopular way of consuming it. Drinking water in the form of mineral water or with ice added may make it more acceptable to some people, but the great majority of people prefer to take their water in the form of a flavoured and usually sweetened beverage – usually a non-alcoholic beverage such as tea or coffee, a fruit juice or a soft drink. Such beverages are more likely to be appreciated for their flavour or stimulating action rather

than for their nutritional value, although most fruit juices are a good source of vitamin C. In recent years, the marketing of sweet, carbonated soft drinks has taken their consumption above that of most more natural forms of drink.

Tea, coffee and cocoa

Tea

Tea leaves, which are the basis of the familiar beverage, come from an evergreen shrub grown extensively in India, China and Sri Lanka, as well as in other countries. The tea shrub is kept small by pruning and only the bud and the two youngest leaves are picked in preparing good-quality tea (Fig. 12.3). Fresh tea leaves contain a number of water-soluble constituents, including polyphenols, which account for about 30 per cent of the dry weight, amino acids (4 per cent), caffeine (4 per cent) and traces of sugars. Tea leaves also contain insoluble materials, mainly fibrous material (e.g. cellulose), proteins and pectins

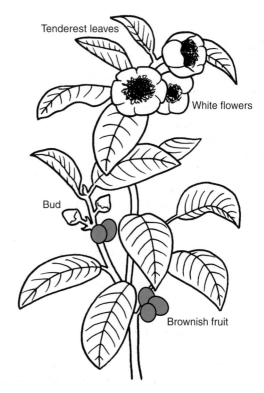

Figure 12.3 *A branch of the tea shrub showing the tenderest leaves and bud, which are used for making good-quality tea*

and a very small quantity (about 0.01 per cent) of essential oils, which contain a large number of volatile components that contribute to flavour and aroma. Tea contains small amounts of the trace elements fluorine and manganese and is a useful source of these elements. It is also high in aluminium.

Caffeine – and the closely related compound theobromine (dimethyl xanthine) – is the most important substance present in tea leaves because it acts as a stimulant to the nervous system. The mild stimulating action of caffeine may help to prevent a feeling of fatigue and some people find that it promotes concentration. It is also a weak diuretic, so that drinking tea (or coffee) stimulates the production of urine more than the same volume of water. Caffeine stimulates the heart and can cause uncomfortable palpitations in some people. It relaxes the airways so can help the symptoms of asthma.

Tannin is another important component of tea leaves. Its astringent properties contribute a certain bitterness to infusions of tea, especially if they have been allowed to brew for a considerable time. Tannin has the property of precipitating milk proteins in tea and it also interferes with the absorption of iron.

After being picked, tea leaves are dried and in addition to loss of moisture this brings about some chemical changes, including an increase in the caffeine and amino acid content. The dried leaves are broken up by passing them between rollers and this process releases enzymes, principally phenolase, which are responsible for the so-called 'fermentation' that follows. Ideally 'fermentation' is carried out at 25°C, at which temperature enzyme activity is at a maximum. The leaves are spread out in layers and in the presence of oxygen in the air phenolase catalyses the oxidation of some polyphenols to *o*-quinones which subsequently react to form coloured compounds, particularly the brownish substances known as thearubigins. The thearubigins contribute most of the colour as well as the astringency, acidity and body to tea infusions. The chemical changes taking place during fermentation are exceedingly complex and the detailed structure of thearubigins is unknown.

After fermentation the leaves are dried further at a temperature which inactivates all enzymes, caramelizes sugars and reduces the moisture content to about 3 per cent.

The popularity of tea as a beverage depends mainly on the mild stimulating effect produced by caffeine,

although a high-grade tea is also prized for its fragrant aroma and delicate flavour. When boiling water is added to tea leaves, the resulting infusion contains a proportion of the soluble constituents of the leaves. An average cup of tea made from 5 g tea contains (in addition to any added milk or sugar): 60–280 mg tannin, 50–80 mg caffeine, 0.2–0.5 mg fluorine, 1 mg manganese, 0.02 mg riboflavin and 0.2 mg niacin.

Caffeine is extracted from tea leaves more readily than tannin, so that the quality of tea is highest after about 5 minutes infusion when most of the caffeine (about 80 per cent), but only some of the tannin (about 60 per cent), has been extracted. Infusion for a longer time increases the proportion of tannin extracted with a consequent increase in bitterness.

Coffee

The coffee plant, like the tea plant, is an evergreen shrub. It originated in Ethiopia and is cultivated as a major cash crop in many tropical countries. The fruit is like a small cherry in appearance and contains two seeds, called 'coffee beans', enclosed in a tough skin or parchment. In order to extract the beans, the outer pulpy part of the fruit is removed and the beans, still surrounded by their skin, are dried in air. The parchment cases are then removed by rolling, so liberating the beans which are green in colour. The beans are roasted, powdered and then extracted using boiling water.

The composition of coffee beans is exceedingly complex, over 300 constituents having been identified, and because of this complexity the chemical basis of coffee flavour and aroma remain largely unknown. The main components of green coffee beans are given in Table 12.2. The figures given are average ones and there is considerable variation in composition between different varieties of coffee. For example, the value given for caffeine refers to Arabica coffee; Robusta coffee, the other main type, contains about twice as much.

Roasting coffee beans reduces the moisture content from about 12 per cent to about 4 per cent, converts some of the sugar into caramel and develops flavour and aroma. Although roasting has little effect on caffeine, chlorogenic acid is broken down to caffeic and quinic acids and trigonelline is largely converted to niacin. Roasted coffee beans are a dark brown colour and brittle, which makes grinding easy.

Table 12.2 The percentage composition of coffee on a dry matter basis

	Green beans	Roasted beans	Soluble coffee
Protein	13	11	15
Sugars	10	1	7
Starch and dextrins	10	12	5 (dextrin only)
Complex polysaccharides	40	46	33
Coffee oil	13	15	<1
Minerals, mainly potassium	4	5	9
Chlorogenic acid	7	5	14
Trigonelline	1	1	4
Phenols	–	2	5
Caffeine (Arabica)	1	1.3	4

When an infusion of coffee is made from ground, roasted coffee beans, about 35 per cent of the constituents of the bean pass into the water. Caffeine is rapidly extracted, especially if very hot water is used; at 95°C about 80 per cent is extracted after 2 minutes and 90 per cent after 10 minutes. A short extraction time of about 2 minutes is ideal as it favours extraction of caffeine but not of less-soluble substances that contribute to bitterness.

A cup of fairly strong coffee contains about 100 mg caffeine together with 100 mg potassium and 1 mg niacin.

French coffee contains added chicory, which is the root of the wild endive. The chicory is roasted before use and although it contains no caffeine it does contribute a bitter flavour as well as a brown colour resulting from caramel produced during roasting. The reason for adding chicory to coffee is that it is much cheaper than coffee but legally the mixture must contain at least 51 per cent coffee.

'Instant' coffee is made by extracting the water-soluble components of roasted beans with hot water and concentrating the resulting liquid extract and converting it to a powder either by spray-drying or by freeze-drying (see Chapter 18). Modern techniques have resulted in the production of 'instant' coffees which retain most of the flavour and aroma constituents of the roasted beans.

Concern about the possible effects of heavy coffee drinking on health has resulted in an increasing demand for decaffeinated coffee. Such coffee is made by removing caffeine with the solvent dichloromethane, which is itself removed by treatment with steam. The resulting coffee must contain less than 0.3 per cent caffeine and less than 10 ppm dichloromethane. The flavour of decaffeinated coffee is poor because other compounds are also lost. It is not known why caffeine is present in the beans and genetically modified coffee plants (with the gene for caffeine synthase eliminated) are likely to find a market.

Cocoa

The processing of cocoa beans to produce cocoa and chocolate has already been described (p. 111). Cocoa powder, unlike tea leaves and coffee beans, has a considerable nutrient content, being approximately 12 per cent carbohydrate, 20 per cent protein and 22 per cent fat (of which about 13 per cent is saturated fats). It also contains small quantities of vitamins A and B and some mineral elements, notably iron (though it is probable that little of the iron is absorbed). Despite its relatively high nutritional value, it makes little contribution to the average diet as it is consumed in small quantities.

In addition to small amounts of caffeine, cocoa also contains the related alkaloid theobromine (dimethyl xanthine) which is a very mild stimulant. An average cup of cocoa contains about 200 mg theobromine and 20 mg caffeine, but these amounts are not sufficiently large to give cocoa a noticeably stimulating effect. Cocoa also contains some tannin.

Drinking chocolate is made from cocoa powder which is treated with alkali to improve solubility and to which sugar and sometimes milk powder, salt and vanilla are added.

Table 12.3 The nutrient content per 100 g of undiluted fruit juices and soft drinks

	Energy (kJ)	Sugars (g)	Vitamin C (mg)	Sodium (mg)	Potassium (mg)
Pineapple juice	177	10.5	11	8	53
Orange juice[a]	153	8.8	39	10	150
Grapefruit juice[a]	140	8.3	31	7	100
Ribena	975	59.1	78[b]	16	92
Tomato juice	62	3.0	8	230	230
Orange squash	399	24.6	25[c]	40	27
Lucozade	256	14.3	8	26	7
Cola	174	10.9	0	5	1
Lemonade	93	5.8	0	7	15

[a] Unsweetened.
[b] When fresh, provides 107 mg vitamin C per 100 g.
[c] Unfortified product contains 2 mg vitamin C per 100 g.

Soft drinks

Soft drinks include fruit squashes, fruit drinks, cordials, carbonated drinks, cola drinks and ginger beer. Soft drinks provide water and usually sugar or an artificial sweetener. Their nutrient value is low, except for the sugar they provide. Some soft drinks contain a little vitamin C derived from the fruit used or added as synthetic vitamin C. Cola drinks contain 50–100 mg caffeine per 330-ml can – about the same amount as a mug of coffee.

In the UK, fruit drinks must contain a stipulated minimum fruit and sugar content. For example, undiluted fruit squash must contain at least 25 per cent fruit juice while comminuted fruit drinks (usually described as made from whole fresh fruit) include both the peel and pulp of the fruit to provide added flavour and must contain at least 10 per cent whole fruit when undiluted.

Fruit-flavoured drinks contain no fruit and usually contain nothing except water, sugar and synthetic fruit flavour; they are often described as an '-ade', such as lemonade. The nutrient content of a variety of soft drinks is given in Table 12.3.

Most carbonated soft drinks are sweetened, with sugar or artificial sweeteners, to the level of a 10 per cent sugar solution, which to those unhabituated is unpleasantly sweet. There is some evidence that their use stimulates the appetite. Those sweetened with sugar contain about 135 kcal/574 kJ per 330-ml can. Drinking two cans per day on top of normal food for energy balance add about 270 kcal, which could ultimately cause over 10 kg weight gain per year.

Fruit juices

Fruit juices are made by extracting the juice from fresh fruit and therefore have a similar nutrient content to whole fruit except that they have lost most of their pectin. Their popularity in Britain is increasing rapidly to the extent that they are now a major source of vitamin C in the average diet. The vitamin C content of fruit juices varies considerably (see Table 12.3), being exceptionally high in Ribena (which is made from blackcurrant juice to which sugar syrup and vitamin C are added), moderately high in citrus fruit juices, somewhat lower in pineapple and tomato juice and very low in apple juice.

Apart from being a pleasant way of receiving useful amounts of vitamin C, fruit juices are of value to people on a low sodium diet as they have a low sodium content but high potassium content (see Table 12.3).

ALCOHOLIC BEVERAGES

Alcoholic beverages are valued on account of their flavour and their stimulating effect and hardly at all as a source of energy; nevertheless, it is worth noting that the energy value of dry wine is about equal to

Table 12.4 Alcoholic beverages

Type	Example	Alcohol content (g/100 mL)	Energy value (kJ/100 mL)
Beers, draught	Bitter	2.9	124
	Mild	3.4	139
Ciders	Dry	3.8	152
	Sweet	3.7	176
Wines			
White	Sauternes	10.2	394
Red	Claret	9.6	283
Fortified	Sweet sherry	15.6	568
Spirits	Whisky	31.7	919
Liqueurs	Cherry brandy	19.8	1099

that of milk. Two glasses of wine or a pint of beer daily add about 630 kJ or 150 kcal/day, so if taken on top of a normal diet will generate a weight gain of about 10 kg. There are three main classes of alcoholic beverages: wines, beers and spirits. They are all made from sources whose main macronutrient is carbohydrate. The particular ingredient used and the way in which it is processed chiefly determines the character of the drink produced. The main types of alcoholic drink and their energy values are shown in Table 12.4.

Manufacture

Alcoholic beverages are made by a process of fermentation. The starting material used depends upon the product required. For example, whisky is made from malt or grain, rum from molasses, wine from grapes, beer from malt and cider from apples. If the starting material is essentially starch (e.g. in the form of barley which is used for making beer and whisky) fermentation occurs in three stages, as follows.

Stage 1: Conversion of starch to maltose and dextrins. This is a hydrolysis which is catalysed by the enzyme diastase. Diastase, a mixture of α- and β-amylases (see p. 94) occurs in malt, which is the name given to germinating or sprouting barley. Malt is obtained by steeping barley in water and then removing it from the water and allowing it to stand in warm air for a few days, before it is very slowly and gently dried. During the germination period amylases and some peptidases are produced, and

these immediately begin their work of hydrolysing the carbohydrate and protein present in the barley. Their action ceases, however, when the malt is dried.

When ground malt is mixed with a mash of starchy materials in water at 50–60°C and allowed to stand for about an hour, the diastase hydrolyses the starch to maltose and dextrins:

$$2(C_6H_{10}O_5)_n + nH_2O \xrightarrow{\text{diastase}} nC_{12}H_{22}O_{11}$$

Starch   Maltose

Stage 2: Conversion of maltose to glucose. This is a hydrolysis catalysed by the enzyme maltase present in yeast which is added:

$$C_{12}H_{22}O_{11} + H_2O \xrightarrow{\text{maltase}} 2C_6H_{12}O_6$$

Maltose   Glucose

After the yeast has been added the process continues for several days, the temperature being kept at about 30–35°C.

Stage 3: Conversion of glucose to alcohol. Zymase (which is the name given to a collection of at least 14 enzymes), also present in yeast, is responsible for the fermentation of glucose into alcohol. Fermentation means boiling and the name arose because during the reaction the liquid is agitated by bubbles of carbon dioxide, which produce a frothing or boiling appearance.

$$C_6H_{12}O_6 \xrightarrow{\text{zymase}} 2C_2H_5OH + 2CO_2$$

Glucose

This equation merely represents the start and finish of a complex series of reactions. The result is a solution of alcohol in water, the alcohol amounting to less than 16 per cent of the whole.

It should be noted that only stage 3 is a true fermentation, as it is only here that a gas is produced. The first two stages are examples of enzymatic hydrolysis although for convenience the whole process is usually referred to as alcoholic fermentation.

If the starting material is molasses (as when making rum) instead of a starchy material the initial hydrolysis (stage 1) is not necessary and if the starting material is a monosaccharide (as when making wine) only stage 3 is involved.

Types of alcoholic beverage

Wines

Wines are made from grapes by a process which involves four stages: pressing, fermentation, casking and bottling.

Grape juice contains the sugars glucose (grape sugar) and fructose (fruit sugar), various acids, tannin and nitrogenous materials. Grapes ferment naturally because they contain all the essential ingredients required, namely sugar, water and yeast, the latter being present as a covering or bloom on the skin. The bloom contains many varieties of yeast including wine yeasts and wild yeasts. When the juice is extracted from grapes by crushing them in a press, sulphites are added in such concentration that the undesirable wild yeasts are destroyed while the desirable wine yeasts can survive.

During the fermentation that follows, glucose and fructose are converted into alcohol. If the fermentation is continued until almost all the sugars are used up the resulting wine is dry, whereas if it is stopped while some sugars remain it is sweet. Since yeasts cannot tolerate an alcohol content greater than 16 per cent, this is the maximum that natural wines can contain; however, most wines contain 9–12 per cent.

After fermentation, wine is transferred to wooden casks or, in modern processes, large containers made of stainless steel. Some wines remain in the cask for several years, during which time a slow secondary fermentation takes place because a few live yeast cells remain from the fermentation stage. The wine slowly matures in the cask, although wines that never come into contact with wood and which are matured for relatively short periods are not necessarily of an inferior quality. Finally, the wine is bottled and maturing continues. In particular, very small amounts of esters are formed which contribute to the final bouquet or fragrance, which is such an attractive feature of a well-matured wine.

Wines are classified by colour as red, white or rosé. The colour of wine is often supposed to depend upon the colour of the grape, although this is not necessarily so since a black grape may produce a white wine. The colour of the grape results from pigment just under the skin, a black grape containing a blue-black pigment that turns red in the presence of the acids in the juice. In making a white wine, only the juice of the grape is used, whereas in making a red wine the skins are added during the pressing stage and the alcohol dissolves out the pigment, which is carried into the wine. Even the so-called white wines usually have a yellow tinge and may even be brown; this coloration is not caused by the grape but is produced while the wine is in the cask, owing to the oxidation of the tannin contained in the wood of the cask. Tannin has an astringent bitter taste and, since it is also present in the skin and stalks of grapes, red wines tend to be more bitter than white. Even so, the amount of tannin in a glass of red wine is not likely to be greater than that in a cup of tea. Tannin is a high molecular weight condensation of small polyphenol molecules. Polyphenols in the skin of grapes are extracted in the presence of alcohol as long as the skins remain in the fermentation mixture. They include flavonoids and the class of anthocyanins responsible for red colours in fruits; some are powerful antioxidants and may contribute to protection against coronary heart disease. Red wine consumption is one factor conferring benefit from Mediterranean diets. The 'French paradox' whereby people in France enjoy high fat foods, and have quite high blood cholesterol but have very little coronary heart disease, has been attributed to the consumption of red wine.

Some wines, such as champagne, sparkle: this is a result of secondary fermentation that occurs in the bottle and is brought about by the addition of a pure culture of yeast and a small amount of sugar. The carbon dioxide so produced is stored within the liquid under its own pressure. A bottle may contain five times its own volume of gas. When the cork is drawn the well-known 'pop' of the champagne is heard, caused by the sudden release of pressure, when about four-fifths of the gas escapes. Special care is taken at every stage in champagne production to ensure that the product is of the highest possible quality.

Wine has many important roles in religious ceremonies, in culture and in literature. Some of the most celebrated are now extinct (the sweet white wine of Shiraz in Persia – now Iran, and the original Tokay from Hungary). However, fabulously expensive specialist wines are still being developed (e.g. Canadian ice-wine – the grapes being harvested when frozen). A great many different wines are made in many countries of the world, although France remains pre-eminent among wine-producing countries, especially in the making of red wines such as the wines of Bordeaux (e.g. St Emilion and Médoc) and Burgundy (e.g. Beaujolais and Mâcon) and champagne. The German white wines of the Rhine and Moselle and the red Chianti of Tuscany in Italy are also renowned. Figure 12.4 shows the different types of wine that are made, with some illustrative examples. High quality wine is also made in other European countries such as Spain, Greece and Hungary, as well as in other parts of the world, notably Australia, Chile, USA (particularly California) and North and South Africa. Indeed, the red wines from Chile and whites from New Zealand (especially from Sauvignon Blanc) have now over-taken the rest of the world for quality and consistency.

Fortified wines   Wines such as port and sherry are said to be fortified because extra alcohol is added to give them an alcohol content of about 15 per cent. This has the advantage that they keep well because the alcohol content is sufficiently high to kill microorganisms that spoil natural wines.

Port, which comes from Oporto in Portugal, is made by adding brandy to wine before fermentation is complete. Genuine sherry is made from a special variety of grape which is grown near Jerez in southern Spain. It is a very dry wine which is fortified after fermentation and it is later blended with sugar if a sweet flavour is required.

Madeira and Marsala are also fortified wines as is Vermouth in which the wine is flavoured with bitter ingredients (and sugar if a sweet wine is desired).

Spirits and liqueurs

Spirits differ from wines in having been distilled after fermentation; brandy is made by distilling wine, rum by distilling fermented molasses, and so on. The special characteristics of these drinks may be associated with a particular ingredient used in the fermentation stage, as with 'Scotch' whisky which is made from barley and is said to owe much of its character to peat fires used in drying the malt. Additional character is imparted by addition of flavouring agents after distillation is complete, as with gin to which juniper berries and other flavouring ingredients are added before a second distillation. Spirits

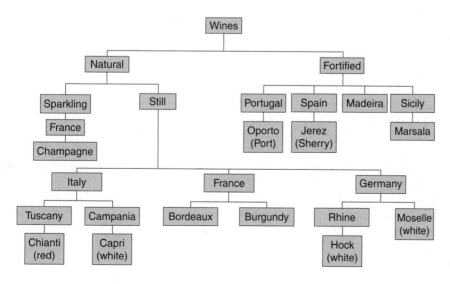

Figure 12.4 *Types of wine*

such as whisky also gain character by being matured in wood casks (usually oak) for several years before they are drunk. Slow chemical changes occur during this time; some ethyl alcohol is oxidized to acetaldehyde, other alcohols are oxidized to corresponding aldehydes, sweet fruity-smelling esters are formed and these changes impart a mellowness of flavour and fragrance of bouquet to the product.

Whisky, and most spirits on sale worldwide, have an alcohol content of about 30–40 per cent (see Table 12.4), but are also described as being 70 per cent proof – an ancient term in which 'proof' spirit was defined as being of such a strength that when mixed with gunpowder it would ignite when a light was applied. In Britain, proof spirit is now defined as containing 57 per cent alcohol by volume and 50 per cent by weight. Cask-strength whisky may contain up to 100 per cent proof spirit.

Liqueurs are made by steeping herbs in strong spirits for a week or two and subsequently distilling. The richly flavoured distillate contains essential oils and other flavouring matters from the plants, and to this is added sugar and colouring matter.

Many of the famous liqueurs originated in monasteries and the methods and materials used in preparing them are kept secret. An aura of romance surrounds even those liqueurs with no monastic associations. Magical health properties are claimed – all without any foundation. The recipe of the renowned Scottish liqueur Drambuie, literally 'the drink that satisfies', is said to have been given to an ancestor of the present manufacturer by Prince Charles Edward Stuart in 1746. The Prince is said to have divulged the secret recipe as a token of gratitude for the help he received in escaping from the Scottish mainland to the island of Skye. It is made from Scotch whisky, Scottish herbs and honey (presumably from Scottish bees). It is very sweet and scorned by aficionados of malt whisky.

Beer

Beer is an alcoholic drink made by the fermentation of malted barley, the other essential ingredients used in its manufacture being hops, yeast and water. Ale, lager, porter and stout are all beers and they are all made by methods which are similar in principle but differ in detail. The essential stages of making beer are the same as those described on p. 179, except that hops are added to the liquor, known as wort which is boiled to extract the flavour of the hops before stage 2 of the process begins. In making typical British beer, a top-fermentation technique is used in which the yeast floats on top of the fermenting liquor. In brewing lager, however, a different strain of yeast is used and a bottom-fermentation technique is used in which the yeast works at the bottom of the tank.

Most beers contain 2.5–6.5 g alcohol/100 mL. They also contain small amounts of riboflavin and niacin. Brown ales are the weakest, containing only 2.2 g alcohol/100 mL and are inferior in flavour because they are matured for only a few days. Bitter ales have more flavour both because they are matured for longer than mild ales and because more hops are used. Lagers are matured for several months at a low temperature. Stout is characterized by a dark colour and often a relatively high alcohol content; a strong stout contains about 4 g alcohol/100 mL. It is made from special malt mixtures which are heated to a high temperature so as to produce some caramel, which imparts a dark-brown colour to the liquor. Stout is no more nutritious than any other beer.

Effects of alcohol on the body

Alcohol must be regarded as a foodstuff because in the body it can be broken down to provide energy. It is a more concentrated source of energy than either carbohydrate or protein, and has an available energy value of 29 kJ/g (7 kcal/g). It also has properties similar to that of a drug and affects the central nervous system. These two effects must be considered together when assessing the desirability of alcohol as a source of energy. The nature of the effects of alcohol on the body, varying from mild stimulation when a small amount is consumed to loss of coordination and even death when a large quantity is taken, as indicated in Fig. 12.5. Consumption of a pint of beer produces a maximum level of about 0.05 per cent alcohol in the blood, which will certainly affect judgement and reaction times, for as long as 24 hours. This effect is not perceived by the drinker.

Unlike most foods, alcohol can be absorbed by the body without prior digestion and this takes place mainly in the small intestine, but also through the walls of the stomach. Absorption may take anything

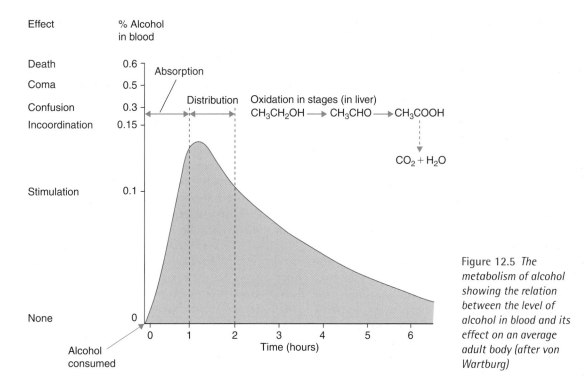

Figure 12.5 *The metabolism of alcohol showing the relation between the level of alcohol in blood and its effect on an average adult body (after von Wartburg)*

from 30 minutes to 2 hours depending on the concentration of alcohol in the beverage consumed, the amount taken and the nature and amount of food eaten with it or immediately beforehand. An average time for absorption is about an hour.

The fate of alcohol in the body is summarized in Fig. 12.5. After absorption the alcohol is distributed through the body in the bloodstream, and thereafter it is broken down in a series of oxidative steps with liberation of energy. The breakdown process is controlled by a series of enzymes, each step being controlled by its own enzymes. Initial oxidation of alcohol to acetaldehyde is mainly controlled by alcohol dehydrogenase and, as its name indicates, this step involves removal of hydrogen. It is followed by further oxidation to acetic acid, the most important enzyme involved in this step being aldehyde dehydrogenase. These initial breakdown steps occur in the liver, and the acetic acid produced then becomes part of the general body pool of this substance and is further oxidized, in a complex process, to carbon dioxide and water. Alcohol is oxidized in the body rather slowly and only about 7 g can be oxidized in an hour. This means that alcohol is removed from

the blood at a slow rate and that it can only make a small overall contribution to energy needs.

Alcohol intake and health

Since 1945 alcohol consumption in the UK has increased rapidly. In a 20-year period between 1962 and 1982 consumption of wine increased by 240 per cent, that of spirits by 95 per cent and that of beer by 22 per cent. It continues to increase, linked most directly to prosperity. In population surveys, the highest intakes are amongst the wealthiest. The effects of such an increase in alcohol consumption are not fully known, but the cost in health and social terms is considerable. The number of deaths caused by alcohol has risen as a result of road traffic accidents – for innocent victims, as well as intoxicated drivers. Deaths caused by cirrhosis of the liver, which is closely linked to alcohol consumption, increased by 60 per cent in the 1970s. It is also recorded that the number of people entering mental hospitals each year as a result of alcoholism or related problems doubled in the 1970s. It is estimated that almost a million people in England and

Wales are either alcoholics or have severe drink problems.

An excessive intake of alcohol has a damaging effect on health, including cirrhosis of the liver mentioned above. If alcohol replaces fat as the main energy source for the liver, metabolism of fat ceases and lipid accumulates in the liver producing what is known as a 'fatty liver'. Prolonged excessive consumption of alcohol, even when it is part of a nutritionally adequate diet, leads to varying degrees of liver damage, ranging from a reversible fatty liver to alcoholic hepatitis and finally irreversible cirrhosis. The same amount of alcoholic drink has proportionally greater effects on women, mainly because they tend to be smaller than men. Thus the limits for healthy drinking are set at 21 units for men, but 14 units for women.

High alcohol consumption also contributes to obesity and may lead to malnutrition as a result of deficiencies of mineral elements and vitamins. While mineral deficiency is relatively uncommon, deficiency of B vitamins – particularly thiamin and folate – is relatively common. Such vitamin deficiency may arise in a number of ways, the most likely being that the high energy content of alcohol consumed reduces the intake of other foods, some of which would have provided the necessary B vitamins. In addition, alcohol may impair absorption of B vitamins (particularly folate) and other nutrients. Conversely, alcohol can increase the absorption of iron, by inactivating the normal controlled pathway. This results in haemosiderosis, with excess iron accumulating in liver, joints, etc., and a variety of toxic consequence.

There is consistent evidence from surveys that modest alcohol intake (1–2 glasses of wine daily) is associated with lower rates of heart disease than occurs in complete abstainers. Some of this effect may be to do with alcohol abstainers, including a number of individuals with poor health who have been advised to stop drinking alcohol, but alcohol does increase plasma high-density lipoprotein (HDL) cholesterol, and high HDL cholesterol is well established to protect against heart disease. It has also been proposed that the phenolic (flavonoid) antioxidants in red wine may help protect against heart disease. In the laboratory, red wine phenolics reduce the oxidation of low-density lipoprotein (LDL) cholesterol (a process believed to accelerate heart disease), and there is some evidence that this happens in the bloodstream after drinking red wine.

> ## Key points
>
> - Water throughput and hydration are critical to human health. The balance between intake and output must always provide enough for kidney function, to excrete toxic waste products
> - Depending on conditions, 2 to 20 litres of water, in drinks, needs to be consumed, but excess intake (over 1.5 litres/hour) can be dangerous
> - Water contributes importantly to the consistency of foods, and small changes can be critical
> - Water provides a vehicle for both water-soluble compounds, and lipids in colloidal form, thereby contributing subtle and complex flavours particularly reflected by the vast range of beverages
> - Water is closely related to alcohol chemically, and alcoholic beverages provide major social and religious functions, as well as a balance between pleasure and the horrors of intoxication or dependency

Chapter summary

Water is the most vital but often the most forgotten nutrient after oxygen. These two are our two nutrients provided directly from the physical environment without the need for processing by plants or other animals. We have sophisticated control mechanisms to regulate our supply of water, to match our needs, and our palates detect very small changes in the water content of foods. Water is beautiful.

FURTHER READING

www.highland-spring.com

www.teacouncil.co.uk

The Natural Mineral Water, Spring Water and Bottled Drinking Water (Amendment) (England) Regulations, 2004, Statutory Instrument 2004 no. 656.

The Natural Mineral Water, Spring Water and Bottled Drinking Water (Amendment) (Scotland) Regulations, 2004, Scottish Statutory Instrument 2004 no. 132.

The Natural Mineral Water, Spring Water and Bottled Drinking Water Regulations, 1999, Statutory Instrument 1999 no. 1540.

13

Mineral elements

The elements which occur most abundantly in food are carbon, hydrogen, oxygen and nitrogen. At least 25 other 'mineral elements' also occur in foods, sometimes in minute amounts, and may find their way into our bodies. About 16 of these are known to be essential to life and must be present in the diet.

The mineral elements which the body requires in largest amounts are listed in Table 13.1. Others, usually known as trace elements, which are required by the body in much smaller quantities, are shown in Table 13.2. The definition of 'trace elements' is arbitrary and not fixed: a trace element is one which is essential for normal cell function, but required only in tiny amounts.

Mineral elements are used by the body in a great variety of ways. They may form part of the rigid structure of the body (e.g. the skeleton). They may be present in the cell fluids (potassium is particularly important) or, like sodium, in extracellular fluids. Their main functions and sources, which are shown in Tables 13.1 and 13.3, are discussed in greater detail below. Trace elements are mostly important as cofactors for enzymes.

The data given in Table 13.1 should be regarded as estimates and not as precisely determined amounts. The quantity of a particular mineral element present in a body will obviously depend on body weight. Whether a person of a given weight is tall, well-built and muscular or short and stout with a comparatively small skeleton will also be relevant. Similarly, the figures for average daily intakes cannot be other than rough averages because of variations in food availability and in individual appetites and tastes.

Average daily intake of minerals must be distinguished from average daily requirement and it should be borne in mind that only part of what is eaten may be absorbed and used by the body. Elements, such as sodium, potassium and chlorine, which form soluble salts, are readily absorbed. Others, such as iron, calcium, magnesium and zinc, may form insoluble compounds which are less readily absorbed by the body. In such cases an allowance has to be made when estimating dietary requirements to take into account the proportion of the intake that is not absorbed by the body. Many mineral elements can be toxic in high concentration, and so the processes of absorption from the gut are regulated to increase absorption when there is low supply or deficiency, and to limit absorption when there is less need. For some, but not all (e.g. iron, but not zinc), there are stores within the body which can accommodate potentially toxic excesses and provide for times of dietary insufficiency.

MAJOR MINERAL ELEMENTS

Calcium and phosphorus

These two elements account for about 75 per cent of the mineral elements in the body, and each of them has a number of essential functions to perform. Hence, the body must receive a sufficient supply of each of them if it is to remain healthy.

Table 13.1 Major mineral elements

Element	Approx. adult daily intake	Approx. adult body content	Functions in body	Main food sources
Calcium (Ca)	1 g	1000 g	Present in bones and teeth. Necessary for blood clotting, muscle contraction and nerve activity	Milk, cheese, bread and flour (if fortified), cereals, green vegetables
Phosphorus (P)	1.5 g	700 g	Present in bones and teeth. Essential for energy storage and transfer, cell division and reproduction	Milk, cheese, bread and cereals, meat and meat products
Sodium (Na)	2–10 g	100 g	Present in body fluids as Na^+. Essential for maintenance of fluid balance in body and for nerve activity and muscle contraction	Main source is salt (sodium chloride, NaCl) used in food processing, cooking and at the table. Bread, cereal products and meat products are the main sources in processed foods
Chlorine (Cl)	3–5 g	100 g	Present in gastric juice and body fluids as Cl^-	
Potassium (K)	2–3 g	140 g	Present in cell fluids as K^+. Similar role to sodium	Widely distributed in vegetables, meat, milk, fruit and fruit juices
Iron (Fe)	10–15 mg	4 g	Essential component of haemoglobin of blood cells	Meat and offal, bread and flour, potatoes and vegetables
Magnesium (Mg)	0.3 g	25 g	Present in bone and cell fluids. Needed for activity of some enzymes	Milk, bread and other cereal products, potatoes and vegetables
Zinc (Zn)	9–12 mg	2.5 g	Essential for the activity of several enzymes involved in energy changes and protein formation	Meat and meat products, milk and cheese. Bread flour and cereal products

Table 13.2 Some trace elements

Element	Approx. average daily intake	Approx. adult body content	Main food sources	Functions in body
Cobalt (Co)	0.3 mg	1.5 mg	Liver and other meat	Required as vitamin B_{12}, for formation of red blood cells
Copper (Cu)	3.5 mg	75 mg	Green vegetables, fish, liver	Component of many enzymes. Necessary for haemoglobin formation
Chromium (Cr)	0.15 mg	1 mg	Liver, cereals, beer, yeast	Contained in all tissues. May be involved in glucose metabolism
Fluorine (F)	1.8 mg	2.5 g	Tea, sea food, water	Required for bone and tooth formation
Iodine (I)	0.2 mg	25 mg	Milk, sea food, iodized salt	Component of thyroid hormones
Manganese (Mn)	3.5 mg	15 mg	Tea, cereals, pulses, nuts	Forms part of some enzyme systems
Molybdenum (Mo)	0.15 mg	?	Kidney, cereals, vegetables	Enzyme activation
Selenium (Se)	0.2 mg	25 mg	Cereals, meat, fish	Present in some enzymes. Associated with vitamin E activity

Table 13.3 Iron content of foods

Food	Iron content (mg/100 g)
Kidney (pig's, fried)	9.1
Liver (lamb's, fried)	7.7
Flour (wholemeal)	4.0
Oats (porridge)	3.8
Beef (cooked)	3.0
Bread (brown or wholemeal)	2.3
Sardines (canned)	2.3
Eggs (boiled)	2.0
Flour (72% extraction)	2.0
Bread (white)	1.7
Spinach (boiled)	1.6
Baked beans	1.4
Cod (fried)	0.5
Cabbage (boiled)	0.4
Cheese (Cheddar)	0.4
Potatoes (boiled)	0.4
Apples	0.1
Milk	0.1

Functions of calcium and phosphorus

Almost all the calcium and 80 per cent of the phosphorus in the body are found in the bones and teeth as calcium phosphate, $Ca_3(PO_4)_2$, or more precisely, as the calcium phosphate derivative calcium hydroxyapatite, $Ca_{10}(PO_4)_6(OH)_2$.

The small amount of calcium (about 1 per cent or 5–10 g) not used for bone or tooth formation is found in the blood and body fluids as calcium ions or in combination with protein. It is mostly bound to albumin in the blood – thus its total concentration varies with albumin – but the active 'ionized' form is held constant. It is involved in muscle contraction (including the maintenance of a regular heartbeat), blood clotting and the activity of several important enzymes. The concentration of calcium in the blood is kept constant by the action of hormones produced by the thyroid and parathyroid glands. The presence of too much or too little calcium in the blood seriously disturbs the function of the muscle fibres and nerve cells.

Most of the phosphorus present in the body is in bones or teeth, but about 100 g is distributed throughout the cells and fluids of the body. Phosphorus is present in the nucleic acids which form part of all cells and are concerned with manufacture of the body's proteins and transmission of hereditary characteristics. Adenosine triphosphate (ATP) plays a key role in the complex processes by which the body obtains energy through the oxidation of nutrients (see p. 103). It also plays an essential part in the metabolism of fats and proteins. Phosphate ions are present in the blood and help with 'buffering' to keep its pH value constant at about 7.4.

Calcium and phosphorus requirements

The reference nutrient intake (RNI) for calcium depends upon age and sex and varies from 350 mg/day to 1000 mg/day. Additional amounts are specified for pregnant and nursing mothers, who require additional amounts to prevent loss of calcium from the mother's bones. Full details are given in Table 13.4. Normally only about 20–30 per cent of the calcium in the diet is absorbed. The rate of absorption may drop to even lower levels if insufficient vitamin D is available. There is some physiological regulation of calcium absorption according to need, so for example, a greater proportion of dietary calcium is absorbed during pregnancy and lactation.

Phytates, which are present in wholemeal bread and wholegrain cereals, may interfere with the absorption of calcium. If wholemeal bread or wholegrain cereals are eaten regularly, however, the body is able to adapt to their presence and the effect of phytates on calcium absorption is less severe than was at one time supposed.

Oxalates, which are present in small amounts in rhubarb and spinach, may react with calcium present in other foods to form insoluble calcium oxalate, thus rendering the calcium unavailable to the body. Luckily, rhubarb and spinach do not constitute a major part of most people's diet, and so we need not be unduly concerned about their detrimental effect on the absorption of calcium.

Some of the calcium absorbed from the diet is subsequently lost in the urine and a smaller amount may be lost in sweat. Such losses must be made up to maintain the concentration of calcium ions in the blood at a level of about 10 mg/100 mL. If dietary sources of calcium are insufficient the calcium required is taken from the bones, and if this continues over a long period serious decalcification may occur. We tend to regard our bones as a fixed and

Table 13.4 Reference nutrient intakes of minerals

Age	Calcium (mg/d)	Phosphorus[a] (mg/d)	Magnesium (mg/d)	Sodium[b] (mg/d)	Potassium[c] (mg/d)	Chloride[d] (mg/d)	Iron (mg/d)	Zinc (mg/d)	Copper (mg/d)	Selenium (µg/d)	Iodine (µg/d)
0–3 months	525	400	55	210	800	320	1.7	4.0	0.2	10	50
4–6 months	525	400	60	280	850	400	4.3	4.0	0.3	13	60
7–9 months	525	400	75	320	700	500	7.8	5.0	0.3	10	60
10–12 months	525	400	80	350	700	500	7.8	5.0	0.3	10	60
1–3 years	350	270	85	500	800	800	6.9	5.0	0.4	15	70
4–6 years	450	350	120	700	1100	1100	6.1	6.5	0.6	20	100
7–10 years	550	450	200	1200	2000	1800	8.7	7.0	0.7	30	110
Males											
11–14 years	1000	775	280	1600	3100	2500	11.3	9.0	0.8	45	130
15–18 years	1000	775	300	1600	3500	2500	11.3	9.5	1.0	70	140
19–50 years	700	550	300	1600	3500	2500	8.7	9.5	1.2	75	140
50+ years	700	550	300	1600	3500	2500	8.7	9.5	1.2	75	140
Females											
11–14 years	800	625	280	1600	3100	2500	14.8[e]	9.0	0.8	45	130
15–18 years	800	625	300	1600	3500	2500	14.8[e]	7.0	1.0	60	140
19–50 years	700	550	270	1600	3500	2500	14.8[e]	7.0	1.2	60	140
50+ years	700	550	270	1600	3500	2500	8.7	7.0	1.2	60	140
Pregnancy	–	–	–	–	–	–	–	–	–	–	–
Lactation											
0–4 months	+550	+440	+50	–	–	–	–	+6.0	+0.3	+15	–
4+ months	+550	+440	+50	–	–	–	–	+2.5	+0.3	+15	–

– No increment.
[a]Phosphorus RNI is set equal to calcium in molar terms.
[b]1 mmol sodium = 23 mg.
[c]1 mmol potassium = 39 mg.
[d]Corresponds to sodium 1 mmol = 35.5 mg.
[e]Insufficient for women with high menstrual losses where the most practical way of meeting iron requirements in to take iron supplements.
DOH 1991. Crown Copyright material is reproduced with the permission of the Controller of HMSO and the Queen's Printer for Scotland.

immutable part of our bodies but, in fact, they are in a state of continuous change. New bone is constantly being formed and old bone lost by exchange of calcium ions between bone and blood. While growth is taking place, calcium is absorbed at a slightly greater rate than it is lost.

The bones of a newborn baby are soft and consist mainly of collagen. They become hard, or calcified, when minute crystals of calcium phosphate (or hydroxyapatite) are deposited in the soft collagen framework. Bone development continues until peak bone mass is achieved, usually sometime between the ages of 20 and 30 years. From this point onwards calcium is gradually lost from the bones which, over a period of time, become less dense. If too much bone loss occurs the condition known as osteoporosis – literally, porous bones – may result. This condition affects many women (and some men) from the age of about 45 years onwards. Bone shrinkage and brittle bones which fracture easily are characteristic of osteoporosis. Osteoporosis is responsible for most bone fractures in older people, especially the vertebra, wrists and hips and many deaths occur as a consequence of these fractures.

Osteoporosis occurs with disease and physical inactivity and shortage of sex hormones, especially the female sex hormone oestrogen. This is why postmenopausal women, whose bodies secrete less oestrogen, are more likely to suffer from osteoporosis than younger women. The onset of the disease cannot be delayed or prevented by increasing the calcium content of the diet in later life but higher calcium intake throughout life may be beneficial. Achievement of high bone mass through good nutrition and exercise during the period of bone growth, however, is beneficial. Studies have also shown that in areas where water has been fluoridated the incidence of osteoporosis is lower. As fluoride increases retention of calcium results in denser, but possibly more brittle bones.

Vitamin D is essential for calcium absorption together with parathyroid hormone. Deficiency of vitamin D, with poor calcium absorption by young children causes the disease rickets, which is characterized by stunted growth and deformed leg bones. A similar condition in adults is known as osteomalacia. This disease was at one time common in underdeveloped countries amongst women whose bones had suffered calcium loss through repeated pregnancies and where for religious reasons women are covered from the sun which prevents synthesis of vitamin D by the skin. Rickets and osteomalacia are still found in some migrant communities in western countries (especially vegetarians who obtain little vitamin D from foods). Kidney disease is another cause, because in order to function vitamin D must be activated by hydroxylation in healthy kidneys.

The average British diet contains about 800 mg (women) to 1000 mg (men) of calcium per day and it is unlikely that normal diets in the UK or other western countries will be deficient in the mineral. Calcium deficiency may still occur, however, even when dietary sources are adequate, if sufficient vitamin D, which is needed for its absorption, is not available. Calcium is absorbed into the blood through the lining of the small intestine by becoming bound to protein. In the absence of vitamin D the calcium–protein complex cannot be formed and absorption of calcium does not occur. The blood concentrations of calcium is not a good guide to whole body statue because calcium is mainly bound to albumin in the blood, and blood concentrations are also affected by movement into and out of bone, under the influence of parathyroid hormone.

Phosphorus is found in almost all foods mainly as phosphate. The average daily intake is about 1.5 g for men and 1.1 g for women and it is unlikely to be lacking in a normal diet. Table 13.4 shows that the RNI varies from 270 to 775 mg/day, with additional amounts for lactating women.

Dietary sources of calcium and phosphorus

Only a few foods are rich in calcium and phosphorus and the most important sources in the British diet are milk, cheese, bread, sea foods and fortified flour. About half the average daily intake comes from dairy foods, one-quarter from bread and other cereal foods and the remainder from meat, seafood, vegetables and drinks (including hard water). Bread and flour in the UK (except wholemeal) are fortified with added chalk (see p. 119) to guard against inadequate calcium intake. The calcium in dairy products is readily absorbed and half a litre of milk contains over three-quarters of the daily RNI for an adult man. The calcium and phosphorus content of some foods is given in Table 13.5.

Strange as it may seem, water may be a good source of calcium in those areas where it is 'hard'

Table 13.5 Calcium and phosphorus content of foods

Food	Calcium (mg/100 g)	Phosphorus (mg/100 g)
Dairy produce and eggs		
Cheese (Cheddar)	739	505
Milk	118	93
Eggs (boiled)	57	200
Butter	18	23
Meat and fish		
Sardines (canned)	540	510
Fish (white, raw)	14	200
Liver (lamb's, raw)	6	390
Beef (raw)	5	200
Cereals		
Bread (white)	177	95
Flour (70% extraction)	140	110
Bread (wholemeal)	106	202
Rice (boiled)	18	54
Vegetables and fruit		
Spinach (boiled)	160	28
Oranges	47	21
Cabbage (Savoy, boiled)	33	25
Potatoes (old, boiled)	5	31
Apples	4	11

(see p. 174). For example, a litre of London tap water contains about 200 mg of calcium – over one-quarter of the daily RNI. Some carbonated drinks made with hard water are good source of calcium.

Vegetables cooked in hard water may pick up some calcium from it. When hard water is used for making tea or coffee, however, most of the calcium is deposited as calcium carbonate in the kettle or percolator.

As already explained, there is no danger of the body going short of phosphorus except on a starvation diet. The muscle, brain and nervous system are rich in phosphorus and become depleted during undernutrition and illness, with many functional consequences. Refeeding after starvation can precipitate the 'refeeding syndrome', including low blood phosphate, if extra phosphate is not provided for recovery of damaged tissue.

Iron

Iron accounts for about 0.1 per cent of the mineral elements in the body and the total amount of iron in the body of a healthy adult is only about 4 g. Over half of this is found in the red blood cells where it is critically important in the pigment haemoglobin which transports oxygen from the lungs to the tissues. Red blood cells have a life of about 4 months, and it has been estimated that some 10 million of these cells are withdrawn from circulation every second. If the iron contained in these cells passed out of the body it would be difficult to replace it from food. Fortunately, most of the iron released is conserved and it is used to form new red corpuscles, which are produced in the bone marrow. In this way, the iron present in haemoglobin is used repeatedly.

A small proportion of the iron in the body is present in the muscle protein myoglobin; some cell enzymes, such as the cytochromes, also contain iron. The remainder of the iron in the body is stored in the liver, spleen and bone marrow in the form of specialized iron-binding proteins called ferritin and haemosiderin. These iron stores may contain up to 1 g iron in men, and about half that amount in women. The iron present can only be released slowly and so it is of no use in combating sudden shortages. The stored iron is of great importance during the first 6 months of a baby's life because only a small amount of iron is present in milk.

Dietary sources of iron

The main dietary sources of iron are meat, bread and other cereal products, potatoes and vegetables. However, even the richest dietary sources of iron contain only very small amounts: lamb's liver, for example, one of the richest sources, contains only about one part iron in 10 000. The main dietary sources of iron are listed in Table 13.3. Bread and other cereal-based foods provide about 40 per cent of the total iron intake in an average British diet. Meat and vegetables each provide about 20 per cent and eggs about 3 per cent. Because of major differences in absorption, dietary sources of haem iron (meat and fish) are much more valuable than non-haem iron in foods of vegetable origin.

Iron is one of the mineral elements which may be lacking in an average diet and for this reason it is added to all flour in Britain, except wholemeal flour, so that its iron content is at least 1.65 mg/100 g. Unfortunately, however, studies have shown that most of the metallic iron added to flour passes through the body unabsorbed. Iron deficiency is one of the major global nutritional deficiencies identified by the World Health Organization (WHO). Its main impact is among young (menstruating) women.

Iron requirements

The body utilizes absorbed iron very efficiently and only a minimal amount is needed each day to replace losses. Only a small portion of the iron present in the diet is absorbed by the body, however, and so dietary intake should be much greater than the amount needed to replenish losses.

Adults usually absorb only about 15 per cent of the iron in their diet, but individuals who have a special need for iron, such as growing children or pregnant women, are able to absorb more. Many factors affect the rate of absorption and the source of iron is among them. The iron in meat or offal – haem iron – is organically bound and is absorbed much more readily than the non-haem iron present in plants. It has been shown, for example, that only a small percentage of the iron added to non-wholemeal flour to replace that lost during milling is absorbed. Similarly, only 2–3 per cent of the non-haem iron present in vegetables may be absorbed.

The presence of ascorbic acid (vitamin C) in the diet can promote the absorption of non-haem iron because it reduces ferric iron to the absorbable ferrous state and helps to keep it as ferrous iron. Absorption of non-haem iron is also promoted by alcohol, but tea, which forms insoluble tannic acid salts with iron, has the opposite effect and can contribute to anaemia if drunk with meals in a vegetarian diet.

The RNI for iron is based on an assumed absorption rate of 15 per cent, and the amounts needed for growth and accumulation of an iron store are 11.3 mg/day and 14.8 mg/day for adult males and females, respectively. Women with high menstrual losses may require more, and this can be ensured by taking iron supplements. The increased needs of pregnancy and lactation can normally be satisfied from the body's iron stores in the absence of losses through menstruation. Supplementation of the dietary intake is usually only required when the maternal iron stores are low at the start of pregnancy. Full details of requirements at different stages in life are given in Table 13.4.

There are relatively large stores of iron in the liver, first to provide for times of dietary insufficiency, or for increased need (e.g. menstruation and pregnancy) and second to be able to avoid excess iron accumulating in the bloodstream or tissues. Stored iron is all in bound form because free iron is very toxic. Ten iron tablets – or less – can be fatal to a young child. In the diseases haemochromatosis and haemosiderosis, there is excess iron accumulation with toxic damage to kidneys, pancreas and heart. Iron tablets, if taken in excess, are very toxic. If the amount of iron provided by the diet is insufficient the deficiency is made up from the body's iron stores. With a prolonged shortage the stores of iron will eventually become so depleted that the amount of haemoglobin in the blood will fall below normal levels – a condition known as anaemia: iron deficiency is one of several dietary causes, others being deficiency of folate, vitamin B_{12} and general malnutrition. Iron deficiency characteristically causes the marrow to produce only very small red blood cells. It is regarded by WHO as one of the most important global nutritional diseases, with many millions affected worldwide. Dietary iron deficiency is relatively common in western countries, especially among vegetarians who do not follow well-balanced diets. Clinical iron deficiency anaemia usually also involves chronic loss of blood (e.g. from an ulcer), but it is most frequent in menstruating women with poor diets.

Sodium and potassium

Sodium and potassium are highly reactive metals – so reactive that they combine vigorously with water. In food or in the body, however, they are present as salts such as sodium chloride, NaCl, or potassium chloride, KCl. In these compounds the sodium and potassium are present as cations, Na^+ and K^+, respectively, and not in the highly reactive metallic form. Sodium chloride is familiar to us all as common salt and it is mainly in this form that sodium is present in foods. In the body, positively charged sodium and potassium ions are accompanied by an equal number of anions (i.e. negatively charged ions) to ensure electrical neutrality. The anions are mainly chloride and phosphate ions, but other anions (e.g. carbonate and bicarbonate ions) may occur in food and they also play an important part in body processes.

Functions of sodium and potassium

Almost all the sodium and potassium in the body is found in the soft body tissues and body fluids. Sodium ions are mainly present in the extracellular tissue fluids and blood plasma, whereas potassium ions are found mainly inside the cells. About 100 g sodium (i.e. about 250 g sodium chloride) and an equivalent amount of potassium salts are present in the body. The volume and osmotic pressure of the blood and tissue fluids are closely related to the concentrations of sodium and potassium ions, which are precisely controlled by the body's regulating mechanisms governing the amount lost in urine and sweat, particularly by the hormone aldosterone.

The average diet is rich in sodium and potassium and both are easily absorbed by the body. Any excess is removed by the kidneys and excreted in the urine. Some loss also occurs in the form of sweat. When sodium and potassium are removed from the body, water is also lost. This is why we become thirsty after eating salty food.

Sodium and potassium are crucially involved in the transmission of nerve impulses and in muscle contraction, including the beating of the heart.

Dietary sources of sodium and potassium

The sodium content of most foods in their natural state is usually quite low, but salt is added to many processed foods. Thus, although the sodium content of fresh meat is low, bacon, sausages, pies and most other meat products contain substantial amounts of added salt. The same is true for fish: fresh fish contains little sodium but kippers or smoked fish may be very salty. Salt is also added to most butter and margarine, canned vegetables, cheese, bread and some breakfast cereals. Indeed, virtually all processed foods are salted to a level of about 1 per cent by weight. Vegetables cooked in salted water contain much more sodium than fresh vegetables. Concentrated foods, such as Marmite, are particularly rich in sodium but if eaten in small quantities it may not greatly affect the total sodium intake.

Despite its presence in so many foods, most people like even more salt and about one-fifth of the salt in the British diet is added during cooking or at the table. One-third comes from cereals and bread, about one-sixth from meat and meat products and the remainder from other foods.

Potassium is present in nearly all fresh or frozen foods, including those of vegetable and animal origin. The main sources in a UK diet are fruit, vegetables, meat and milk. Fruit and fruit juices contain much more potassium than sodium. In canned and processed foods, much potassium is replaced by sodium.

Sodium and potassium requirements

Sodium chloride (or other sodium salts) must be present in our diet to replace sodium lost through sweating and in the urine, where sodium is excreted for exchange for potassium (as well as the excess consumed). The daily requirement varies a little according to how much a person perspires, but salt concentration in sweat falls with increased sweating, or if body sodium content falls. A daily salt intake of 2–3 g should provide sufficient sodium for most people. These variable requirements make it difficult to recommend individual daily intake levels.

The average daily salt intake in Britain is estimated to be about 9–10 g, although many individuals consume more than this. It is difficult to consume much less because so much salt is added to so many foods. Thus, it is virtually impossible to consume less than the minimum requirement. Very active people who lose more sodium in sweat more than compensate from the salt in their increased food intake. The main concern, therefore, in recommending daily amounts of sodium, is to avoid high intakes.

Babies less than about 1 year old are unable to deal effectively with excess sodium because their kidney functions are not fully developed. An infant fed only on breast milk will receive only about 0.5 g salt/day, but two or three times as much may be consumed if cow's milk is used. The salt content of powdered milk for babies and other baby foods is kept low to avoid an excessive intake. Salt should never be added to home-prepared baby food and salty spreads, such as Marmite, should not be given to very young babies.

Strong evidence has accumulated recently for a causal link between high salt intake and the development of high blood pressure, or hypertension, in later life. Some studies indicate that about 10–20 per cent of the population, who show special sensitivity to salt, are particularly likely to be affected. Others find that exposure of young children to high sodium intakes can have permanent, long-term effects on blood pressure. High blood pressure is one of the risk factors associated with coronary heart disease and cerebrovascular disease or 'stroke'. These serious and common diseases would be markedly reduced by quite modest reductions in sodium consumption in the population. The Scientific Advisory Committee on Nutrition (UK) has reviewed the evidence on the association between salt and high blood pressure and recommended that consumption of salt should be decreased to no more than 6 g/day (2.3 g sodium). This can only be achieved by an informed public provided with foods and meals which contain much less salt than at present. High salt intake is a special problem for obese people because they need to eat more calories in order to stay obese, and most of their food is salted in manufacture.

The RNIs for sodium specified in the 1991 Committee on Medical Aspects of Food Policy (COMA) report on Dietary Reference Values are given in Table 13.4. The RNI for an adult – i.e. 1600 mg/day – is equivalent to 4069 mg of sodium chloride, which is roughly one teaspoonful daily.

Potassium is present in such a wide variety of foods, and is so readily absorbed, that a dietary deficiency is unlikely to occur outside the context of undernutrition or from the use of some drugs (e.g. diuretics). The RNIs, which range from 700 to 3500 mg/day, are given in Table 13.4.

Magnesium

A human adult contains about 20–25 g magnesium and most of it is found in the bones as magnesium phosphate. Magnesium is also present in ionic form in all tissues where it plays a part in many reactions involved in energy utilization, and in nerve muscle and brain function.

Magnesium occurs widely in foods. It is present in green vegetables as a part of the chlorophyll molecule but vegetables provide less than 10 per cent of the magnesium in an average British diet. Meat is a good source, providing around 12 per cent but the greatest contribution is from cereals and cereal products (27 per cent).The body regulates magnesium absorption very efficiently. Dietary intakes above 2 g/day pass through the body unabsorbed: below this level, the absorption rate increases as the intake decreases and hence a deficiency rarely occurs. The RNI for adult males and females is 300 and 270 mg/day, respectively; details of RNIs for other age groups are given in Table 13.4. Magnesium can be lost from the body when there is tissue damage, diarrhoea with diabetes and with the use of diuretic drugs. Alcoholics may suffer from dietary magnesium deficiency. In these situations, extra magnesium may be required. However, supplements of magnesium (e.g. milk of magnesia) cause diarrhoea, which actually aggravates the problem, so repletion usually has to be slowly, from foods.

During recovery from severe weight loss growing tissues use up blood magnesium rapidly and extra must be provided to avoid serious consequences (part of the 'refeeding syndrome').

Zinc

An adequate intake of zinc is essential for the maintenance of good health. It forms part of the enzyme carbonic anhydrase found in red blood cells, which assists in releasing carbon dioxide from venous blood passing through the lungs. Zinc is also important as a necessary constituent of over 100 other enzymes, and it plays a part in protein and carbohydrate metabolism. Prolonged shortage of zinc can lead to retarded physical and mental development in adolescents.

Zinc is present in a wide variety of foods, including meat and meat products, milk, bread and other cereal products and the estimated daily average intake in Britain is 10–15 mg. The RNI for adult males and females is 9.5 mg/day and 7.0 mg/day, respectively; RNIs for other age groups are given in Table 13.4.

Usually only about 30 per cent of the zinc present in the diet is absorbed but if dietary intake is low the absorption rate may rise to 50 per cent. There are no body stores of zinc, so it is needed every day.

OTHER MINERAL ELEMENTS

The body requires small quantities of other mineral elements in addition to those already considered. They are sometimes referred to as trace elements and the more important of them are listed in Table 13.2.

Some trace elements form part of enzyme and hormone molecules which regulate the complex biochemical processes taking place within the body. Dietary requirements of most trace elements are not known with certainty, but RNIs have been specified for copper, iodine and selenium, and these are given in Table 13.4.

Normal diets supply a sufficiency of all the trace elements, except iodine, fluorine and selenium which are affected by geographical variation in the soil and water supply. For this reason these two elements warrant separate consideration.

Iodine

Iodine is the heaviest member of the halogen group which comprises the chemically related elements fluorine, chlorine, bromine and iodine. They all occur in nature in the form of salts and are all found in seawater. All the halogens are found in the body and are all essential except bromine. Iodine is carried round the body in blood as iodide and is absorbed in the thyroid gland in the neck where it is converted to the hormones thyroxine and its most active form, tri-iodothyronine. These two important hormones are involved with the general metabolic activity of the body and control the rate of energy production in all cells.

Selenium is needed by the enzyme which converts thyroxine into tri-iodothyronine. The body normally contains only about 20–50 mg iodine and the amount required daily in the diet is very small indeed (about 0.15 mg being sufficient for normal needs). When the diet provides insufficient iodine, the thyroid gland may increase in size in an attempt to compensate for the deficiency. The characteristic swollen neck, or goitre, was at one time known in the UK as 'Derbyshire neck' because of the prevalence of the condition there. Goitre still occurs in some parts of the world, especially mountainous and inland areas, where iodine levels in the soil, and hence in vegetation, are low. Its incidence in developed countries, where preventive measures can be taken, and where food comes from a wider area are low.

Iodine, in thyroid hormones, is essential for brain development and deficiency in early life *in utero* can result in cretinism. Small amounts of iodine may be present in drinking water, and it is also obtained from food, with sea foods being the richest sources. Thus, cod, salmon and herring are all useful sources of iodine, although the best marine source is cod-liver oil. Milk and other dairy products are important dietary sources of iodine in many countries as a result of iodine-enrichment of cattle feed. Vegetables grown on iodine-rich soil also contain available iodine but most cereals, legumes and roots have a low iodine content.

Some vegetables are said to be goitrogenic (i.e. capable of causing goitre). Cabbage, cauliflower and Brussels sprouts all contain compounds (goitrogens) which can interfere with the uptake of iodine by the thyroid gland and cause it to enlarge, as a 'goitre'. This is only likely to occur, however, if substantial amounts are eaten and when the iodine content of the diet is very low.

Some seaweeds concentrate iodides from seawater and are, therefore, a useful reservoir of combined iodine. In some parts of the world, certain seaweeds are regarded as valuable foods for humans and cooked seaweed, known as laver bread, is eaten in southwest Wales.

In areas where the iodine content of the diet is low, a satisfactory way of increasing the intake of iodine is the use of 'iodized salt'. This is prepared by adding about one part of potassium iodide to about 40 000 parts of salt. Potassium iodide is soluble in water and is rapidly absorbed into the blood, any surplus being quite harmless. The use of iodized salt is a simple and harmless way of supplementing the iodine obtained from food. Dietary iodine deficiency is one of the three biggest dietary deficiency diseases worldwide (with iron deficiency and vitamin A deficiency) and iodized salt as a major part of the solution being orchestrated by WHO.

Fluorine

Fluorine is the lightest and most reactive member of the halogen group of elements. It is so reactive that it never occurs naturally in the free state: in the body and in foods it occurs in the form of salts, i.e. fluorides. Traces of fluoride in the diet are important for dental enamel development in protecting teeth against decay, especially in children under 8 years of age. Dietary fluoride hardens tooth enamel by combining with calcium phosphate to form calcium fluorapatite.

Minerals containing combined fluorine have a wide distribution in nature, although they only occur in small quantities. Small amounts of fluorides are, therefore, usually present in natural water. Water in the UK nearly always contains fluorides, though their concentration rarely exceeds one part per million (ppm) parts of water. Drinking water is the main source of fluoride in the diet as very few foods contain more than 1 ppm, the main exceptions being sea fish, which contain 5–10 ppm, and tea which may contain up to 100 ppm.

The average daily intake of fluoride in Britain from food and beverages is about 0.6–1.8 mg, but this average is misleading because of large geographical variations. In areas where drinking water contains very little or no fluoride, the intake of fluoride is too low to provide protection against dental decay. This situation can be remedied by regular use of fluoride-containing toothpaste or if controlled amounts of fluoride are added to drinking water. This may be done by adding sodium fluoride or sodium silicofluoride, Na_2SiF_6, or hydrofluorosilicic acid in such quantities that the total fluoride content of the water is 1 ppm. The amount of fluoride added must be carefully controlled because if it exceeds 1.5 ppm, teeth may become mottled in appearance for children with exceptionally high water consumption. Their teeth are still protected against caries.

Experiments carried out over many years in the USA, UK and other countries prove beyond reasonable doubt that fluoridation of water to increase the fluoride content to 1 ppm is enough to correct dietary fluoride deficiency and reduces the incidence of dental caries, particularly in young children. Recent debates and evidence strengthen the consciousness of an authoritative report by the Royal College of Physicians (1976) that:

1 The presence of fluoride in drinking water substantially reduces the incidence of dental caries throughout life.
2 A level of 1 ppm of fluoride in drinking water is completely safe irrespective of the hardness of the water.
3 Alternative methods of taking fluoride, such as using fluoridated toothpaste or taking fluoride tablets, are less effective than fluoridation of water supplies.
4 Fluoridation to 1 ppm does not harm the environment.
5 Where the natural fluoride content of water supplies is less than 1 ppm, dietary deficiency becomes likely (manifest as dental caries), and fluoride should be added to bring it to this level.

In areas where water supplies have been 'fluoridated' to this very low level, childrens' dental decay has fallen dramatically. The fact that these steps have not been taken in all areas (to the detriment of many millions of teeth) has to do with a conflict between people's legal right to 'pure' water, and people's right to protection against disease. It also has to do with ignorance about nutritional requirements and the impact on social inequalities in health (because children in low socio-economic families are less likely to brush their teeth). The failure to correct fluoride deficiency nationally is one of the biggest health scandals of the twentieth and twenty-first centuries.

Other minerals

A number of other mineral elements may be essential, or important nutritionally, in addition to those already discussed or listed in Table 13.2. Aluminium, arsenic, antimony, boron, bromine, cadmium, caesium, germanium, lead, lithium, mercury, nickel, silicon, silver, strontium, sulphur, tin and vanadium are all present common foods, and it is probable that some of them are involved in body metabolism. Their importance in the diet, however, is not sufficient to merit further consideration here.

Key points

- Most essential minerals are required in only tiny amounts, and present only in tiny amounts in the body, functioning as cofactors in enzymes
- Some minerals are needed in large amounts and used in major body structures (Ca, P, Ng, in bone, teeth) or as major electrolytes (Na, K)
- Most minerals are biochemically active, and potentially toxic in free form. Few are stored within the body and those which are, e.g. iron, iodine, are stored in organic complex form
- Dietary supplements of minerals are not of any value outwith clinical deficiency states
- Although required in very small amounts and present in trace amounts in the water supply, most essential minerals need to be provided in forms naturally concentrated from the environment by plants, or in food from animals which have in turn consumed plant foods

Chapter summary

An exception is salt (NaCl) where pure mineral extracted from the environment is the main source of dietary supply. However, it is debatable whether additional salt is in fact required if natural sources such as milk and sea foods are eaten, and current links are several-fold greater than needed. Minerals are provided in most foods and dietary deficiencies are rare, with the exceptions of iron and iodine, which are commonly added to fortify foods. It is possible that large K and Mg intakes would benefit health, but little evidence for higher intakes of Se.

FURTHER READING

THE SCIENTIFIC ADVISORY COMMITTEE ON NUTRITION (2003). *Salt and Health*. London: The Stationery Office.

BRITISH NUTRITION FOUNDATION (1995). Iron BNF Task Force report.

MOYNIHAN P, PETERSEN PE (2004). Diet, nutrition and the prevention of dental diseases. *Public Health Nutr* 2004; 7(1A):201–226.

MURRAY JJ (1986). *Appropriate Use of Fluorides for Human Health*. Geneva: World Health Organization

WORLD HEALTH ORGANIZATION (1996). *Trace Elements in Human Nutrition and Health*. Geneva: World Health Organization. New reports on salt, DRVs, Fluoride, WHO on FE, Iodine.

ROYAL COLLEGE OF PHYSICIANS (1976). *Fluoride: Teeth and Health*. London: Pitman Medical.

14

Vitamins and other bioactive food constituents

Vitamins are organic compounds found in small amounts in many foods; their presence in the diet is 'essential' because, the body is unable to synthesize them from other nutrients and they are required for normal growth and function. Various deficiency diseases are associated with shortages of specific vitamins. Deficiency diseases have caused much suffering and death in the past, but now that they are understood better they can largely be prevented and cured by ensuring that the diet contains a sufficient quantity and variety of vitamins.

Most vitamins have complex chemical structures; they do not belong to one chemical family but are all quite different from each other. However, the structures of all of them are known and they can be prepared synthetically. Before their structures were determined the vitamins were designated by letters as vitamin A, vitamin B, and so on. They are now known by names which give some indication of their chemical structure or function and, in general, these names should be used in preference to the letters. In many cases, however, the letters by which they were originally known are still widely used.

Foods contain only very small quantities of vitamins, but these small amounts carry out some most important tasks in the body. Members of the 'B group' of vitamins, for example, form part of several coenzyme molecules which are necessary for the maintenance of good health. The other vitamins are equally essential, although in some cases their exact job in the chemistry of the body is not known.

Only small amounts of vitamins are needed by the body and the quantities present in a balanced diet of common foods are usually sufficient for people's needs. They are, however, distributed among many types of food and to ensure that all the vitamins are present in the diet it is important that a variety of different foods is eaten. The vitamin content of a single type of food can vary quite considerably. This is especially so with fruit and vegetables, where the vitamin content depends, among other things, on the freshness and variety of the fruit or vegetable and climatic conditions during its growth. The figures for the vitamin content of foods given in this chapter are average values and this must be borne in mind when consulting them.

It is so important that sufficient quantities of vitamins are consumed that in some cases extra vitamins are added to food. Examples have already been encountered in connection with flour, to which the vitamins thiamin and niacin are added to replace losses that occur during milling, and margarine, to which vitamins A and D are added. Similarly, most brands of breakfast cereals are 'fortified' with added B-group vitamins often to compensate for the low vitamin content of the cereal and sugar from which they are made.

Table 14.1 Vitamins (the reference nutrient intake of vitamins are shown in Table 14.2)

Name	Main sources	Functions in the body and effect of shortage
Fat-soluble vitamins		
Vitamin A or retinol	*Milk, dairy products, margarine, fish-liver oil. Also made in the body from carotenes found in green vegetables and carrots*	*Necessary for healthy skin and for normal growth and development. Deficiency will slow down growth and may lead to disorders of the skin, lowered resistance to infection and disturbances of vision such as night blindness*
Vitamin D or cholecalciferol	*Margarine, butter-milk, fish-liver oils, fatty fish*	*Necessary for the formation of strong bones and teeth. A shortage may cause bone diseases or dental decay*
Vitamin E or tocopherols	*Plant-seed and oils*	*Antioxidant*
Vitamin K or naphthoquinones	*Green vegetables*	*Assists blood clotting*
Water-soluble vitamins **The B vitamins**		
Thiamin, B_1 *Riboflavin, B_2* *Niacin* *Pyridoxine, B_6* *Pantothenic acid* *Biotin*	*Bread and flour, meat, milk, potatoes, yeast extract, fortified cornflakes (see text for details)*	*Function as coenzymes in many of the reactions involved in making use of food. Shortage causes loss of appetite, slows growth and development and impairs general health. Severe deficiency causes disease such as pellagra or beriberi.*
Cobalamin, B_{12}	*Offal, meat, milk, fortified cornflakes*	*Necessary for formation of nucleic acids and red blood cells. Shortage leads to megaloblastic anaemia and (for cobalamin) to neuropathy in severe pernicious anaemia (see text)*
Folate	*Potatoes, offal, green vegetables, bread, Marmite, fortified cornflakes*	
Vitamin C or ascorbic acid	*Green vegetables, fruits, potatoes, blackcurrant syrup, rosehip syrup*	*Necessary for the proper formation of teeth, bones and blood vessels. Shortage causes a check in the growth of children and if prolonged may lead to the disease scurvy*

When vitamins are taken as supplements as pills, or added to foods synthetic vitamins (i.e. man-made vitamins) are often used rather than the naturally occurring compounds. Synthetic vitamins are identical in structure to the naturally occurring vitamins and behave in the body in the same way. However, their absorption may be different, and their effects may be different when presented to the body in isolated form and in high doses. For example, folic acid is more readily absorbed than folate in food, β-carotene (a pro-vitamin A compound in vegetables) is associated with protection against coronary heart disease (CHD) and cancers, but when taken as a capsule, β-carotene is associated with higher rates of this disease.

The main sources and functions of the vitamins are summarized in Table 14.1. It is convenient to divide the vitamins into a fat-soluble or water-soluble group. The fat-soluble vitamins, namely vitamins A, D, E and K, are mostly found in fatty foods; fish-liver oils are particularly rich in vitamins A and D. These last two vitamins are also found in human liver; if the diet contains more vitamin A or D than is immediately required the surplus is stored in the liver. Enough of these vitamins are stored in the liver of a well-nourished person to satisfy the body's needs for several months if they are absent from the diet. If the diet contains too much vitamin A or D, however, the surplus will accumulate in the liver and may be harmful. Such excessive intakes are most unlikely to result from over-eating but may occur through over-enthusiastic use of vitamin pills or dietary supplements.

The water-soluble group of vitamins is made up of several B vitamins and ascorbic acid (vitamin C). The body is unable to build up a store of these vitamins and if the diet contains more than is immediately required the surplus is excreted in the urine. If an increased amount is demanded then there needs to be surplus in the diet. Nevertheless, a well-nourished person can remain apparently healthy for several weeks on a diet which contains little vitamin C. Vitamin B_{12} is an exception in that there are large stores in the liver, enough for many months or even years. In general, however, adequate and regular dietary supplies of the water-soluble vitamins are necessary for the maintenance of good health.

Although 'essential' means that vitamins cannot be synthesized by the body, there are special circumstances for two vitamins. Vitamin D is formed throughout the animal kingdom by the action of sunlight on skin, which activates the final biochemical transformation of a relatively inactive pro-vitamin to the most active form 1,25-dihydroxycholecalciferol. Only if one has virtually no sun exposure (e.g. heavily covered Moslem women) is one dependent on dietary vitamin D, from other animals which have better sun exposure. Heavily covered Moslem women who are vegetarian are at risk of rickets and osteomalacia (the vitamin D deficiency disease). Vitamin B_{12} may be provided from synthesis by bacteria living in the bowel.

The optimum daily intake for each vitamin cannot be stated with certainty. Precise requirements vary from person to person and with the nature of the rest of the diet. Despite these uncertainties, various national and international bodies have recommended desirable vitamin intakes for certain groups of the population. In Britain, the Department of Health through a specialist panel of the Committee on Medical Aspects of Food Policy (COMA) has published reference nutrient intakes for food energy and nutrients, and Table 14.2 gives details of the reference nutrient intake (RNI) for vitamins. The RNIs are specified as daily amounts but it should perhaps be emphasized that it is not necessary to regard these as strict daily allocations. They are defined as the amount that is enough, or more than enough for about 97 per cent of people in a group, but the precise amount required will vary from person to person and from time to time. Although prolonged shortage of a particular vitamin will be harmful, the body has a sufficient reserve of vitamins to enable it to cope easily with day-to-day variations in need or in intake.

FAT-SOLUBLE VITAMINS

Retinol (vitamin A) and the carotenoids

Retinol is a pale yellow solid which dissolves freely in oils and fats but is only very slightly soluble in water. It is a fat-soluble vitamin and so it is found in the fatty parts of foods, for example, in the fat of milk and butter, fish-liver oils and the small amount of fat present in green vegetables and carrots. It is able to circulate in the bloodstream by being bound to a specific transport protein (retinol-binding protein).

Retinol is a fairly complex unsaturated alcohol of molecular formula $C_{20}H_{29}OH$. In animal tissues it is stored and transported as an ester formed with a long-chain fatty acid such as stearic acid or palmitic acid, which is bound to a protein, 'retinol binding protein', which is synthesized in the liver.

Retinol has been synthesized and is now produced industrially on a fairly large scale for the enrichment of margarine.

Vegetables contain no retinol as such, but pigments called carotenoids, which are chemically related to it, are present. Carotenoids can be converted to retinol in the wall of the small intestine during absorption and hence vegetables have considerable vitamin A activity. Several carotenes are known; the most important is β-carotene which is often referred to as pro-vitamin A. β-Carotene is a red solid which was first isolated from carrots; indeed, it owes its name to this relationship. Solutions of β-carotene are yellow in colour and it is used for colouring margarine. The molecule of β-carotene is almost exactly twice as big as that of vitamin A, but it is an unsaturated hydrocarbon, not an alcohol.

The vitamin A activity of carotenes is not as great as that of retinol itself. β-Carotene, for example, is only about one-sixth as effective as an equal weight of retinol. Other pro-vitamin A carotenoids present in vegetable foods are converted to retinol even less efficiently and have half the activity of β-carotene.

Table 14.2 Reference nutrient intakes (RNI) for vitamins

Age	Thiamin (mg/day)	Riboflavin (mg/day)	Niacin[a] (mg/day)	Vitamin B₆[b] (mg/day)	Vitamin B₁₂ (µg/day)	Folate (µg/day)	Vitamin C (mg/day)	Vitamin A (µg/day)	Vitamin D (µg/day)
0–3 months	0.2	0.4	3	0.2	0.3	50	25	350	8.5
4–6 months	0.2	0.4	3	0.2	0.3	50	25	350	8.5
7–9 months	0.2	0.4	4	0.3	0.4	50	25	350	7
10–12 months	0.3	0.4	5	0.4	0.4	50	25	350	7
1–3 years	0.5	0.6	8	0.7	0.5	70	30	400	7
4–6 years	0.7	0.8	11	0.9	0.8	100	30	500	–
7–10 years	0.7	1.0	12	1.0	1.0	150	30	500	–
Males									
11–14 years	0.9	1.2	15	1.2	1.2	200	35	600	–
15–18 years	1.1	1.3	18	1.5	1.5	200	40	700	–
19–50 years	1.0	1.3	17	1.4	1.5	200	40	700	–
50+ years	0.9	1.3	16	1.4	1.5	200	40	700	c
Females									
11–14 years	0.7	1.1	12	1.0	1.2	200	35	600	–
15–18 years	0.8	1.1	14	1.2	1.5	200	40	600	–
19–50 years	0.8	1.1	13	1.2	1.5	200	40	600	–
50+ years	0.8	1.1	12	1.2	1.5	200	40	600	c
Pregnancy	+0.1[d]	+0.3	e	e	e	+100	+10	+100	10
Lactation:									
0–4 months	+0.2	+0.5	+2	e	+0.5	+60	+30	+350	10
4+ months	+0.2	+0.5	+2	e	+0.5	+60	+30	+350	10

[a]Nicotinic acid equivalent.
[b]Based on protein providing 14.7 per cent of estimated average requirement (EAR) for energy.
[c]After age 65 the RNI is 10 µg/day for men and women.
[d]For last trimester only.
[e]No increment.
DOH 1991. Crown Copyright is reproduced with the permission of the Controller of HMSO and the Queen's Printer for Scotland.

To allow for this variation in availability the vitamin A activity of foods is usually expressed in 'retinol equivalents'.

Carotenoids have another very important function in the diet which is quite separate from their role as a pro-vitamin. Many are antioxidant and help to protect easily oxidized nutrients, such as polyunsaturated fatty acids (PUFAs), from oxidation and also able to combat the harmful effects of free radicals in the body. Free radicals are highly reactive molecules or groups of atoms containing unpaired electrons (see p. 55). They can be produced inside cells by normal metabolic processes or outside cells through the action of harmful substances brought into the body in food, air pollutants or in tobacco smoke, and in many other ways. Because free radicals have unpaired electrons they are very unstable and highly reactive. A free radical can achieve stability by acquiring an electron from another molecule, for example, a molecule in a cell membrane, to form a pair with its own unpaired electron. The molecule from which the electron has been captured is itself converted into a new, highly reactive free radical which repeats the process of achieving stability by electron capture. By so doing, another free radical is formed and the process will continue in a chain reaction until it is terminated by, for example, pairing of a free radical with another free radical. Free radical chain reactions occur very rapidly and many thousands of reactions can occur within seconds of initiation of a chain by one free radical.

Free radical chain reactions are highly damaging to living cells. They can cause serious and irreversible harm to cell membranes and so reduce their capacity to carry out their essential tasks of transport of nutrients, oxygen, water and cellular waste products. Complex metabolic processes may be disrupted and damage caused to nucleic acids may increase the likelihood of abnormal cell replication and growth. Free radicals may be implicated in the initiation of many serious diseases, including some forms of cancer, impaired immune function and coronary heart disease. The body has a complex antioxidant system within its cells which protects cell membranes, nucleic acids and other cell constituents against damage or destruction through free radical attack by scavenging the free radicals before they are able to attack cells. This is capable of dealing effectively with free radicals generated within cells but may not be sufficiently powerful to cope with additional demands posed outside the cells by pollutants and dietary sources of free radicals. Antioxidants present in the diet are able to supplement the body's own defence mechanism and thus ensure that minimum damage is done by free radicals. Vitamin C is the best known water-soluble dietary antioxidant and vitamin E is the most potent fat-soluble one. Most carotenoids also behave as an antioxidant by scavenging or 'mopping up' free radicals and by generating other antioxidants. The most potent antioxidant carotenoid is lycopene, followed by lutein, cryptoxanthine α- and β-carotenes. The most important pro-vitamin A carotenoids tend to be least potent as antioxidants. Vitamin A itself does not display antioxidant properties.

Sources of retinol and carotenes

Retinol is found in animal tissues (especially liver) and dairy products. Fish-liver oils are the richest source and consumption of cod-liver or halibut-liver oil is a simple way of ensuring that a sufficient supply of the vitamin is obtained.

Carotenes are found in plant tissues and about one-third of the vitamin A activity of the average British diet is contributed by carotenes. Carrots, dark-green vegetables and yellow fruits are all good sources of carotenes. Some green vegetables are rather poor sources, however. Lettuce, with its pale-green leaves, cabbage (especially the paler inner parts) and peas are not good sources but spinach, with its dark-green leaves, is well endowed with carotene. When vegetables are eaten not all the carotene they contain is absorbed and only a fraction of that absorbed may be converted into retinol. The source of carotene may affect its availability; for example, carotene is obtained from green vegetables more easily than from carrots, which have a comparatively fibrous structure.

Milk and milk products are also good sources of vitamin A, but the amount present depends upon the amount of carotene or retinol in the food eaten by the cow and so dairy produce is usually a richer source of the vitamin in summer, when fresh grass is available, than in winter. Cod-liver oil or synthetic retinol is incorporated into many animal foodstuffs, however, and so the difference is not as great as one might expect.

Table 14.3 Average values for vitamin A content of foods

Food	Retinol equivalents (μg/100 g)
Foods supplying retinol	
Halibut-liver oil	90 000
Cod-liver oil	18 000
Liver, lamb's fried	19 710
Herring	45
Sardines, canned	7
Butter	1059
Margarine	819
Cheese, cheddar	388
Eggs, boiled	190
Milk	36
Foods supplying carotene	
Red palm oil	20 000
Carrots	2233
Spinach, boiled	1100
Lettuce	171
Tomatoes	94
Bananas	4
Foods with negligible vitamin A activity	
Potatoes	
Cooking fats, lard and suet	
Bacon, pork, beef (trace) and mutton (trace)	
Bread, flour and other cereals	
Sugar, jams and syrups	
White fish	

Table 14.3 shows the main sources of vitamin A activity in the diet. Retinol and carotenes are highly unsaturated and so they are easily destroyed by oxidation, especially at high temperatures. They are much more susceptible to oxidation after extraction from foods than when in animal or plant tissues. Losses from oxidation during normal cooking processes are small, but considerable loss may occur during storage of dehydrated food if precautions are not taken to exclude oxygen. Apart from this sensitivity to oxidation, retinol and carotenes are reasonably stable and are only slowly destroyed at the temperatures used in cooking food. They are also almost insoluble in water and so there is little or no loss by extraction during the boiling of vegetables.

Dietary requirements of vitamin A

The RNIs for vitamin A are expressed in terms of retinol equivalents, to allow for the fact that much of the vitamin A activity in a mixed diet is provided by carotenes. The RNI for adult men and women is 700 μg and 600 μg/day, respectively. The amounts are increased by 100 and 350 μg/day for pregnant and lactating women, respectively. Details of the RNIs for other age groups are given in Table 14.2.

Retinol is not soluble in water and an excess above the body's need is not excreted in the urine but accumulates in the liver. This is why animal liver is such a valuable source of the vitamin. The liver of a well-nourished person may contain sufficient retinol to permit subsistence for several months without further intake of retinol or carotene. Because retinol accumulates in this way an excessive intake should be avoided. Mothers who give their babies vitamin A supplements in the form of fish-liver oil should take particular care not to exceed the recommended dose. Adults are not immune from the ill-effects of grossly excessive vitamin A intake: vitamin pill and vitamin pill enthusiasts should be warned that most of these preparations have quite unnaturally high levels, and their safety and efficacy have not been established. Vitamin A toxicity can result in liver and bone damage, hair loss, double vision, vomiting and headaches. It is recommended that pregnant women should avoid vitamin A supplements (unless deficient) because excess can accumulate in and damage the fetus. Because the livers of farmed animals are so rich in vitamin A (partly the result of medicating cattle) it is also recommended that pregnant women should avoid liver.

The RNIs of vitamin A are expressed in terms of a daily amount, as with other nutrients. Day-to-day deficiencies of the vitamin are normally of no consequence, however, because of the liver's capacity to store the vitamin. A normal mixed diet which provides adequate amounts of other nutrients will almost certainly provide sufficient vitamin A to meet the recommended intake levels over a period, even if it does not do so every day.

Effects of retinol deficiency

A long-term deficiency of vitamin A may lead to blindness. An early stage is known as 'night blindness' which makes it difficult to see in a dim light. Normally, one's eyesight is able to adapt to changes in illumination. This is why one is able to see one's surroundings after a short while in a cinema which at first seems very dark. Night blindness is caused by a shortage of a retinol derivative called rhodopsin (or visual purple) which is essential for the proper functioning of the retina at the back of the eye. Night blindness is common in some parts of Asia and Africa where the diet is deficient in vitamin A. It recovers with vitamin replacement.

Long-term deficiency results in xerophthalmia, in which dead cells accumulate on the surface of the eyes causing them to become dry and opaque. The cornea may become ulcerated and infected – a condition known as keratomalacia – and blindness is a common sequel. Although the cause of the condition is known and preventive measures can easily be taken, it is estimated that up to 20000 children become blind in this way every year in underdeveloped countries. An adequate intake of vitamin A or pro-vitamin A carotenoid is essential for the maintenance of healthy skin and other surface tissues such as the mucous membranes. Retinol deficiency is one of the world's most widespread and damaging dietary deficiency. It is closely associated with infections and there is evidence that giving retinol (or carrots) will prevent many infections, especially in children in areas of poor nutrition. During acute infections, retinol-binding protein is not made by the liver, so circulatory retinal levels fall and tissues may lose access to retinol.

Shortage of vitamin A in infancy during the formation of teeth may produce poor teeth and even after they have been formed, a lack of vitamin A may affect the enamel.

Cholecalciferol (vitamin D)

Naturally occurring vitamin D is more precisely referred to as vitamin D_3 or cholecalciferol. Another form of vitamin D, known as vitamin D_2 or ergocalciferol, can be made by exposing the compound ergosterol, which is found in fungi and yeasts, to ultraviolet light. The name vitamin D_1, which was at one time used for a mixture of substances displaying vitamin D activity, is not now used. Cholecalciferol is the only one of these compounds of dietary importance and in what follows it will be referred to simply as vitamin D.

Vitamin D is a white crystalline solid which, like vitamin A, is freely soluble in oils and fats but insoluble in water. Vitamin D is stored in the liver, and

Table 14.4 Average values for vitamin D content of foods

Food	Vitamin D (μg/100 g)
Halibut-liver oil	up to 10 000
Cod-liver oil	210
Margarine	8
Herrings, sardines	5–45
Salmon	5–20
Egg yolk	4–10
Shreddies	2.8
Butter	up to 2
Eggs, whole	1–1.5
Cheese	0.3
Milk (summer)	0.1

since it is insoluble in water, an excess cannot easily be removed in the urine and it accumulates in the liver. Too much vitamin D can be harmful and in this respect also it resembles vitamin A.

Sources of vitamin D

Vitamin D is not widely distributed and it is found almost exclusively in animal foods. Fish-liver oils are the richest natural source. The main sources in an average British diet are margarine, vitamin-fortified breakfast cereals, butter, eggs and fatty fish. Synthetic vitamin D is added to all margarine sold in Britain, except that used by the baking industry, and in many baby foods. Table 14.4 summarizes the important sources of vitamin D.

Vitamin D is not destroyed to any significant extent during normal cooking processes.

As well as being obtained from the diet, vitamin D is produced in the body by the action of sunlight on a chemically related compound present in the skin.

Functions and reference nutrient intakes of vitamin D

Vitamin D is needed for the absorption of calcium and phosphorus by the body. In its absence, the body is unable to make use of these elements and they are lost in the faeces. Phosphorus and calcium are both needed to form bones as explained earlier (see p. 188). Deficiency of vitamin D causes rickets in the young and the related bone disease osteomalacia in those in whom bone growth has ceased. Rickets is characterized by curvature of the bones in the limbs and other symptoms of improper bone formation caused by loss of calcium from the bones and its replacement by softer tissue. At one time it was common in Britain but is now rare except among children of some immigrant groups.

It has been recognized for about 90 years that rickets is more prevalent in industrial areas in the temperate regions where sunlight is deficient. The disease has been successfully treated by exposure to the maximum amount of sunlight and later it was shown that any other source of ultraviolet light (e.g. a 'sun-lamp') is also efficient. The reason for this is now clear; it is because the ultraviolet light converts a pro-vitamin present in the tissues of the skin into the vitamin, which is then able to carry out its function.

No amount of vitamin D or exposure to sunlight will prevent the development of rickets if the diet contains insufficient calcium. The disease may be caused by calcium shortage, vitamin D shortage or lack of sunlight, but usually a combination of factors. Vegetarian, heavily covered Moslem women are at high risk.

Rickets is often found in conjunction with dental caries because vitamin D is also necessary for proper calcification of teeth. Not only does vitamin D assist in the formation of healthy teeth but it can also help to prevent the development of dental caries in existing teeth (although other factors are also involved). Most people obtain sufficient vitamin D through the action of sunlight on their skin, and for this reason there is no RNI for adults under the age of 65 years. The RNIs for other age groups are given in Table 14.2.

A high intake of vitamin D can be harmful. Too much calcium is absorbed from the diet and the excess is deposited in the kidneys, where it causes damage and eventually death may result. There is a particular danger that babies who are given extra vitamin D in the form of fish-liver oil could receive an excessive intake unless the recommended dosage is carefully observed.

Tocopherols (vitamin E)

Vitamin E is the name given to α-tocopherol (a light yellow oil with the formula $C_{29}H_{50}O_2$) and a group of fat-soluble saturated and unsaturated alcohols closely related to it.

Vitamin E is a powerful fat-soluble antioxidant with a vital physiological role in plants to protect lipids (especially PUFAs) in membranes, etc., from oxidation. This is particularly important for seeds and fruits. Most plant tissues contain some vitamin E and vegetable oils extracted from seeds or fruits such as corn oil (maize oil), soya bean oil and wheatgerm oil, and olive oil which are rich in polyunsaturated acids, are good sources. Meat and other foods of animal origin are poor sources.

Naturally occurring vitamin E is the α-isomer and its presence in heavily unsaturated oils probably indicates that its function in plant tissues is to protect these easily oxidized oils from oxidation. It performs a similar function in the body where it is the major lipid-soluble antioxidant. Similar to β-carotene, it scavenges free radicals and prevents them from damaging cell membranes and their contents. Vitamin E also protects easily oxidized nutrients such as PUFAs, vitamin A and vitamin C from oxidation. Epidemiology evidence suggests that dietary vitamin E may also be protective for diseases, such as some types of cancer, arthritis and ischaemic heart disease in which free radicals are thought to be involved.

There is evidence that vitamin E can help to prevent the occurrence of a serious eye disease called retrolental fibroplasia which affects premature babies. This disease is caused by the action of oxygen on the developing blood vessels in the baby's eyes.

Lack of vitamin E renders male rats sterile: female rats deficient in the vitamin can conceive but the pregnancy is interrupted and no live young are born. There is no conclusive evidence that vitamin E influences human fertility, although various claims have been made. Vitamin E supplements are sometimes taken in the optimistic belief that the vitamin will delay ageing, improve the condition of the skin or enhance sexual capabilities. All of these hopes are unfounded and there is no reliable evidence of beneficial results.

The dietary requirement of vitamin E is related to the PUFA content of the diet, and it is estimated that 0.4 mg of the vitamin is required for each gram of PUFA. On this basis, a man with a dietary energy intake of 2550 kcal – the estimated average requirement (EAR) for an adult (see p. 9) – where 6 per cent of the energy is supplied by PUFAs would require 7 mg of vitamin E per day. Similarly, the requirement a woman of the same age range and dietary PUFA ratio (EAR 1940 kcal) is 5 mg of vitamin E per day.

In general, bigger, and more active people need more vitamin E in absolute forms. The amount of PUFA in the diet varies greatly, and for this reason, no RNI values have been specified. Foods rich in PUFAs are also normally rich in vitamin E and so an increase in the PUFA content of the diet is usually accompanied by a corresponding increase in the vitamin E intake. Normal diets contain sufficient vitamin E and there is little danger of a deficiency. Tocopherols are used in the food industry as anti-oxidants and they are permitted food additives (E307–309; see Chapter 20). Bigger, more active people generally tend to eat more anyway. The high levels in cheap oils and margarine are thought to have contributed to the decline in heart disease observed over recent decades in many countries.

Because it is so lipophilic, vitamin E can only be transported around the bloodstream, to tissues where it is needed, in lipoproteins closely associated with cholesterol – specifically low-density lipoprotein (LDL) cholesterol. Vitamin E thereby protects cholesterol esters and lipoproteins from oxidation (oxidized LDL is a potent toxic factor involved in CHD development). In a rare genetically inherited disease called a-β-lipoproteinaemia, there is a complete deficiency of LDL cholesterol. Sufferers never get CHD but, sadly, they cannot transport vitamin E, and critical tissues such as the brain and eyes suffer progressive damage. The only treatment is with massive injections of vitamin E, but even this does not work well.

Naphthoquinones (vitamin K)

Vitamin K comprises several closely related fat-soluble compounds derived from menadione (2-methyl-1,4-naphthoquinone) all of which display vitamin K activity. It is essential for normal clotting of the blood; without vitamin K, the liver is unable to synthesize prothrombin which is the precursor of the blood-clotting enzyme thrombin.

Vitamin K is present in most foods but green leafy vegetables are the richest source. Bacterial synthesis in the bowel provides humans with vitamin K in addition to that obtained from foodstuffs.

In most cases, the amount made available in this way is sufficient to supply the body's requirements. There is little danger of vitamin K deficiency in a person who eats a normal diet and, while there are no specified dietary reference values, a daily intake of 1 µg/kg of body weight is thought to be both safe and adequate for adults. Newborn infants lack the bacteria which produce vitamin K in the gut and are commonly given an injection soon after birth to prevent deficiency and the possible occurrence of life-threatening intracerebral haemorrhage in the early post-partum stage. Some concerns have been raised about this practice.

WATER–SOLUBLE VITAMINS

The B group of vitamins

The B group of vitamins comprises several vitamins which have similar functions and which are often found together in foods. In the body they are largely concerned with the release of energy from food. They are all soluble, to a greater or lesser extent, in water and since the body lacks the capacity for storing them any excess over immediate requirements is excreted in the urine. The members of the B group of vitamins are: thiamin, or vitamin B_1; riboflavin, or vitamin B_2; niacin (nicotinic acid and nicotinamide); pyridoxine, or vitamin B_6; pantothenic acid; biotin; cobalamin, or vitamin B_{12} (formerly called cyanocobalamin); folate (provided as folic acid in supplements).

Thiamin (vitamin B_1)

This is a white, water-soluble crystalline solid. The thiamin molecule has a complex structure which includes an amino ($—NH_2$) group and a hydroxyl group. Like all amines, thiamin forms salts with acids. Thiamin hydrochloride is made on quite a large scale for use in fortifying flour. The hydroxyl group can be esterified and thiamin is found in foods and in the body as its pyrophosphate ester.

Sources of thiamin

Thiamin plays an essential part in the utilization of carbohydrates by living cells. As a result it is present in all natural foods to some extent. Unfortunately, it is often absent from processed foods because it has been removed or destroyed in the preparation of

Table 14.5 Average values for thiamin content of foods

Food	Thiamin (mg/100 g)
Marmite	4.10
Cornflakes (fortified)	1.20
Oats (porridge)	0.90
Pork (cooked)	0.60
Bacon (fried)	0.86
Kidney (pig's, fried)	0.41
Peas (frozen, boiled)	0.26
Bread (wholemeal)	0.26
Bread (brown)	0.24
Bread (white)	0.24
Mutton or lamb (cooked)	0.10
Eggs (raw or boiled)	0.09
Potatoes (boiled)	0.20
Milk (pasteurized)	0.05
Cheese (Cheddar)	0.04

the food for the market. Polished rice and low extraction rate flour from which thiamin has been largely removed, sugar, refined oils and fats and alcoholic beverages are examples of foods which contain little or no thiamin. Nevertheless, thiamin is still present in a fairly wide range of foodstuffs as Table 14.5 shows. Most of the thiamin in an average British diet comes from bread and fortified cereal products, potatoes, milk and meat.

Because thiamin is so soluble in water, as much as 50 per cent may be lost when vegetables are boiled. Potatoes boiled in their skins retain up to 90 per cent of their thiamin compared with a retention of about 75 per cent in the case of peeled boiled potatoes. Thiamin decomposes on heating, though it is fairly stable at the boiling point of water and little loss occurs at this temperature in acid conditions. In neutral or alkaline conditions breakdown is more rapid. Foods which have been subjected to higher temperatures, as in roasting, or in 'processing' during canning, may have a large proportion of their thiamin destroyed. Meat loses about 15–40 per cent of its thiamin when boiled, 40–50 per cent when roasted and up to 75 per cent when canned. When bread is baked some 20–30 per cent of thiamin present in the flour may be destroyed by the moist heat. In cakes made with baking powder all the thiamin may be destroyed by reaction with the baking powder. Some preservatives also destroy thiamin

and sulphites – those used in sausages are particularly likely to cause thiamin breakdown.

The deficiency disease beriberi, which is caused by a deficiency of thiamin, is almost unknown in the UK, but it is still common in some Far Eastern countries where the standard of living is very low. In these countries, the main article of diet is polished rice, which contains little thiamin. The husk and silverskin of the rice grains are removed to improve its palatability and keeping properties. Unfortunately, this process also removes most of the thiamin. If the rice grains are parboiled before the husks are removed much of the thiamin is absorbed and retained by the endosperm. Loss of thiamin occurs in the same way during the milling of wheat to produce flour of low extraction rate and it is for this reason that synthetic thiamin is now added to all such flour produced in Britain. Enriched flour provides about 25 per cent of the thiamin in the average diet in the UK.

Functions and recommended intakes of thiamin

Thiamin is esterified with pyrophosphoric acid in the body to give thiamin pyrophosphate, which is an essential coenzyme involved in the utilization of carbohydrates, alcohol and fats. A deficiency of thiamin restricts the growth of children together with loss of appetite and other symptoms such as irritability, fatigue and dizziness. Prolonged and severe deficiency can cause the disease beriberi. Several types of this disease are known but all of them are associated with loss of appetite, leading to reduced food intake and, in time, emaciation. An enlargement of the heart occurs with high cardiac output heart failure in 'wet beriberi'. In 'dry beriberi' the nervous system is badly affected and this may produce partial paralysis and muscular weakness. Alcoholics with poor food intake develop a neuropathic syndrome affecting legs, balance and cognitive function. The most dramatic presentation of vitamin B_1 deficiency is a loss of memory-making capacity (Korsakoff's psychosis) together with acute paralysis of the muscles which move the eyes (ophthalmoplegia). This full syndrome known as Wernicke's encephalopathy responds only partly to treatment with thiamine in high doses. Memory-making capacity may be lost permanently. However, it is preventable with adequate dietary thiamine.

Dietary requirements of thiamin are proportional to the amount of carbohydrate, fat and alcohol in the diet and, consequently, it is difficult to arrive at dietary reference values for the vitamin. The situation is made more complicated by the fact that some thiamin is synthesized by bacteria in the small intestine and the amount available from this source varies from person to person and from time to time. In the UK, the RNI is based on total energy intake and it is considered that 0.4 mg thiamin/1000 kcal is the appropriate amount for all groups of people, except babies in their first year of life. Thus, for a man whose diet has an energy content of 2550 kcal the RNI is 1 mg/day.

In common with other water-soluble vitamins, thiamin is not stored by the body and any excess over immediate requirements is rapidly excreted in the urine. A regular and adequate supply of the vitamin is thus essential.

Riboflavin (vitamin B$_2$)

This is a yellowish-green fluorescent solid which, like thiamin, has a complex chemical structure. The molecule contains a complex heterocyclic ring system of carbon and nitrogen atoms combined with the sugar ribose. Riboflavin is synthesized commercially and is used in some countries for enrichment of food.

Sources of riboflavin

Riboflavin is widely distributed in plant and animal tissues and the more important sources are shown in Table 14.6. The main sources of riboflavin in the British diet are milk, cheese, meat, fortified breakfast cereals and eggs. It is found in beer, but it is present in such small amounts that about eight pints per day would be required to provide the RNI for a man.

Riboflavin is only very slightly soluble in water and losses by solution during cooking are small. Heating causes little breakdown of riboflavin and little or no loss occurs during canning. Meat loses about one-quarter of its riboflavin during roasting. Greater losses occur if riboflavin is heated under alkaline conditions such as occur when sodium bicarbonate is added to the water used for boiling vegetables.

Although riboflavin is very stable to heat, it is sensitive to light. This is not important with solid

Table 14.6 Average values for riboflavin content of foods

Food	Riboflavin (mg/100 g)
Marmite	11.9
Liver (lamb's, fried)	5.65
Kidney (pig's, fried)	3.70
Cornflakes (fortified)	1.30
Cheese (Cheddar)	0.39
Eggs (boiled)	0.35
Beef (cooked)	0.33
Milk	0.23
Bread (white)	0.08
Bread (brown)	0.06
Bread (wholemeal)	0.06
Beer (keg bitter)	0.03
Cabbage (boiled)	0.01
Potatoes (boiled)	0.02

foods such as meat, but serious losses can occur in milk. Up to three-quarters of the riboflavin present in milk may be destroyed by exposure to direct sunlight for 3.5 hours. The substances produced when riboflavin breaks down in this way are oxidizing agents capable of reacting with, and totally destroying, the ascorbic acid (vitamin C) present in the milk. In addition, the fats present in milk may be partly oxidized with the production of unpleasant 'off' flavours. Obviously, it is not good practice to allow bottles of milk to remain for too long on the doorstep or, for that matter, in a brightly illuminated supermarket display cabinet.

Functions and dietary requirements of riboflavin

In the body, riboflavin is esterified with phosphoric acid or pyrophosphoric acid and forms part of two coenzymes involved in a variety of oxidation reduction processes concerned with the release of energy from proteins, fats and carbohydrates in living cells. A deficiency of riboflavin limits the growth of children and lesions on the lips and scaliness at the corners of the mouth may occur. The tongue and eyes may also become irritated.

When riboflavin is eaten it is stored temporarily in the liver until it is needed by the body. It is not possible to store large amounts in this way, however, and it is necessary for regular and adequate amounts to be eaten. The quantity of riboflavin needed for the maintenance of health is not known with certainty, but it is believed to be related to the basal metabolic rate rather than (as with thiamin) to total energy content of the diet. The RNI for adult males is 1.3 mg/day, and for adult females 1.1 mg/day. Details of the RNIs for other age groups are given in Table 14.2.

During pregnancy and lactation, the RNI is increased by 0.3 and 0.5 mg, respectively. The riboflavin in the diet may be supplemented to a small extent by that produced by bacterial synthesis in the large intestine but not all of this is absorbed.

Niacin (nicotinic acid and nicotinamide)

The B group vitamin known as niacin exists in two forms: a pyridine carboxylic acid, nicotinic acid, and its amide, nicotinamide. Unlike most other members of the B group of vitamins, these two substances have simple chemical structures. The acid and the amide are equally effective as vitamins.

Nicotinic acid   Nicotinamide

Nicotinic acid was first prepared long before its importance as a vitamin was realized, from nicotine. In food, however, it is not derived from nicotine, neither is it produced during tobacco smoking. The name niacin is used to refer to both nicotinic acid and nicotinamide, although the latter is also sometimes called niacinamide. Niacin is manufactured on a fairly large scale for use in enriching flour.

Sources of niacin

Niacin is found in both animal and vegetable tissues. The main sources of the vitamin in the average British diet are meat and meat products, potatoes, bread and fortified breakfast cereals. In the UK all flour (except wholemeal) is 'fortified' with added niacin to a content similar to that of white flour) (see p. 119) and about one-quarter of

Table 14.7 Average values for niacin equivalent content of foods

Food	Niacin equivalent (mg/100 g)
Yeast extract (Marmite)	75.0
Beef extract (Bovril)	90.0
Liver (lamb's, fried)	24.7
Cornflakes	21.9
Kidney (pig's, fried)	20.1
Tuna (canned)	18.8
Chicken (roast)	11.5
Sardines (canned)	11.3
Bacon (grilled)	11.0
Lamb (roast)	11.0
Pork chop (grilled)	11.0
Beef (roast)	10.2
Corned beef	9.1
Cheese (Cheddar)	6.9
Cod (fried)	4.9
Eggs (boiled)	3.7
Peas (frozen)	2.6
Bread (brown)	4.9
Bread (white)	3.6
Bread (wholemeal)	6.1
Potatoes	1.5

the average daily intake is obtained from bread and cereal products.

Some cereal products are fairly rich in niacin but, unfortunately, it is bound up in a complex with hemicelluloses called niacytin. This is not broken down during digestion and so the niacin is not available to the body. For this reason, therefore, unfortified cereal products must be regarded as poor sources of niacin. The amino acid tryptophan, which is present in cereals, can be converted by the body to niacin but the amount made available from cereals in this way is normally small.

Milk and eggs contain little niacin but their proteins are especially rich in tryptophan and so they serve as good sources of the vitamin. To allow for the presence of tryptophan in the diet the niacin content of foods is conveniently expressed in terms of niacin equivalents and for this purpose 60 mg of tryptophan are taken to be equivalent to 1 mg of niacin. The values given in Table 14.7 are expressed in this way.

Niacin is not easily decomposed by heating and it is only moderately soluble in water so that losses in cooking are small.

Functions and dietary requirements of niacin

Nicotinamide occurs in the body as part of two essential coenzymes required in a large number of oxidation processes involved in the utilization of carbohydrates, fats and proteins.

The amount of niacin required for the maintenance of good health is related to the energy content of the diet and to the amount of tryptophan also present. The RNI for all ages and both sexes (except lactating women) is 6.6 mg niacin/ 1000 kcal. Thus, for an adult man with a diet of energy content 2550 kcal the RNI is 16.8 mg/day, and for an adult woman with a 1940 kcal diet it is 12.8 mg/day. The RNI is increased by 2 mg per day for lactating women. Additional amounts are not required by pregnant women because they are able to convert tryptophan to niacin about twice as efficiently as usual. Full details are given in Table 14.2. Most diets with enough high-quality protein to maintain nitrogen balance will contain enough tryptophan to satisfy the body's needs for niacin, and in such cases there will be no need for the preformed vitamin.

A severe deficiency of niacin can cause the disease pellagra which is characterized by dermatitis, diarrhoea and symptoms of mental disorder, which can culminate in dementia. (Pellagra is known colloquially as the disease of 'd's.) Less severe deficiencies can produce one or more of these symptoms. Pellagra has long been associated, like many other deficiency diseases, with a low standard of living. In particular, pellagra results from subsistence on a diet consisting mainly of maize, and for this reason it was in the past particularly prevalent in the southern states of the USA, where maize was a staple food. The niacin present in maize is not available for reasons already given and its proteins are deficient in tryptophan. Pellagra is not associated solely with consumption of maize, however, and it may occur whenever the intake of nicotinamide, or its precursor tryptophan, is insufficient. Some nicotinamide may be synthesized by microbial action in the large intestine but the amount absorbed is small.

Pyridoxine (vitamin B_6)

Pyridoxine or vitamin B_6 is the name given to a group of three pyridine derivatives which have the structures shown:

Pyridoxol

Pyridoxal

Pyridoxamine

All three compounds are interconvertible in the body and they are equally potent as vitamins. Vitamin B_6 is found in foods which contain the other B vitamins. The main sources in the diet are potatoes and other vegetables, milk and meat. The vitamin B_6 content of some foods is shown in Table 14.8.

Table 14.8 Average values for vitamin B_6 content of foods

Food	Vitamin B_6 (mg/100 g)
Wheat germ	3.30
Bananas	0.29
Turkey (cooked)	0.63
Chicken (cooked)	0.63
Fish (white) (cooked)	0.41
Brussels sprouts (boiled)	0.19
Beef (cooked)	0.27
Potatoes (boiled)	0.33
Baked beans	0.12
Bread (wholemeal)	0.12
Peas (frozen)	0.10
Bread (white)	0.07
Milk	0.06
Oranges	0.10

Symptoms of vitamin B_6 deficiency in animals can be produced by feeding them with a diet devoid of the vitamin. It is not easy, however, to do the same thing with humans although various skin lesions are reputed to be caused by vitamin B_6 deficiency. Infants fed on milk powders deficient in vitamin B_6 were found to suffer from convulsions but responded rapidly to treatment with the vitamin.

Vitamin B_6 functions as a coenzyme for a large number of enzymes involved in amino acid metabolism and hence requirements are related to dietary protein intake. The protein content of the average diet is known from a comprehensive survey of UK diets carried out in 1990, and the RNI values shown in Table 14.2 have been calculated on the assumption that the appropriate relationship is $15\,\mu g$ of vitamin B_6 per gram of protein. The RNI for a man is $1.4\,mg/day$ and for a woman it is $1.2\,mg/day$. Because of the variability of the protein content of the diet, and because some vitamin B_6 synthesized in the gut supplements dietary sources, the RNI figures, despite their apparent precision, can only be regarded as approximate.

Pantothenic acid

This vitamin is a pale yellow oil with the structure shown:

$$HOCH_2C(CH_3)_2CHOHCONHCH_2CH_2COOH$$
Pantothenic acid

It is found in a wide variety of plant and animal tissues, indeed the name is derived from Greek words meaning 'from everywhere'. It is soluble in water and is rapidly destroyed by treatment with acids or alkalis or by heating in the dry state.

Pantothenic acid is an essential constituent of coenzyme A which is concerned in all metabolic processes involving removal or addition of an acetyl group ($-COCH_3$). Such processes are of great importance in the many complex transformations occurring within the human body, especially those concerned with the release of energy from carbohydrate, protein and fat.

Pantothenic acid is undoubtedly of fundamental importance as a coenzyme and symptoms of deficiency of the vitamin have been produced in numerous species of animals and also in man by diets devoid of pantothenic acid. The daily requirements are not

known with certainty and no dietary reference values have been specified. It is so widely distributed that a normal diet, which contains $10–20\,mg$, should be adequate and there is no danger of a deficiency.

Biotin

Biotin is another widely distributed vitamin which is required in minute amounts as a coenzyme involved in the metabolism of fats and carbohydrates. Many foods contain biotin. Liver and kidney are good dietary sources (but see below) and smaller amounts are found in egg yolk, milk and bananas.

Such small amounts of biotin are required by the body that sufficient may be produced by the microorganisms present in the large intestine. Consequently, dietary sources are not of great importance and there is no evidence of biotin deficiency. Current intakes of $10–200\,mg/day$ are considered to be both safe and adequate and dietary reference values have not been specified.

Raw egg white contains a protein or protein-like substance called avidin which combines with the biotin of the yolk to form a stable compound. This is not absorbed from the intestinal tract and so the biotin is not available to the body. Avidin can also render unavailable the biotin in other foods. This avidity for biotin is not shown by cooked egg white.

Cobalamin (vitamin B_{12})

Cobalamin is a deep red crystalline substance with molecular formula $C_{63}H_{90}O_{14}N_{14}PCo$, and it has by far the most complex chemical structure of any vitamin. The presence of a cobalt atom in the molecule is a noteworthy feature. It is the only function of cobalt, which is not technically an essential nutrient itself, since cobalamin cannot be synthesized in the body.

Cobalamin is found in small amounts in all animal tissues but it is absent from foods of vegetable origin. It is required by the body in extremely minute amounts and vegetarians usually obtain sufficient from eggs and milk. Vegans, who abstain completely from foods of animal origin, including dairy foods, may suffer from a deficiency. Fortunately, cobalamin can be made from a mould used to produce the

Table 14.9 Average values for cobalamin content of foods

Food	Cobalamin (µg/100 g)
Liver (lamb's)	83.0
Liver (pig's)	23.0
Eggs	2.5
Cheese (Cheddar)	2.4
Beef, lamb, pork	2.0
Fish (white)	2.0
Cornflakes (fortified)	1.0
Marmite	1.0
Milk	0.9

antibiotic streptomycin and supplies are available for vegans from this source.

Cobalamin plays a part in the production of nucleic acids and in the complex process of cell division in the body. It is especially important, in conjunction with folate and iron, for the formation of red blood cells. It is also involved in the formation of the myelin tube or sheath which surrounds each nerve fibre.

The amount of cobalamin required for the maintenance of good health is exceedingly small and the RNI for those over 15 years of age is 1.5 µg per day. Even smaller amounts are specified for younger age groups (see Table 14.2). These very small amounts are almost certain to be present in all diets except the rigorous vegetarian dietary regime of vegans. Milk, for example, which is not a particularly rich source, contains over 2 µg per pint (568 mL). The liver holds good reserves of cobalamin and it has been estimated that enough is usually present to last for up to 5 years in the absence of a dietary intake. Deficiency syndrome therefore develops very slowly.

Table 14.9 shows the average cobalamin content of some foods: the main sources in the average British diet are meat, offal and milk. Cobalamin is fairly stable to heat and is only slightly soluble in water so losses during cooking are small.

People who are unable to absorb cobalamin from their diet suffer from a serious disease known as pernicious anaemia, in which macrocytic anaemia is subsequently accompanied by degeneration of the nerve tracts in the spinal cord. At one time this disease was invariably fatal, but it is now treated very successfully by injection of hydroxocobalamin at 3-monthly intervals. Pernicious anaemia is caused by the absence

from the gut of an intrinsic factor which is essential for the absorption of cobalamin. It is not a dietary deficiency disease because, if the intrinsic factor is absent, it will occur even when the diet contains sufficient cobalamin.

Folate

Folate is the name given to a group of closely related compounds derived from folic acid (pteroylglutamic acid). Folates are involved in the body, in conjunction with cobalamin, in the production of nucleic acids and, in particular, in the formation of red blood cells. A western diet is only just adequate in folates because of low intake of fruit and vegetables, so deficiency is relatively common in people with even lower intakes of these foods than usual, and this commonly results in a degree of anaemia. Chronically low serum folate allows serum homocysteine concentrations to rise, and this is a factor involved in the development of coronary heart disease. Low folate levels are also linked to higher rates of colonic cancer.

A deficiency of folate may cause a particular type of anaemia called megaloblastic anaemia. This is identical to the anaemia caused by cobalamin deficiency but it is not accompanied by degeneration of the nerve cells, which is a feature of pernicious anaemia. Pregnant women are prone to folate deficiency because the physiological demand increases during pregnancy. Folate deficiency during pregnancy may lead to premature birth and low birthweight. Some women, for genetic reasons, need much more folate than is usually possible from foods, and they are prone to having babies with neural tube defects such as spina bifida, unless they have supplements of folic acid (the synthetic form of folate).

The RNI for folate for those over 11 years of age is 200 µg/day, with smaller amounts being specified for younger age groups and larger amounts for pregnant or lactating women (see Table 14.2).

Folates are found in small amounts in a wide variety of foods; liver, green vegetables, potatoes, Marmite, orange juice and fortified cornflakes are good sources. Fruit and vegetables contribute about 40 per cent of the folate in an average British diet and bread and flour products about 26 per cent. Folates are easily destroyed during cooking and a good deal can be lost in the water used for cooking vegetables. Even greater losses occur if sodium bicarbonate is added to the water to preserve the colour of green vegetables. Alcohol interferes with folate absorption, so deficiency is common in alcoholics.

In some countries, notably the USA, Canada and most South American countries, it is now obligatory to fortify all flour and other cereals with folic acid. This measure aims to reduce neural tube defects in babies, and may help reduce colon cancer and CHD by suppressing blood homocysteine concentrations. High alcohol users are at particular risk. Given that folate deficiency is so common, and that there are no hazards associated with food fortification, the failure of European governments to demand folate fortification is now becoming a scandal. One could argue for fortifying alcoholic drinks with folate, but this idea has not yet been adopted by manufacturers, who hate to admit that alcohol can be hazardous.

Ascorbic acid (vitamin C)

Ascorbic acid, or vitamin C, is a white water-soluble solid with the formula $C_6H_8O_6$. Despite the name ascorbic acid the molecule does not contain a free carboxyl group. It is really a lactone formed from the free acid by loss of water between a carboxyl group on one carbon atom and a hydroxyl group on another. It has the structure:

$$
\begin{array}{cc}
\begin{array}{c}
\text{HO} \quad \text{OH} \\
| \quad | \\
\text{C}=\text{C} \\
| \quad | \\
\text{HOCH}_2\text{CHOH} - \text{HC} \quad \text{CO} \\
\diagdown \diagup \\
\text{O}
\end{array}
&
\begin{array}{c}
\text{HO} \quad \text{OH} \\
| \quad | \\
\text{C}=\text{C} \\
| \quad | \\
\text{HOCH}_2\text{CHOH} - \text{HC} \quad \text{CO} \\
| \quad | \\
\text{HO} \quad \text{OH}
\end{array}
\\
\text{Ascorbic acid} & \text{Free acid corresponding to} \\
& \text{ascorbic acid}
\end{array}
$$

Lactones behave much like acids and for many purposes can be regarded as such. Ascorbic acid has the sharp taste usually associated with acids and will form salts. It is optically active and is dextrorotatory; laevorotatory ascorbic acid is also known but it has little or no vitamin activity. Ascorbic acid is a good reducing agent and consequently it is easily oxidized. The oxidation product dehydroascorbic acid is easily reconverted into ascorbic acid by mild reducing agents, and because this reduction can be accomplished by the body, its vitamin activity is as

high as that of ascorbic acid itself. It is, however, less stable than ascorbic acid and only small amounts are present in foods.

Ascorbic acid is one of the most unstable nutrients, and it is easily destroyed by oxidation, exposure to light or high temperatures, alkalinity and metal ions. In extracts, juices and foods with cut surfaces it may be oxidized at room temperatures by exposure to air. The oxidation is enzymically catalysed by oxidases which are contained within the cells of foodstuffs and are set free on cutting or crushing. The rate of oxidation is greatly accelerated by heat (provided that the temperature is not high enough to destroy the oxidases), by alkalis and especially by traces of copper, which catalyse the oxidation. The rate of oxidation is diminished in a weak acid solution and by storage at low temperatures.

Because ascorbic acid is so easily oxidized it is able to protect other substances from oxidation (i.e. it acts as an antioxidant in the body, in plants and in foods). Synthetic ascorbic acid is available cheaply, and the acid and its sodium and calcium salts and palmityl ester are used as permitted food additives, as antioxidants (see p. 279) by the food industry. In body tissues ascorbic acid protects easily oxidized nutrients and, like β-carotene and vitamin E, is effective in 'mopping up' free radicals. It may also have a preventive function for the large number of diseases in which free radicals are involved. However, this is not the reason for its essential 'vitamin' status.

Sources of ascorbic acid

Ascorbic acid occurs mainly in foods of plant origin. Most fruits are good sources but many popular eating apples, pears and plums supply negligible amounts. Green vegetables, potatoes and fruit are the most important sources of ascorbic acid in the British diet. Table 14.10 lists the average ascorbic acid content of the more important sources.

The amount of ascorbic acid present in vegetables is greatest in the periods of active growth during spring and early summer. Storage decreases the ascorbic acid content and this can be clearly seen in the values given for potatoes in Table 14.10.

Potatoes contain less ascorbic acid than green vegetables, but such large quantities of them are eaten that they constitute an important source of this vitamin. A normal serving of boiled new potatoes

Table 14.10 Average values for vitamin C (ascorbic acid) content of foods

Food	Vitamin C (mg/100 g)
Blackcurrants	150–230
Rosehip syrup	175
Sprouts (raw)	115
Sprouts (boiled)	60
Cauliflower:	
Raw	43
Cooked	27
Cabbage:	
Raw	49
Boiled	20
Spinach:	
Raw	26
Boiled	8
Watercress (raw)	62
Strawberries	77
Raspberries	32
Oranges (raw)	44–79
Lemons (juice)	58
Grapefruit (raw)	36
Peas:	
Raw	25
Boiled	15
Dried, boiled	trace
Tomato (raw or juice)	17
Liver (lamb's, fried)	19
Potatoes:	
Raw, new	16
Raw, Oct–Nov	20
Raw, Dec	15
Raw, Jan–Feb	10
Raw, March onwards	8
Boiled	6
Apples (eating, raw)	3–20
Lettuce (raw)	5
Bananas (raw)	10
Beetroot (boiled)	5
Onions:	
Raw	5
Boiled	3
Carrots:	
Raw	6
Boiled	2
Plums:	
Raw	4
Stewed	3
Pears:	
Raw	6
Stewed	3
Canned	2
Milk:	
Cow's (fresh)	2
Human	5

provides about 90 per cent of the EAR of ascorbic acid and about one-sixth of the ascorbic acid in the British diet is derived from potatoes – a little less than that from all other vegetables. For many years potatoes were the main source of ascorbic acid in the UK, but fruit and fruit juices are now the main source.

As much as 75 per cent of the ascorbic acid present in green vegetables may be lost during cooking. This loss can be avoided by eating raw green vegetables in salads but the amounts which can conveniently be eaten in this way are comparatively small and more ascorbic acid may be obtained by eating a larger quantity of cooked vegetables. For example, 25 g of lettuce, which is a convenient serving, provides about 1 mg of ascorbic acid compared with about 20 mg provided by 100 g of cooked cabbage. Raw cabbage is a much better source of ascorbic acid than lettuce, as 25 g provides about 13 mg of the vitamin.

Cow's milk has only about one-quarter or one-third the ascorbic acid content of human milk and some of this is destroyed during pasteurization. Presumably, evolution did not involve human infants eating grass as an extra source. Exposure of milk to sunlight also decreases its ascorbic acid content and this change is brought about by the breakdown products of riboflavin (see p. 208). It is important that babies, and particularly those fed on cow's milk which has been boiled, should be provided with other sources of the vitamin. Concentrated orange juice, rose-hip syrup or blackcurrant juice are attractive additional sources of the vitamin. When babies progress to a mixed diet, there is less need for such supplements and at 2 years of age a normal diet should provide sufficient ascorbic acid.

Canned fruits and vegetables vary considerably in their ascorbic acid content, but some more acidic vegetables and fruits, for example, tomatoes, are good sources of the vitamin. Some loss of ascorbic acid is inevitable in canning, but good quality canned fruits and vegetables often contain more of this vitamin than 'fresh' fruit and vegetables cooked at home. This is because they are canned while fresh and cooked under carefully controlled conditions.

Foods such as yeast, egg yolk, meats and cereals, which are rich in B vitamins are usually devoid of ascorbic acid, but liver and kidney are exceptions. Vitamin C is concentrated in the eye, but eyes are not popular as food.

Loss of ascorbic acid in cooking

It has already been mentioned that losses of ascorbic acid occur during storage of fruits and vegetables. Some loss also occurs during the preparation and cooking of foods. This is due partly to oxidation and partly to solution in the water used for cooking. To avoid excessive losses, vegetables and fruit should not be crushed or finely chopped before cooking, as this sets free oxidases which catalyse the oxidation of ascorbic acid by the air. There is evidence to show that loss of ascorbic acid is greater when vegetables are cut with a blunt knife than with a sharp one, because the former ruptures more cells by crushing and hence sets free more oxidases than the latter.

If vegetables are put in cold water which is brought to the boil the dissolved oxygen in the water will, in the presence of the oxidases, destroy a substantial amount of the ascorbic acid present. The oxidases are most active at about 60–85°C and above this temperature are quickly inactivated. It is best to place vegetables in boiling water because this contains no dissolved oxygen and the oxidases are rapidly destroyed at this temperature. With potatoes, for example, it has been found that cooking in this way causes only half the reduction in ascorbic acid content experienced with the normal method of cooking.

A minimum quantity of water should be used when cooking vegetables, so that large amounts of the vitamin are not dissolved. This is particularly important with leafy vegetables, such as cabbage, because of the large surface area from which vitamin losses may occur. Vegetables which are completely immersed in water when being cooked may lose up to 80 per cent of their ascorbic acid. If they are only one-quarter covered by water, only about half as much ascorbic acid is lost. With potatoes, which have a smaller surface area per unit weight, and in which gelatinization of the starch prevents diffusion of the ascorbic acid, the quantity of water used in cooking does not greatly affect the amount of ascorbic acid lost. Alkaline conditions should be avoided during cooking and the addition of bicarbonate of soda to green vegetables to preserve or intensify their colour should be avoided, although small quantities may be used to reduce the sourness of acid fruits without serious diminution in the ascorbic acid content.

Microwave cooking may help to preserve ascorbic acid in vegetables owing to the use of less water and rapid heating, but a controlled comparison using the same amount of water and length of cooking showed no differences between the amounts of ascorbic acid retained in boiling or microwaving broccoli.

Because ascorbic acid is very rapidly oxidized in the presence of trace amounts of copper, copper or copper-alloy cooking vessels should not be used for cooking foods rich in vitamin C.

Finally, cooked food should not be kept hot longer than is absolutely necessary before serving because this can destroy almost all the ascorbic acid. It has been shown that a loss of 25 per cent of the ascorbic acid of hot cooked food occurs in 15 minutes and 75 per cent in 90 minutes. This is likely to be the greatest cause of loss of ascorbic acid in restaurants and hotels and in canteens where cooked food is received from a central kitchen.

Functions and requirements of ascorbic acid

The functions of ascorbic acid in the body are not all known with certainty, but it has been shown to be necessary for the formation of the intercellular connecting protein collagen. The cells of the body concerned in the formation of bone and the enamel and dentine of teeth lose their normal functional activity in the absence of ascorbic acid.

A lack of ascorbic acid in the diet causes a condition known as scurvy, which is characterized by a mechanical breakdown of collagen, weakening ligaments and reopening scars and wounds, haemorrhages under the skin and in other tissues, and swollen and spongy gums from which the teeth are easily dislodged or may fall out. Scurvy in infants is associated with great tenderness and pain in the lower limbs together with changes in the bone structure which are not found in adult scurvy. The disease has been known for hundreds of years and was formerly rife among sailors and others whose diet was deficient in ascorbic acid. The cause of the disease was not known but in the course of time it was noted that consumption of fresh foods, particularly vegetables and fruits, could prevent and cure it. Scurvy is almost unknown in the UK, at present, although it still occurs occasionally in alcoholics and in deprived elderly people.

A deficiency of ascorbic acid not severe enough to cause scurvy is thought to increase the susceptibility of the mouth and gums to infection and to slow down the rate at which wounds and fractures heal. Increased susceptibility to many kinds of infection, including the common cold, has been attributed to a shortage of ascorbic acid, but although this is known to be true for guinea-pigs, it is not at all certain that the same applies to human beings. Some evidence suggests reduced symptoms from colds in people who take large supplements, but infection rates are not reduced. It is known, however, that increased amounts of the vitamin are needed by the body when suffering from infectious diseases. Ascorbic acid also assists in the absorption of iron by promoting its reduction to the ferrous state.

The optimum dietary intake of ascorbic acid is not known with certainty. Most animals, unlike humans, are able to synthesize it and so its presence in their diet is not essential. Their tissues are saturated with ascorbic acid, and for this reason it has been suggested that the desirable daily intake for humans should be sufficient to ensure tissue saturation. This occurs at an intake level of about 100 mg/day: above this level the excess is excreted in the urine. However, a lower level of intake – as little as 10 mg/day – has been found to be enough to prevent scurvy and to promote wound healing. The RNI for ascorbic acid has been based on a lower level than that required for tissue saturation but exceeds the very low level at which its anti-scorbutic effect first appears. For those over 15 years of age the RNI is 40 mg/day; smaller amounts are specified for younger age groups and larger amounts for pregnant or lactating women. Full details are given in Table 14.2.

OTHER BIOACTIVE FOOD CONSTITUENTS

The characteristics of vitamins are that they are 'bioactive' (i.e. they have direct and specific effects on the biochemical processes of body cells), and they are 'essential' (i.e. they cannot be made within the body and without them a specific deficiency disease develops).

There are a number of other compounds within foods which are bioactive, but not essential. Some of these compounds may, however, contribute valuably

to health. The distinction between a bioactive food constituent and a drug is not absolute. Some foods contain compounds which are also purified and sold as drugs. For example, caffeine, a normal constituent of tea, coffee and cocoa is marketed as theophylline for the treatment of asthma and heart failure. Some bioactive compounds have multiple actions, with a variety of effects – some valuable or pleasant, others unpleasant or even hazardous. Again, caffeine is a good example: it can produce intolerable palpitations, sleeplessness, anxiety and urinary frequency in some people but provide a valuable mental stimulus for many. These are all the results of biochemical actions of caffeine, which have nothing to do with food allergy. A food allergy is a reaction of the body to a molecule in foods to which antibodies have developed. The unpleasant effects of food allergy are caused by the antibody binding and are not specific to the food molecule.

PLANT POLYPHENOLS

A large number of compounds, found widely in plants, but especially in fruits, are based on groups of phenol rings. A variety of polyphenols are found in food, usually termed flavonoids, but including several main classes (e.g. flavonols, flavonones and anthocyanins). Some of these polyphenols are very powerful antioxidants, and they appear to be produced in plants for this purpose. They are particularly plentiful in leaves and fruits exposed to high levels of oxidizing ultraviolet light. Many polyphenols are yellow, orange or red in colour (e.g. anthocyanins in raspberries) and so absorb blue and ultraviolet light. They have many free hydroxyl groups able to neutralize free radicals produced by ultraviolet light (or other noxious stimuli).

Polyphenols are stable in foods, although under some conditions over time there may be some condensation to larger molecules (e.g. to form tannins in tea and wine). They withstand cooking. Many polyphenols are absorbed from the intestine, but are rapidly metabolized in the gut and liver. Because of their known antioxidant and vasodilatory actions, a variety of health benefits has been proposed, and epidemiological evidence shows associations between consuming flavonols (or high flavonol foods) and protection against coronary heart disease.

Polyphenols are among the most powerful antioxidants, and therefore potentially toxic, so they are usually found in plants and foods bound to other molecules, e.g. sugars. They may have a role in regenerating antioxidant vitamins (e.g. vitamins C and E) whose antioxidant actions are important but subsidiary to other essential roles. At one time, flavonoids were called 'vitamin P' (P for protection) but they proved not to be essential, so did not qualify as vitamins.

Histamine

Histamine is a monoamine compound which some plants produce in response to noxious stimuli (e.g. stinging nettles), but which can occur in response to plant injury. Histamine is involved in allergic reactions (eczema, asthma, hay fever) and if consumed can sometimes mimic part of these effects. It has no beneficial actions.

Caffeine

Caffeine (and the closely related theobromine found in tea) are unusual compounds in that they are synthesized and accumulate to high levels in certain specific foods (coffee beans, cocoa beans, tea leaves) but have no known function in plant physiology. They are valued for their stimulatory effect on mental functions, increasing alertness and mental agility. This arises from a stimulation of the intracellular messenger, cyclic AMP in the brain. The same action accounts for a variety of unwanted effects on brain (sleeplessness, anxiety) heart (fast pulse, ectopic 'missed' beats) and kidneys (increased urine flow). There is also a stimulatory effect on muscle function and respiration which athletes have found to enhance performance in short events. Caffeine is banned by the International Olympic Committee. It causes tremor when taken in large amounts.

Caffeine extracted from plants, or more usually synthesized commercially, is marketed as a drug called theophylline to relax bronchial muscle and relieve asthma, and to enhance the pumping action of the heart in patients with heart failure.

A cup of coffee or a strong cup of tea contains about 50 mg caffeine. A similar amount is added to 'cola' drinks and is probably responsible for many of the unwanted effects in children which are attributed

to 'food additives'. Caffeine is not a permitted additive, but can be incorporated in recipes since it qualifies as a food product.

Phytoestrogens

It has been known for many years that certain diseases are much less common among the Chinese and Japanese, but increase when these people adopt western diets and lifestyles. Coronary heart disease, breast cancer, uterus cancer and osteoporosis are all lower on traditional eastern diets, and women suffer less from menopausal symptoms. The explanation is believed to lie in high levels of flavonoids in beans (particularly soya) which have weak oestrogen-like action. All these diseases are lower in 'oestrogenized' pre-menopausal women. Several specific compounds (e.g. genistein) in legumes (peas, beans, lentils) bind to oestrogen receptors, and are grouped together as 'phytoestrogens'. Despite the epidemiological association, and the clever rationale, intervention studies have produced little direct proof of these effects.

Creatine

Creatine is a small molecule found in muscle and involved in the conversion of chemical energy – derived from macronutrient oxidation but stored temporarily as adenosine triphosphate (ATP) – to mechanical work in muscle contraction. Although creatine is made by the human body, athletic performances can be slightly enhanced by taking extra creatine as a supplement. This has been demonstrated for athletes and for patients with chronic lung disease. The amount of creatine in meat is not sufficient to affect performance even if very large amounts are consumed.

Plant sterols and stanol esters

A small group of these compounds, extracted from pine trees, specifically block the absorption of cholesterol from the bowel. They reduce plasma LDL cholesterol by about 10–15 per cent and so have a role in coronary prevention. One compound, Benecol, is now widely available in oils and spreads, but expensive. Dietary saturated fatty acids, not dietary cholesterol, are the main factor increasing plasma cholesterol and so should be addressed before taking measures to reduce cholesterol absorption.

Other potentially bioactive compounds

From the text above, it can be seen that the evidence for biological effects of food-derived molecules in humans is weak. A number of other compounds present in foods have biological effects in test systems, in large doses, and they are widely marketed as 'nutritional aids' to gullible consumers, without evidence. While we can be sure that compounds such as taurine or coenzyme Q are not essential – so not vitamins – it is hard to prove that they have no effect. At present, we can only say that these compounds have not been shown to have any effect to the satisfaction of any reputable scientific authority (Department of Health, 1991) and health claims made about them should be regarded as fraudulent and illegal.

Key points

- Vitamins are essential, i.e. required from foods for health because they cannot be synthesized within the body, and bioactive as cofactors in enzyme systems
- Water-soluble vitamins (B, C) have no body stores and dietary inadequacy can rapidly lead to deficiency diseases
- Fat-soluble vitamins (A, D, E, K) can be stored in the body and so deficiency states develop more slowly
- A range of plant-derived molecules (e.g. polyphenols, caffeine) have biological effects, but are not required for life or health
- Vitamin D is synthesized by skin exposed to sunlight

Chapter summary

Vitamins were the first described 'essential' nutrients. The apparently magical effects of tiny amounts led to a huge industry attempting to promote supplements and megadoses, but they have not been shown to provide benefits, and in some cases profiles of vitamin and other bioactive compounds in foods vary enormously and the effects of cooking and storage can be damaging. The food and catering industries need to be aware of this and minimize losses during food processing and preparation.

FURTHER READING

BENDER DA (2003). *Nutritional Biochemistry of the Vitamins*, 2nd edn. Cambridge: Cambridge University Press.

BRITISH NUTRITION FOUNDATION (1991). *Antioxidant Nutrients in Health and Disease. BNF Briefing Paper No. 26*. London: BNF.

DEPARTMENT OF HEALTH (1991). *Dietary Reference Values for Food Energy and Nutrients for the United Kingdom – Department of Health Report on Health and Social Subjects 41*. London: HMSO.

FOOD AND AGRICULTURE ORGANIZATION (1988). *Requirements of Vitamin A, Iron, Folate and Vitamin B_{12}. Report No. 23*. Rome: FAO.

FOOD STANDARDS AGENCY (2002). *McCance and Widdowson's The Composition of Foods*. 6th (Summary) edn. London: Royal Society of Chemistry, Food Standards Agency and Institute of Food Research.

HENDERSON L *et al.* (2003). *National Diet and Nutrition Survey: Adults aged 19–64 Years. Volume 3 Vitamin and Mineral Intake and Urinary Analysis*. London: HMSO.

ZHANG D, HAMAUZU Y (2004). Phenolics, ascorbic acid, carotenoids and antioxidant activity of broccoli and their changes during conventional and microwave cooking. *Food Chemistry*, 88(4): 503–509.

15

Fruits, nuts and vegetables

Fruits and vegetables form an important part of the diet and are usually regarded as 'good' foods. They are major sources of vitamin C, folates and non-starch polysaccharides but, as Tables 15.1 and 15.2 show, they are not, in general, rich in other nutrients. They are low energy-density, and are low in fats. Fruits tend to be relatively bulky, and can displace other desserts in meals, such as higher energy, higher fat foods. There is plenty of evidence to recommend eating more fruits and vegetables, for a range of health reasons. Most countries have adopted the WHO recommendation to consume *a minimum* of five 80 g portions each day (excluding potatoes).

FRUITS

Botanically, a fruit is a matured ovary of a flower, including the seed (or seeds) and any part of the flower remaining attached to it. Fruits which conform strictly to this definition are called true fruits and they include nuts, legumes, berries and drupes (see below). Fruits such as apples, pears and strawberries, which include some other part of the flower that has enlarged as well as the matured ovary, are called false fruits. This botanical distinction has no relevance to nutrition or food science.

Botanists regard peas, tomatoes, peppers, aubergines and cucumbers as fruits but most people have a more restricted idea of what constitutes a fruit and look upon them as vegetables. We have come to regard as fruits the succulent parts of plants which are characterized by a sweet or acid taste and a distinct flavour. This somewhat vague description – it hardly merits being called a definition – is more suitable for our hybrid scientific/culinary interests than the more restrictive botanical definition.

Types of fruit

Hundreds of different edible fruits are known and each may exist in a number of varieties. There are over 6000 different varieties of apples, for example, all originating from the wild crab apples, *Malus pumila* and *Malus silvestris*.

Fruits can be classified in a number of ways but a simple method, which is satisfactory for our purposes, is based on their physical characteristics:

- *Pomes* have a seed-bearing compartmented core surrounded by a firm fleshy body: apples and pears are pomes.
- *Drupes* have a single stone or nut embedded in edible flesh: cherries, plums, peaches and olives are obvious examples.
- *Berries* have seeds enclosed in a pulp: grapes and oranges are berries.

Pomes

The most important members of this class of fruit are apples and pears, both of which are members of the same botanical family – the rose family or Rosaceae. The core of an apple or pear is really the matured ovary consisting of five carpels each containing two seeds or 'pips'.

Apples are grown almost everywhere, except in the very hottest and coldest areas of the world. Most apples are eaten raw and dessert apples, or eating apples, are usually small and sweet with a fragrant aroma and flavour. Cooking apples are usually large and green; they have a sharper taste than eating apples owing to the presence of more acid and they pulp easily on cooking. Apples are not particularly good sources of nutrients but they contain some vitamin C and about 2 per cent non-starch polysaccharide (NSP). About one-third of the NSP is in the form of pectin which is commercially extracted from apple pulp for use as a gelling agent (see p. 97). Large quantities of apples are converted to cider.

Pears are closely related to apples but they differ in flavour and often have gritty particles or 'stone cells' embedded in their flesh. Pears are roughly equivalent to apples nutritionally. Just as apple juice is used for making cider, pear juice is made into perry.

Drupes

Drupes are juicy fruits containing one seed surrounded by a hard woody layer which together form a pip or stone.

Plums grow in most parts of the world and are eaten as a fresh dessert fruit and used for jam manufacture or canning. Dried plums are known as prunes.

Cherries vary in colour from yellow to black and in acidity from sour to sweet.

Peaches occur in two main varieties. Freestone peaches have a stone which can be easily separated from the flesh. The more popular cling peaches are firmer, more deeply coloured and less easily damaged than the freestone variety. The nectarine is a type of peach but it is smaller and hairless.

Blackberries, raspberries and strawberries are usually grouped together as soft fruits. Despite their names they are not berries. The first two are drupelets (i.e. aggregates of several 'mini-drupes' which are attached to the swollen tip, or receptacle, of the fruit stalk). Strawberries are false fruits: the true fruits are the tiny seed-like achenes or 'pips' on the outside of the fruit.

These fruits grow wild in most parts of Europe and worldwide, but they are also cultivated commercially.

They are used mainly in cooking and for jam and jelly manufacture. Large table varieties have been produced by selective plant breeding. There is scientific interest in their high content of antioxidants (vitamin C and flavonoids) which may help prevent heart disease and cancers.

Berries

Blackcurrants are notable for their high vitamin C and flavonoid content and one of their main uses is for the manufacture of blackcurrant juice, for use in fruit drinks rich in this vitamin. Large quantities are also made into jam or sun-dried to produce fruit for use in cakes. Currants also occur in red and white varieties.

Forest berries – cranberries, lingonberries, blueberries, blaeberries and others – have been regular features of human diets in high latitudes since prehistoric times. They are gathered from the wild in huge amounts in Nordic countries, and increasingly cultivated. These berries are extremely rich sources of vitamin C and a variety of other antioxidant compounds (polyphenols and flavonoids). They are used fresh, frozen and processed for their flavour and colour in both savoury and sweet dishes, as well as preserved in jams and in drinks, and regular consumption has been related to freedom from a range of illnesses including coronary heart disease (CHD), cancer and urinary infection.

Grapes are probably the world's most widely cultivated fruit crop. Only a small proportion of the grapes grown is used as food, the bulk being converted to wine by fermentation of the juice as explained in Chapter 12. Most of the grapes grown are varieties of a single European grape *Vitis vinifera*. Sun-dried grapes or *raisins* are usually made from seedless grapes. Grapes have a high content of glucose (utilized in wine-making). They contain only about one-tenth as much vitamin C as oranges, but are rich in other antioxidants including flavonoids.

Bananas are cultivated in most tropical countries but those imported into the UK come mainly from Central America and the Caribbean islands. The fruit is picked while it is unripe and during transportation to the UK by ship it is kept at about 12°C in ventilated holds to retard ripening. Before sale the fruit is ripened in temperature-controlled warehouses at

15°C. During ripening the banana skin changes from green to yellow and the fleshy part of the fruit becomes softer and sweeter as its starch is almost completely converted to sugar.

Bananas are not particularly important as a food in Britain and they are normally eaten raw as a sweet dessert fruit. In some other parts of the world, however, boiled or steamed green bananas serve as an important source of starch.

Ripe bananas are little more than easily digested sources of carbohydrate. They provide energy and some vitamin C but very little else. They are roughly equal in nutrient density to potatoes, but as much smaller quantities are eaten they are not important as providers of nutrients.

Citrus fruits

The most important citrus fruits are oranges, lemons, limes and grapefruit. Their seeds are contained in segmented sections or carpels of juicy flesh which are surrounded and protected by a tough skin or peel. Citrus fruits are rich in vitamin C, particularly in the pithy white layer or albedo found under the peel. Orange juice contains only about 20–30 per cent of the fruit's vitamin C and grapefruit juice has an even smaller proportion. Citrus fruits have a refreshing taste because of their high water content and the presence of citric acid and sucrose. The relative amounts of these two substances determines whether the fruit is sharp or sweet to the taste.

Oranges are by far the most important citrus fruit and orange juice is a major source of vitamin C in the British diet. Oranges can be grown in tropical and subtropical countries but they develop their characteristic colour only where night temperatures are below 10°C during the ripening period. Green (but ripe) oranges may be treated with ethylene gas which artificially stimulates them (see p. 223) and brings out their orange colour. Bitter, or Seville, oranges are used for marmalade manufacture. There are many different varieties of orange and also orange-like fruits such as tangerines, mandarins and satsumas which have characteristic flavours and a soft, loosely adherent skin. Some 'soft-citrus' fruits are hybrids of oranges and tangerines or mandarins.

Lemons are not eaten as dessert fruits because of their high citric acid content and consequent sharp taste.

Grapefruit derives its name from the fact that the fruit grows in vine-like clusters containing 3–18 fruits. Over 25 grapefruit varieties are known, some of which have a pink or reddish flesh which is caused by the presence of the carotenoid lycopene.

Nutritional value of fruit

Fruit is refreshing to eat and adds colour and flavour to the diet. Most fruits consist largely of water, however, and hence their nutrient content is low, as Table 15.1 shows. Their main importance is as a source of vitamin C and NSP. About 40 per cent of the vitamin C content of the average British diet is provided by fruit and fruit juices. Most of this comes from citrus fruit and, especially, fruit juices and little from bananas, apples and pears which are the most popular fruits. Some fruits also contain vitamin A; they also make a small contribution to the mineral content of the diet. Despite their sweetness, fruits contribute only about 5 per cent to the energy content of the average British diet.

Fruit contains NSP in the form of cellulose, hemicellulose, pectin and protopectin. In fact, a good deal of what is left after the juice has been completely expressed from a fruit consists of NSP. If we discount those parts not normally eaten – such as pips, cores and the peel of citrus fruits – the actual dry weight of NSP is quite small and usually amounts to less than 2 per cent of the weight of the fruit. Nevertheless, about 10 per cent of the NSP in the average British diet comes from fruit. Consumption of additional fruit is a pleasant (but expensive) way of increasing the intake of NSP.

When fruit is stored there is a progressive loss of vitamin C and up to 20 per cent of that present in citrus fruit may be lost in 1 month. There is usually also a loss of thiamin, but as only small amounts are present initially the loss is not nutritionally significant. Small amounts of carotene may also be lost. Flavonoid levels are more stable. These changes are pathophysiological, rather than decay, since the cells in fresh fruit remain alive.

Frozen fruit retains most of its nutrients during the freezing process and subsequent storage.

Canned fruit can be a good source of vitamin C, despite losses of 20–30 per cent that may occur during the canning process. This is because canning

Table 15.1 Average values or nutrient content of fruit per 100 g of edible portion

Type of fruit	Energy (kJ)	Protein (g)	Sugars and starch (as monosaccharide) (g)	Water (g)	Calcium (mg)	Iron (mg)	Sodium (mg)	Vitamin A (retinol equiv.) (μg)	Thiamin (mg)	Riboflavin (mg)	Niacin (equiv.) (mg)	Vitamin C (mg)
Apples	196	0.3	11.9	84	4	0.3	2	5	0.04	0.02	0.1	5
Bananas	326	1.1	19.2	71	7	0.4	1	33	0.04	0.07	0.8	10
Blackcurrants	121	0.9	6.6	77	60	1.3	3	33	0.03	0.06	0.4	200
Cherries	201	0.6	11.9	82	16	0.4	3	20	0.05	0.07	0.4	5
Dates (dried)	1056	2.0	63.9	15	68	1.6	5	10	0.07	0.04	2.9	0
Figs (dried)	908	3.6	52.9	17	280	4.2	87	8	0.10	0.08	2.2	0
Gooseberries (cooked)	62	0.9	2.9	90	24	0.3	2	25	0.03	0.03	0.5	31
Grapes	268	0.6	16.1	79	19	0.3	2	0	0.04	0.02	0.3	4
Grapefruit	95	0.6	5.3	91	17	0.3	1	0	0.05	0.02	0.3	40
Melon	97	0.8	5.2	94	16	0.4	17	175	0.05	0.03	0.3	50
Oranges	150	0.8	8.5	86	41	0.3	3	8	0.10	0.03	0.3	50
Orange juice	161	0.6	9.4	88	12	0.3	2	8	0.08	0.02	0.3	25–45
Peaches	156	0.6	9.1	86	5	0.4	3	83	0.02	0.05	1.1	8
Pears	175	0.3	10.6	83	8	0.2	2	2	0.03	0.03	0.3	3
Pineapple (canned in juice)	194	0.5	11.6	77	12	0.4	1	7	0.08	0.02	0.3	20–40
Plums	137	0.6	7.9	85	12	0.3	2	37	0.05	0.03	0.6	3
Prunes	686	2.4	40.3	23	38	2.9	12	160	0.10	0.20	1.9	0
Raspberries	105	0.9	5.6	83	41	1.2	3	13	0.02	0.03	0.5	25
Strawberries	109	0.6	6.2	89	22	0.7	2	5	0.02	0.03	0.5	60

takes place promptly after picking when vitamin C content is at a peak. The carotene and thiamin content of fruit is not much reduced during canning. If canned fruit is stored for a long period some loss of vitamin C may occur, but less than 15 per cent is usually lost during 1 year's storage.

When fruit is dried to produce raisins, sultanas, prunes or dried currants, its vitamin C content and about 50 per cent of its thiamin are destroyed. The carotene content is little affected.

Ripening and storage of fruit

Ripening

Much of our food can be eaten at any time in its life cycle: it does not pass through a period when its appeal to the palate is outstandingly greater than at other times. This is not so with fruit, however. Some unripe fruit is inedible but when it ripens (at the time when the seed is ready for planting) it changes dramatically to a condition in which flavour, colour and texture are all at a peak. Unripe fruit is often green but during ripening the green colour may be replaced by a yellow or reddish hue. The flesh softens and becomes sweeter and juicier and a characteristic 'ripe' flavour and odour develops. Extreme examples of this process are provided by fruits that are powerfully astringent when unripe, such as pears, plums and most dramatically persimmon (also known as kaki or 'sharon fruit').

The changes that occur during ripening are, in part, consequences of enzymic conversion of complex substances to simpler ones. Hard starch-packed cells are softened by conversion of starch to sugars which dissolve and enhance the sweetness and juiciness of the fruit. At the same time, insoluble protopectin, which cements the plant cells tightly together, is converted to soluble pectin, which connects them more flexibly.

When a fruit is harvested, it is cut off from a supply of nutrients and growth ceases. Ripening may continue, however, and sometimes the fruit ripens more rapidly than if it had been allowed to continue growing.

Citrus fruits and other fruits that do not store starch obtain their sugar from the leaves of the plant on which they grow. Thus, they do not become sweeter after picking.

Some fruits produce minute amounts of the unsaturated hydrocarbon ethylene (or ethene), $H_2C{=}CH_2$, during their growing period. Larger amounts are produced when the fruit is passing through the critical ripening period when cell activity is at a maximum. Not only is ethylene produced during ripening but it has been shown that it actively promotes ripening. If unripe fruit is exposed to small amounts of ethylene in air (less than one part per million) it initiates ripening and, in addition, stimulates the fruit to produce its own ethylene. This has been commercially exploited by using the gas to accelerate the ripening of fruit which has been harvested unripe for transport, and stored in conditions that retard ripening. Citrus fruits do not produce ethylene when they ripen naturally, but even these can be artificially ripened by using an ethylene-enriched atmosphere. In this way, green but ripe oranges which, understandably enough, have little market appeal can be converted into the familiar orange-coloured fruit. Green bananas can be ripened in the same way.

Storage

Ripeness marks the end of a fruit's growth and the beginning of its death. Fruits which have a soft flesh and a thin skin pass rapidly from ripeness to rottenness and they can hardly be said to have a storage life at normal temperatures. Harder fruits, however, and those protected by a tough skin, can remain in good condition for several months.

Stored fruit deteriorates through normal ageing and shrinkage caused by loss of water. Undamaged fruit may remain edible for some time but eventually it will decay as a result of the continued activity of its own enzymes and attack by microorganisms. Soft fruit usually becomes inedible owing to the growth of moulds and yeasts on its surface. Mould and yeast spores are always present in the air (see Chapter 18) and on the skin of fruit and they are especially numerous near other mouldy fruit. As fruits age and shrink, especially if the skin has been damaged, sugary juice escapes and coats the skin with an ideal growth medium for moulds and yeasts. In general, fruit is not attractive to bacteria because of its acidity and lack of protein but mould growth occurs with ease.

Dark patches may appear on the surface of fruit which has been roughly handled. Ruptured cell membranes allow the contents of cells to mix and soft spots develop. The enzyme phenolase (or polyphenoxidase) oxidizes phenolic cell components to compounds that polymerize to dark-coloured polymers. This is how the familiar brown 'bruises' on the surface of damaged fruit are produced. Phenolase is not present in citrus fruits, melons or tomatoes and thus they do not develop brown bruises. Nevertheless, when cell rupture occurs and juice leaks they are prone to attack by moulds and can rapidly become inedible.

Fruit should be stored in conditions that slow down the action of its own destructive enzymes and the growth of moulds. It should be kept cool and in conditions where loss of moisture is minimized. Humidity should be high enough to prevent undue loss of water, but not so high as to encourage mould growth. Temperatures just above freezing point are best for slowing down enzyme action and mould growth but are too low for many tropical fruits. Bananas, for example, can be irreversibly damaged if kept below 10°C for more than a few hours. The 'crisper' compartment of a refrigerator, where neither temperature nor humidity is too low, provides good conditions for storing most fruits.

Unblemished apples can be kept for long periods in cool surroundings but some varieties are damaged if the temperature falls below 3°C. Commercially their storage life can be considerably extended if they are kept in an atmosphere containing little oxygen (1–3 per cent) and added carbon dioxide (1–5 per cent). Ethylene production is suppressed and post-harvest ripening is delayed by this treatment.

Freezing changes the structure and taste of many fruits, although nutrient contents are well retained. Some fruits are considered to have better eating qualities after freezing (e.g. raspberries, cranberries and lingonberries).

NUTS

Nuts are the seeds of trees, which are frequently packaged naturally in a hard shell to withstand hostile environments. As seeds, they contain all the nutrients necessary to start the growth of roots and stem into a new tree. They therefore contain relatively high contents of proteins, and of energy to provide for the time before the new tree can survive by photosynthesis.

To conserve volume and weight, evolution has arranged for nuts (like all seeds) to contain rather more fat (or oil) than fruits or vegetables.

Nuts are eaten in relatively modest quantities intact, and used as garnishes for desserts. Some, such as almonds, are used extensively in the manufacture of specific nut-based foods, such as marzipan. Others are cultivated as sources of oil, such as walnuts.

The chestnut is remarkable in having a relatively high carbohydrate content, and is used to make a variety of sweetened purées and savoury stuffings, as well as being eaten intact when in season. The chestnut is an interesting crop as it has a very high yield per acre and it grows well in extremely rocky land where other forms of agriculture are difficult. In the past, chestnuts were ground into flour to make bread.

Nuts have been promoted as health-giving, and there is some evidence to favour their use. Of course, eating large amounts of nuts will displace other foods – including those with higher saturated fat contents – so plasma lipids will tend to improve. Nuts tend to contain unsaturated fatty acids, but also some saturated fats (e.g. walnuts) which are less liable to raise cholesterol. Nuts (like all seeds) are rich in vitamin E and contain valuable amounts of selenium.

Some foods, called nuts, are not nuts at all. The coconut technically is a nut and contains a relatively high amount of saturated fat. Peanuts (ground nuts), however, are not nuts. They are the seeds of a leguminous plant, and so much more closely related to peas or beans, and more similar to them nutritionally.

VEGETABLES

The word 'vegetable' is used in several ways. In one sense – as employed in the phrase 'animal, vegetable or mineral' – it includes all substances of plant origin, including fruit. Here, however, we shall be more restrictive and concern ourselves only with those plants or parts of plants which are regarded as vegetables from a culinary and nutritional point of view. The term 'vegetables' is usually applied to plant foods eaten as part of a savoury dish. This still covers a large and somewhat miscellaneous collection of plants, including leafy plants (cabbage and lettuce), stalks (celery) roots and tubers (carrots, parsnips and potatoes), flowers (cauliflower, broccoli and artichoke) and buds (asparagus). The members of one entire group of 'vegetables' (tomatoes, peppers, aubergines and cucumbers) are, in fact, fruits, and a variety of fruits and seeds can be eaten in savoury dishes.

Vegetables in the diet

Most vegetables are edible raw, but in northern cultures commonly cooked before they are eaten. Those that are never cooked are sometimes referred to as 'salad vegetables'. The distinction is far from hard and fast, however, as many vegetables that are normally cooked before eating are eaten raw in salads and, conversely, 'salad vegetables' may be cooked. Thus, grated carrot is often eaten in salads and tomatoes in soups and sauces. Some root vegetables in particular are more-or-less inedible until they are cooked. Cooking softens them by dissolving pectins and hemicelluloses and gelatinizing starch (see p. 95). Uncooked starchy vegetables are difficult to digest because the starch granules resist the action of the digestive enzymes.

Vegetables constitute such a diverse group that it is difficult to generalize about their nutrient content. Table 15.2 lists some of the common vegetables and from this it will be seen that, in general, green leafy vegetables and potatoes are good sources of vitamin C and legumes are good sources of protein and soluble dietary fibre (NSP). Like fruits, however, vegetables are mainly composed of water. Nevertheless, because large quantities of vegetables are eaten, they provide about half the vitamin C, 15–20 per cent of the vitamin A, thiamin, niacin and iron and about 10 per cent of the protein and energy in the average British diet. They also provide about half the NSP.

Some common vegetables

Green vegetables

Green leafy vegetables, such as cabbage and Brussels sprouts, are nutritionally important as sources of vitamin C, β-carotene (pro-vitamin A, see p. 201), folate and iron. The dark green outer leaves contain more vitamin C and β-carotene than the paler inner leaves. Cabbage and Brussels sprouts contain 3–4 per cent fibre, but lettuce has only about one-third

as much. Green vegetables rapidly lose vitamin C when they are kept, and if they are cooked in boiling water up to half their vitamin C can be leached out. Whenever possible, therefore, fresh raw green vegetables should be eaten in preference to those that have been cooked.

Broccoli and spinach are good sources of vitamins A and C. Cauliflower is also rich in vitamin C but contains little vitamin A except in the green outer leaves. Onions and leeks qualify as green vegetables, because their leaves are green. The white parts we eat contain a little vitamin C but no vitamin A and are chiefly of value for their flavour. Onions are rich in the polyphenol quercetin. Celery consists of leaf stalk and, apart from NSP, contains little of nutritional value.

Root vegetables

Carrots, turnips, Swedes and parsnips are the more important root vegetables. The potato is also commonly regarded as a root vegetable although it is a tuber (see below). Root vegetables are good sources of NSP, often too good in the case of Jerusalem artichokes. Carrots are an important source of vitamin A (as β-carotene). The colourless turnips, Swedes and parsnips contain no β-carotene, but they are much richer than carrots in vitamin C.

Potatoes

Potatoes are tubers, that is, swollen tips of underground stems which store energy as starch to feed new stems that grow from the 'eyes'. Potatoes are easily grown and give good yields. They have played an important part in the British diet for over 200 years. Apart from cheapness, ease of cultivation and culinary versatility, one of their advantages is the fact that they have a dormant period after harvesting. Thus, they can be stored and used during the winter months when other vegetables are in short supply. Potatoes can be processed into a flour for use in baked goods or dehydrated to give a product that is easily rehydrated with hot water to produce 'instant' mashed potato. Most dehydrated potato contains added vitamin C and thiamin to replace that destroyed during processing.

Potatoes, like all vegetables, consist principally of water. Apart from water, they are mainly made up of starch and for this reason they are often looked

Table 15.2 Average values for nutrient content of vegetables per 100 g of edible portion

Type of vegetable	Energy (kJ)	Protein (g)	Fat (g)	Sugars and starch (as monosaccharide) (g)	Water (g)	Calcium (mg)	Iron (mg)	Sodium (mg)	Vitamin A (retinol equiv.) (µg)	Thiamin (mg)	Riboflavin (mg)	Niacin (equiv.) (mg)	Vitamin C (mg)
Baked beans	345	4.8	0.6	15.1	74	48	1.4	550	12	0.08	0.06	1.3	0
Beans, runner (boiled)	83	1.9	0.2	2.7	91	22	0.7	1	67	0.03	0.07	0.8	5
Beetroot (boiled)	189	1.8	0	9.9	83	30	0.4	64	0	0.02	0.04	0.4	5
Brussels sprouts (boiled)	75	2.8	0	1.7	92	25	0.5	2	67	0.06	0.10	0.9	40
Cabbage (raw)	92	2.8	0	2.8	88	57	0.6	7	50	0.06	0.05	0.8	55
Cabbage (boiled)	66	1.7	0	2.3	93	38	0.4	4	50	0.03	0.03	0.5	20
Carrots (old)	98	0.7	0	5.4	90	48	0.6	95	2000	0.06	0.05	0.7	6
Cauliflower (cooked)	40	1.6	0	0.8	95	18	0.4	4	5	0.06	0.06	0.8	20
Celery	36	0.9	0	1.3	94	52	0.6	140	0	0.03	0.03	0.5	7
Cucumber	43	0.6	0.1	1.8	96	23	0.3	13	0	0.04	0.04	0.3	8
Lentils (cooked)	420	7.6	0.5	17.0	72	13	2.4	12	3	0.11	0.04	1.6	0
Lettuce	51	1.0	0.4	1.2	96	23	0.9	9	167	0.07	0.08	0.4	15
Onion	99	0.9	0	5.2	93	31	0.3	10	0	0.03	0.05	0.4	10
Parsnips (cooked)	238	1.3	0	13.5	83	36	0.5	4	0	0.07	0.06	0.9	10
Peas (frozen)	307	6.0	0.9	10.7	78	35	1.6	2	50	0.30	0.09	1.6	12
Peas (canned, processed)	366	6.9	0.7	18.9	70	33	1.8	380	10	0.10	0.04	1.4	0
Potatoes	315	2.0	0.2	7.1	79	8	0.4	8	0	0.2	0.02	1.5	8–19
Potatoes (boiled)	322	1.8	0.1	18.0	80	4	0.4	7	0	0.2	0.02	1.2	5–9
Potato crisps	2224	6.3	35.9	49.3	3	37	2.1	550	0	0.19	0.07	6.1	17
Potatoes (fried as chips)	983	3.6	10.2	34.0	44	14	0.84	41	0	0.2	0.02	1.5	6–14
Spinach (boiled)	128	5.1	0.5	1.4	85	136	4.0	120	1000	0.07	0.15	1.8	25
Tomatoes (fresh)	60	0.9	0	2.8	93	13	0.4	3	100	0.06	0.04	0.8	20

Table 15.3 Retention of vitamin C in cooked potatoes

Method of cooking	Vitamin C content (percentage of raw value)
Boiling	55–65
Baking	70–80
Roasting	60–70
Frying (chips)	75–85

upon merely as a cheap source of energy. However, when eaten in large amounts potatoes can be a major source of vitamin C, thiamin, folate and NSP.

Table 15.2 shows that potatoes are by no means rich in vitamin C and about half of what is present is lost when potatoes are cooked (see Table 15.3). Nevertheless, they are an important source of vitamin C because we eat so many of them. Such a wide variation exists in the amount eaten, however, that statements about the contribution of potatoes to the average British diet (both here and elsewhere) must be interpreted with caution.

The data given in Table 15.2 indicate that potato crisps and chips are richer sources of vitamin C than boiled potatoes. Their water content is considerably lower, however (especially for crisps), and on a dry-weight basis their vitamin C content is also lower.

The vitamin C content of freshly dug new potatoes can be as high as 20 mg/100 g but it declines sharply to about half that value after 3 months' storage. Loss of vitamin C continues, but much more slowly, during longer storage. Substantial losses of vitamin C occur when potatoes are cooked (as shown in Table 15.3). Losses during cooking occur through oxidation and solution. If boiled potatoes are kept hot for a period of time before serving, or if air is beaten into them by mashing or creaming, further substantial losses of vitamin C may occur.

Only about 4 per cent of the protein in an average British diet is provided by potatoes, but its biological value (see p. 143) is high and almost equals that of egg protein. People that eat large amounts of potatoes often have a diet that is far from ideal and in these circumstances the protein provided by potatoes is valuable. A daily intake of 1 kg of boiled potatoes or 0.5 kg of 'chips' will provide enough of all the essential amino acids except methionine (which can come from fish, meat or from legume).

Potatoes are a major source of thiamin and folate. They supply about 20 per cent of the thiamin in the average diet and are second only to green vegetables as a source of folate. Modern methods of analysis have shown that the folic acid content of cooked potatoes can be as high as 45 µg/100 g.

The iron content of potatoes is by no means high, but a kilogram provides about half the reference nutrient intake (RNI) for an adult. Potatoes provide about 5 per cent of the iron in an average British diet and they are the third most important dietary source. The iron present in potatoes is well absorbed, possibly because vitamin C is also present, and this may also promote the absorption of iron from other foods eaten at the same time.

Potatoes contain about 1 per cent NSP and provide about 15 per cent of the average NSP intake. About half the NSP is classified as soluble fibre (see p. 98). It is sometimes suggested that potatoes cooked in their jackets contain substantially more fibre than those that have been peeled but the difference is actually insignificant.

In the past, potatoes were seldom included in 'slimming' diets and they acquired an undeserved reputation as a 'fattening food'. It is true that they are a cheap form of energy but they are no more 'fattening' than any other food and, as we have seen, they provide the diet with appreciable quantities of valuable nutrients. Although we eat so many potatoes, they contribute only about 5 per cent to the energy content of the average British diet. In fact, because of their high water content their 'energy density' (i.e. the amount of energy available per unit weight) is quite small. If they are cooked or served with large additions of fat, as in crisps, chips or mashed potatoes with added butter then, of course, the energy density of the product bears little relation to that of the potato itself. In general, potatoes have a high water content, so low enough density and, they are suitable for wider use in weight management. The carbohydrate in some potatoes is largely unavailable, but cooking releases a rather pure form of starch, which is rapidly absorbed and hydrolysed in the small intestine. Freshly cooked potatoes therefore have a high glycaemic index and have again received adverse comment in relation to diabetes and blood lipid management. If eaten in large amounts and in isolation, potato increases blood glucose rapidly. However, after cooking, the starch becomes 'retrograded' forming larger complexes which are again more slowly absorbed.

When potatoes are exposed to light the poisonous alkaloid solanine may be formed at their surface. Fortunately, they also become green at the same time, and this coloration serves as a warning that solanine may be present. Green parts of potatoes and all shoots and eyes (which may also contain solanine) should be removed when potatoes are being prepared for cooking. It is illegal to sell green potatoes.

Legumes or pulses

Peas, beans and lentils, which grow as seeds inside a pod, are referred to collectively as legumes or pulses. As mentioned earlier, peanuts are also members of this botanical family. Normally only the seeds are eaten but sometimes, as with runner beans, green ('haricot') beans and the aptly named 'mangetout' peas the pod also is eaten. Pulses have a high protein content and are rich in lysine but poor in methionine. This is the opposite of cereal proteins and so a combination of a cereal-based food with pulses provides an amino acid mixture of high biological value. (The undoubted popularity of baked beans on toast embraces sound nutritional principles!)

On a worldwide basis, many traditional diets compile legumes and cereal products to provide a sustainable, nutritionally balanced basis for the overall diet. Fresh or frozen peas and beans eaten in their pods supply vitamin C, thiamin, niacin and carotene. Many pulses are eaten after they have been dried and stored, however, and this destroys their vitamin C content. Canned peas (which are often canned dried peas) contain no vitamin C. (It is a good plan to enjoy fruit with beans on toast!)

Peas are popular as a green vegetable in the UK and well over half those sold are frozen peas. A large proportion of the green beans sold have also been frozen. Freezing often takes place within hours of harvesting and the vitamin C content of frozen peas and beans is often higher than that of their 'fresh' counterpart because of the time that the latter take to reach the market.

Over 200 types of bean are known and they are grown all over the world. Most of them are varieties of the species *Phaseolus vulgaris*. Kidney beans (green beans or runner beans) are widely popular and many other types are available. Baked beans are more popular in Britain than anywhere else. They are made from 'pea beans' or 'navy beans' by soaking them in water, baking them and canning them in a sweet tomato sauce. Baked beans, like all pulses, are a good source of protein and iron. Soya beans form part of the staple diet (with rice as the cereal) in most of the Far East, and are of great importance worldwide. The beans are rich in protein of high biological value and contain over 20 per cent fat. Soya bean oil, which is rich in PUFAs, is extensively used in the manufacture of margarine and as a cooking oil. The beans are also used for making textured vegetable protein (TVP; see p. 166). Soya beans, and to a lesser extent other legumes, contain compounds known as phyto-oestrogens. These compounds bind weakly to oestrogen receptors in the body, and they are claimed to protect against osteoporosis, breast cancer, heart disease and menopausal symptoms.

Soya beans and red kidney beans contain an anti-trypsin factor which interferes with the action of the protein-splitting enzyme trypsin in the small intestine. Some beans notably red kidney beans contain lectins, which interfere with the absorption of nutrients in the small intestine, and haemaglutinins, which cause red blood cells to cling together. Fortunately, all these toxins are destroyed by heating and beans which have been thoroughly cooked are not harmful.

Pulses are richer in B vitamins and NSP than green vegetables and root vegetables.

Pulses sometimes cause digestive problems, or flatulence through intestinal gas production if consumed in large amounts without adaptation. They contain fairly high quantities of NSP, which has characteristics similar to gel-forming 'soluble' fibre. They contain NSP trisaccharides and tetrasaccharides, which are not digested by enzymes in the small intestine. These pass unchanged to the large intestine, or bowel, where they are broken down by bacteria to smaller molecules, including the gases carbon dioxide, methane and hydrogen. The NSP content of legumes is valuable for control of blood lipids and glucose, but measured consumption of legumes needs to be introduced gradually.

Storage of vegetables

Most hard vegetables can be stored for long periods after they have been harvested. Potatoes, for example, deteriorate only slowly and they remain in good condition for many months. Some other vegetables, however, have a much shorter storage life. Broccoli, for example, is harvested while the plant is still developing and must be eaten before the flowers open.

The storage life of a particular type of vegetable depends mainly upon its quality at the time it was harvested but storage conditions, of course, are also important. Most vegetables mature gradually and, unlike fruits, they do not have a critical ripening period. They are often harvested before their growth is complete to ensure that tenderness and flavour are at a peak. If harvesting is delayed for too long, vegetables may become tough or stringy through thickening of the cell walls. Their sugar content may also fall, leading to a reduction in sweetness and flavour. Careful judgement is needed to ensure that vegetables are harvested at such a time that they are in peak condition when they are eaten or upon arrival at a freezing or canning plant.

Once vegetables are harvested, they begin to lose water by diffusion through the cell walls. This causes shrivelling or wilting as the cell membranes draw away from the walls and the vegetable becomes less firm.

When raw vegetables are eaten, the contrast between fresh and 'not-so-fresh' is striking. A fresh vegetable offers an initial resistance to biting followed by release of copious juice. A vegetable which has begun to deteriorate, on the other hand, will be less firm and juicy. Leafy vegetables are particularly likely to wilt, because water loss occurs more readily owing to their large surface area.

For maximum storage life, leafy vegetables should be kept in cool and fairly moist conditions. Dry conditions obviously encourage water loss and wilting. The 'crisper' compartment of a refrigerator provides good conditions because the temperature is low and the humidity in the closed compartment is higher than on the shelves of the refrigerator.

Potatoes should not be kept in a refrigerator because they begin to convert their starch to sugar below about 8°C. They develop a sweet taste and chips or crisps made from them tend to be dark in colour. At temperatures below 0°C cell rupture occurs and an inedible 'flabby' potato, which decays rapidly, is obtained on thawing.

In general, vegetables are not as easily damaged as fruits during storage and transportation. Nevertheless, they can be bruised and develop brown patches through the action of phenolase in the same way as fruits (see p. 224).

Stored vegetables gradually lose vitamin C as they age but the rate of loss may be slow if they are undamaged. Whole cabbages, for example, lose little or no vitamin C in a week. Vegetables which have an 'open' structure and wilt quickly, such as spinach and lettuce, lose vitamin C fairly quickly. Their storage life is not very long, however, so that they are usually eaten before serious loss of vitamin C has occurred. The other vitamins present in vegetables are not greatly affected by storage, although some loss of thiamin may occur. There may be advantages to storing green vegetables in the light, to retain both colour and antioxidant content. Root vegetables on the other hand should be stored in the dark and that is particularly important for potatoes, which synthesize the poisonous solanin if kept in the light.

If stored in damp conditions, peanuts are susceptible to a mould which produces a toxin, aflatoxin, which is responsible for liver disease and even liver cancer.

SENSORY QUALITIES OF FRUITS AND VEGETABLES

A preference for a particular type of fruit or vegetable is more likely to depend on its taste, smell and colour than on a knowledge of its nutritional qualities. Taste and smell both contribute to flavour and these qualities are so closely related that it is difficult to distinguish between them or to define them. All of them are of chemical origin inasmuch as they are caused by the presence of specific compounds in the fruit or vegetable. Beyond that, however, it is not always possible to say with confidence exactly why a particular fruit or vegetable should have the characteristic taste, smell and flavour we associate with it. In general, repeated exposure to fruit and vegetables leads people to develop a taste for them (like tea or beer). Some people with profound dislike of particular vegetables may have unusual, specific, taste buds, possibly genetically determined.

Taste and smell

The taste of a fruit is a subtle blend of sweetness and acidity (combined in some cases with astringency or bitterness) delicately complemented by the flavour of the particular fruit. Fruits are sweet because of the presence of sugars which are formed when a fruit ripens and if 'fruit acids' are also present they will produce a sharp taste. The relative amounts of sugar and acids present largely determine whether a particular fruit is sweet or sour.

The chemical structures of some acids which commonly occur in fruit are shown below. All of them contain a carboxyl group (—COOH). Oxalic acid, malic acid and tartaric acid are dicarboxylic acids because their molecules contain two carboxyl groups and, similarly, citric acid and isocitric acid, where there are three carboxyl groups, these are tricarboxylic acids. With the exception of oxalic acid

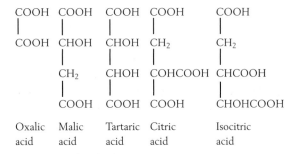

| Oxalic acid | Malic acid | Tartaric acid | Citric acid | Isocitric acid |

they are all hydroxy acids because their molecules contain hydroxyl (—OH) groups.

The fruit acids are colourless, odourless, water-soluble solids. Citric acid, as its name makes clear, is present in the juice of citrus fruits but it also occurs in other fruits. Malic acid also is present in most fruit juices and it is mainly responsible for the acidity of apple juice. Tartaric acid is the main acid in grape juice, but citric and malic acids are also present. Blackberries owe their acidity mainly to isocitric acid. Oxalic acid occurs in unripe tomatoes and strawberries in very small amounts, but rhubarb stalks may contain as much as one part in 200. The presence of oxalic acid is undesirable because it combines with calcium present in other foods to form insoluble calcium oxalate and thus renders it unavailable to the body.

Bitterness and the closely related taste characteristic, astringency, are not related to pH or the presence of fruit acids and both sweet and sour fruits can be bitter or astringent. Bitterness (e.g. in Seville oranges) is caused by the presence of complex phenolic substances known as flavonoids or tannins.

A low level of astringency contributes to the taste of many fruits and much higher levels are found in unripe fruit and some grapefruit.

Flavour is a more subtle property than taste, consisting as it does of a combination of taste and smell. Fruit owes its smell to the presence of a variety of volatile sweet-smelling organic compounds including acids, alcohols, esters (which are formed by reaction between acids and alcohols), aldehydes, ketones and hydrocarbons. A large number of such compounds may contribute to the flavour of a particular fruit and over 200 have been identified in ripe bananas. Some of these may be present in exceedingly small amounts but they can still be detected by the palate. It has been shown, for example, that the smell of ethyl 2-methylbutyrate can be detected in concentrations as low as one part in 10 000 000 000. The simpler compounds are present in many ripe fruits and they provide a common background of ripeness and fruitiness, but a single compound may be responsible for the characteristic flavour of a particular fruit. For example, the presence of benzaldehyde characterizes the flavour of cherries and almonds and ethyl 2-methylbutyrate that of ripe apples. When fruits ripen, there is an increased production of volatile compounds and the proportions in which the various substances are present also changes.

Blends of esters with alcohols and other fragrant compounds are used in cooking and in manufactured foods as synthetic flavours or 'essences' as substitutes for genuine fruit flavours (see p. 304).

Vegetables do not, in general, have such pleasant tastes, smells and flavours as fruits. No one has found it worthwhile to produce artificial cabbage or onion flavour for use in soft drinks or jellies, neither do we have vegetable-flavoured sweets. Nevertheless, vegetables do have tastes, smells and flavours which, although less prominent than fruit flavours, are equally distinctive.

Many of the less attractive (and perhaps more pronounced) vegetable smells are caused by sulphur compounds. Cabbage, Brussels sprouts and cauliflower owe their smell to a group of sulphur compounds known as isothiocyanates or mustard oils. In raw and undamaged vegetables these offensive compounds are bound to sugar and are thereby rendered odourless. When plant tissues are damaged by cutting, bruising or chewing, an enzyme catalyses the breakdown of the complex sulphur-containing compounds and the pungent isothiocyanates are released. The tastes and smells thus produced vary in intensity from the acrid odour of crushed mustard seed to the relatively mild smell of shredded cabbage. Some people are more sensitive than others to these odours.

When cabbage-type vegetables are cooked in boiling water, the complex sulphur compounds break down and combine with other plant materials. New powerfully smelling sulphur compounds are produced, including the gas hydrogen sulphide.

Garlic, onions, leeks and chives also owe their similar but different smells and flavours to the presence of sulphur compounds. They contain a compound derived from the amino acid cysteine which is odour-free while inside the plant tissues. When the cells are broken by crushing, however, this odourless compound is converted enzymatically to other sulphur compounds. Some of these have powerful odours while others are lachrymators (i.e. substances that cause a burning sensation in the eyes and make them water). The compound chiefly responsible for the well-known odour of garlic is diallyl sulphide, $(CH_2{=}CH{-}CH_2)_2S$.

Colour

There are three main groups of compounds which give colour to fruit and vegetables:

- Chlorophylls – green colours
- Carotenoids – yellow, orange and red colours
- Anthocyanins – red, purple and 'bluey' colours

Chlorophylls

These are the green colouring matter of leafy vegetables and unripe fruit where their presence is essential for the conversion of carbon dioxide to simple carbohydrates by photosynthesis. Two types are present in fruit and vegetables – chlorophyll a, which is bright green in colour, and chlorophyll b, which is less brightly coloured. The two versions differ slightly in structure but they both have large molecules, as can be appreciated from the molecular formula of chlorophyll a which is $C_{55}H_{72}O_5N_4Mg$. Usually about three times as much chlorophyll a is present in plant tissues as chlorophyll b. From our point of view they are both equivalent and in the

text that follows they will be referred to simply as chlorophyll.

The chlorophyll molecule has a large and complicated ring structure that in some respects resembles the molecule of haemoglobin, the red colouring matter of blood. The chlorophyll molecule, however, has a magnesium atom at its centre instead of the iron atom present in haemoglobin. It also has a long 'tail' containing 20 carbon atoms, derived from the alcohol phytol, $C_{20}H_{39}OH$, and this makes it fat-soluble.

The chlorophyll molecule is not particularly stable and both the central magnesium atom and the phytyl side chain are easily removed when fruit or vegetables are cooked or processed. The magnesium atom is displaced by heating in acid conditions and chlorophyll derivatives, which are brownish in colour, are produced. This is what happens when cabbage is overcooked. If sodium bicarbonate is added to the water in which 'greens' are cooked it 'preserves' their green colour by preventing or slowing down the loss of magnesium. This practice is not to be recommended, however, because it causes loss of vitamin C.

Displacement of the central magnesium atom from the chlorophyll molecule causes canned green vegetables to lose their natural colour. This may occur when they are canned or during subsequent storage and it is probably caused by release of organic acids from the plant tissues. The loss of colour cannot be prevented by adding sodium bicarbonate because when this is done the vegetables become soggy during processing and storage. To compensate for the loss of natural colour artificial dyestuffs are usually added to canned green vegetables (see p. 301).

The phytyl side chain may split off from a chlorophyll molecule during blanching, cooking or processing. The remainder of the molecule, which retains its green colour, is more soluble in water and colour loss may occur through leakage into the surrounding water.

Carotenoids

Most yellow or orange (and some red) foods owe their colour to the presence of carotenoids, which are the most widespread of all plant colouring matter. Over 300 carotenes are known and they are all related to lycopene, the red colouring matter of tomatoes and pink grapefruit. Carotenoids occur with chlorophyll in all green plants: they play an indirect role in photosynthesis by absorbing sunlight of certain wavelengths and making it available to chlorophyll.

There are many carotenoids but they fall into two categories: the carotenes that are hydrocarbons (i.e. contain only carbon and hydrogen) and the xanthophylls, that also contain oxygen. Carotenes are mainly found in orange- or reddish-coloured plants and xanthophylls in yellow plants.

Carotenoids have large molecules and they are highly unsaturated and fat-soluble. Their molecules contain numerous carbon–carbon double bonds and they are therefore susceptible to oxidation. β-Carotene, for example, has the molecular formula $C_{40}H_{56}$ and its molecule contains 11 carbon–carbon double bonds. In plant tissues, however, they are in a protected environment and only small losses occur during storage or normal cooking operations.

Several carotenes function as antioxidants and some can be converted to retinol (vitamin A, see p. 201) in the small intestine. They therefore have nutritional significance in addition to their role in making food more visually attractive.

Anthocyanins

The anthocyanins belong to a class of compounds known as flavonoids and they impart red, purple and blue colours to fruit, vegetables and wine. There are a variety of anthocyanins which differ slightly in chemical structure but they all possess the same basic skeleton. In plant tissues they are combined with sugars and the number of different combinations, and hence different colours, is very large.

Anthocyanins are soluble in water and they easily leak out of fruit and vegetable tissues during cooking. They are sensitive to changes in acidity which cause them to change colour. Red colours predominate in acidic conditions (i.e. at low pH), but at higher pH the colour changes to yellow or blue. In most cooking operations, however, anthocyanins are quite stable and they retain their colour because the pH is kept low by plant acids. More severe conditions occur when fruit is canned and many coloured fruits are bleached or become discoloured. Artificial colouring matter is often added to canned fruit to compensate for loss of natural colour.

BIOACTIVE COMPOUNDS IN FRUITS AND VEGETABLES

A variety of compounds present in plant foods have biological or biochemical actions on cells in the human body, with possible consequences for health. As with drugs, these effects may be beneficial or toxic, and this may depend on dosage. They can be classified within four groups: terpenoids, phenolics, alkaloids (which contain nitrogen) and sulphur-containing compounds. The number of bioactive compounds identified are staggering: 25 000 terpenes, over 10 000 polyphenols and 250 different sterols exist in plants, many of which are eaten. These compounds have physiological functions in plants. Carotenoids are central to photosynthesis and therefore present in all green plants; sterols regulate membrane fluidity and permeability, phenolics are involved in protection against attack by insects, bacteria and even browsing animals, and provide colours, glucosinolate help protects against microbial attack, and terpenoids function to attract or repel insects; salicylic acid is produced by plants in response to injury, to initiate defence mechanisms.

Among the potentially hazardous effects of bioactive food compounds are the goitrogens – which interfere with iodine metabolism and can lead to enlargement of the thyroid gland (goitre). These compounds are in the class of glucosinolates, and found exclusively in brassicas (cabbage, kale etc.). Cyanogens (which can release cyanides after hydrolysis are present in tiny amounts in kernels of almonds, apricots, peaches, etc., but also in pears. Cyanogens are present in potentially dangerous amounts in raw cassava. Exposure to sunlight and fermentation are necessary to denature these poisonous alkaloids and make this staple food safe to eat.

Celery and related plants contain a small molecule called psoralen that causes skin sensitization to sunlight, such that in some people skin that has been in contact with raw celery can burn and blister after exposure to sunlight; this is not an allergy. Psoralen's function is to protect the plant against insect attack and tends to be higher in strains suitable for organic cultivation.

Some bioactive compounds in plant foods are unequivocally beneficial to health, for example, the vitamins and carotenoids, but there are many others for which the evidence is mixed, or for which the dose and context of consumption may lead to different effects. Thus, the glucosinolate glucobrassicin in foods of the cabbage family is an example of a group of compounds that induce 'Phase II enzymes' involved in tumour genesis. They appear to protect against cancers if consumed in small amounts, but at high doses can promote mutations.

Even within the vitamins and carotenoids, which are generally protective when consumed in normal foods, several studies have shown increased heart disease and cancer if they are taken as high-dose supplements.

Polyphenols, particularly flavonoids, have recently been promoted as health-promoting. Many are potent antioxidants which can share this function with vitamin C, and there is evidence that some classes of polyphenols can protect LDL and DNA from oxidative damage. Effects on health are much more difficult to ascertain and even the epidemiological evidence is mixed, based often on incomplete self-report consumptions of foods, some of which have had measurements of some phenolic compounds. Some studies suggest protection against heart disease by dietary flavonoids, and some suggest adverse effects. This is in keeping with the patchy mechanistic literature on laboratory studies. Potentially hazardous effects are only seen at very high concentrations. Among the most promising groups of phenolics are the flavan-3-ols (including catechins) and anthocyanidins found in tea and red wine. They have antioxidant and vascular relaxant effects which could explain generally beneficial, if weak, associations with heart health in the literature. These compounds also provide a bitter taste. They combine to form insoluble tannins which contribute to bitter taste by binding to salivary proteins, but their biological effects in humans are uncertain.

Few foods contain alkaloids in significant amounts, notable exceptions being the purine alkaloids caffeine and theobromine. Sulphur-containing compounds especially glucosinolates in brassicas have generated recent research interest, but without clear health conclusions.

Key points

- Fruits are mature ovaries of flowers, which become edible to attract animals and thereby dispense the seeds inside fruits, which escape digestion
- Fruits may be astringent before the seeds are fully formed, but when ripe are rich in free sugars
- Nuts are seeds whose fruit is usually inedible and protective
- Nuts contain enough energy for tree seeding growth before photosynthesis, so tend to be rich in fats
- All fruits, nuts and vegetables contain antioxidant vitamins (C, E) and/or carotenoids, which act as natural preservatives, and are important sources of potassium and dietary fibre (NSP)

Chapter summary

Fruits and vegetables are mainly water, so not concentrated sources of nutrients, but if eaten in recommended amounts (at least 5 x 80 g portions daily) they contribute most of several essential vitamins and minerals and a variety of other bioactive compounds. People who eat less than this risk multiple deficiencies, and higher rates of cancers and cardiovascular diseases. Bad cooking and storage (e.g. boiling, canning) can deplete them, as well as making inherently attractive foods horribly unattractive.

FURTHER READING

DUCKWORTH, R.B. (1966). *Fruit and Vegetables*. Oxford: Pergamon Press.

HOLLAND, B. *et al.* (1992). First supplement to McCance and Widdowson's *The Composition of Foods*, 5th edition: *Fruit and Nuts*. Cambridge: Royal Society of Chemistry.

HOLLAND, B. *et al.* (1992). Second supplement to McCance and Widdowson's *The Composition of Foods*, 5th edition: *Vegetable Dishes*. Cambridge: Royal Society of Chemistry.

YAWIAGUCHI, M. (1984). *World Vegetables – Principles, Production and Nutritive Values*. Chichester: Ellis Horwood.

16

Methods of cooking

WHY COOK?

It was a very long time ago that humans relied entirely on raw food. Even before harnessing fire, humans may well have cooked food using hot springs, as New Zealand Maoris have until recent times; sun-drying or baking is another ancient way to alter texture and flavour. However, the mastering of fire, and cooking of food, are two characteristics which set humans apart from all other species. Very few such unique characteristics exist in all cultural settings. A sense of humour is often cited as a unique human quality, but commonly seems lacking in certain northern European settings.

Some foods are best eaten when freshly harvested without further preparation or cooking. Some vegetables, such as lettuce, tomatoes and radishes, and some fruit, such as strawberries, peaches and melons, come into this category. Their characteristic flavour and texture can best be appreciated when they are fresh and raw; cooking can only cause deterioration of these qualities. Many foods, however, are greatly improved by cooking which, if properly carried out, enhances appearance, flavour, texture and digestibility. Indeed, some foods are inedible or indigestible without cooking. Cooking may also promote the safety and keeping qualities of food by killing moulds, yeasts and bacteria that are pathogenic or cause spoilage. Cooking, however, needs to be distinguished from the use of heat treatment to preserve food – a subject which is discussed in Chapter 18.

The preparation and cooking of food is both an art and a science. The art of cooking food has developed over centuries and in refining cooking techniques and recipes cooks have unwittingly developed the necessary scientific skills of careful experimentation and precise observation. The knowledge accumulated in this way has been passed down through many generations and represents the results of numerous experiments. Today, by applying scientific principles, we can understand the changes that occur during cooking and in this way we can improve the cooking process both in terms of the quality and the nutritional value of the food produced.

Cooking may be simply defined as the heat treatment of food carried out to improve its palatability, digestibility and safety. Cooking involves transfer of both heat and mass.

Traditional methods of cooking, such as boiling and baking, are all developments of the original method which used an open fire. The only cooking methods that are not derived from the open fire technique are microwave and electromagnetic induction methods of cooking.

METHODS OF HEAT TRANSFER

Food is a relatively poor conductor of heat. In traditional cooking methods the food is heated at its surface and heat is then transferred into the body of the food by conduction and/or convection. In methods using a high temperature source, such as grilling or toasting, heat is transferred to the surface of the food directly by radiation. More usually, heat is transferred from the source of heat to the surface of the food using some intermediate medium such as water, steam, air or oil. Microwave cooking differs from traditional methods, in that heat is generated within the food. Even so, the heat so generated is then transferred to regions of lower temperature by means of conduction and convection.

Radiation involves the emission of heat from a high temperature source in the form of waves. Such waves, which are similar in nature to light waves, pass through air in straight lines to reach the surface of the food without any intermediate medium being involved. The energy of the radiation is absorbed by the surface of the food which, in consequence, heats up rapidly. Methods of cooking which utilize radiant heat, such as grilling and infrared cooking, are therefore liable to overcook the outside of a food while leaving the inside underdone. Where such a result is desirable, as in cooking steaks, grilling may be the preferred method of cooking.

While radiation involves direct heat transfer from heat source to food, conduction and convection are both indirect means of heat transfer. Convection is the transfer of heat as the result of the movement of a fluid, such as air or water, from a higher temperature region to one at a lower temperature. Thus, when food is placed in a heated oven, the heated air in the oven rises and when it reaches the surface of the food some of the kinetic energy of the air molecules is transferred to the food surface as heat energy. The rising hot air displaces the cooler air from the top of the oven forcing it downwards so that it is reheated by the heat source. In such an oven there is therefore a circulation of heated air, the top of the oven being some 50°C hotter than the bottom. Convection heating in ovens depends upon the flow of hot air over the food, and this can be improved by increasing the rate of flow using a fan. This is the principle used in forced convection ovens which allow an even temperature to be achieved throughout the oven.

Conduction of heat occurs when a metal pan is placed on a heat source. Metals are good conductors of heat, meaning that they transfer heat energy rapidly and efficiently. In boiling, for example, the pan conducts heat from the heat source to the water in the pan. The heated water circulates, heating the surface of solid food by convection. Heat is then transferred to the interior of the food by conduction.

One other method of cooking by conduction involves electromagnetic induction. The principle of this method is that some metals, particularly aluminium alloys, can absorb electric currents of certain frequencies and generate from them eddy currents in the metal which produce a heating effect. The advantage of this technique is that heat for cooking is generated within the cooking vessel so eliminating the transfer of heat from its source to the pan used for cooking. Consequently, this technique is both more efficient and safer than traditional methods; at present it is also more expensive.

The rate of heat transfer involved in cooking can be considered in two stages:

1   The rate at which heat is absorbed by the surface of the food;
2   The rate of conduction of heat to the centre of the food.

The art of cooking is to control these two rates so as to produce the desired result. The factors which affect the first rate are the rate of conduction if the heat source is in direct contact with the food, as in contact grills, or the rate of convection if the food is immersed in a fluid such as air or water, as in baking or boiling. The factors that affect the second rate are the temperature of the surface of the food, the thickness of the food, the rate of evaporation from its surface and its thermal conductivity.

TRANSFER OF MASS

In addition to transfer of heat, cooking involves transfer of mass, mainly the transfer of water through the food as cooking proceeds. During cooking, water travels from the centre of the food to the surface, where it evaporates. Soluble nutrients and flavours also travel with the water, and in moist heat cooking methods may be lost from the surface of the food into the cooking water – a process which is known as leaching. Fat is also transferred during cooking and may either be added to the food, as during frying, or lost from the food as 'cooking drip' in grilling or roasting.

GENERAL EFFECTS OF COOKING

The transfer of heat and mass produces many of the changes of colour, flavour, volume, texture and digestibility that occur during cooking. The art of cooking is to promote the desirable changes while minimizing the undesirable ones. For example, in the baking of pastry the rate at which heat is absorbed by the surface of the pastry determines the extent of browning, which is brought about partly by the caramelization of sugar and partly by non-enzymic browning caused by the interaction of sugar and lysine. If the rate of heating is too low the product will have an uncooked whitish appearance; if it is too high its colour may be too brown (or even black!) and there will be severe destruction of lysine because of excessive non-enzymic browning.

In addition to the changes mentioned, there are also changes in nutritional value during cooking. Some specific effects may be beneficial, for example, destruction by heat of the substance that inhibits the enzyme activity of trypsin in many raw legumes, such as groundnuts and soya beans. Other specific effects may be detrimental, such as non-enzymic browning mentioned above. Some cooks, in attempting to improve the colour of green vegetables by the addition of sodium bicarbonate, cause destruction of vitamin C. Table 16.1 summarizes the main types of nutrient loss that occur during preparation and cooking of food.

Some specific hazards from chemical changes during cooking have been identified. High temperature, e.g. barbecuing or frying of proteins, can generate heterocyclic polycarbon compounds which are implicated in cancers. The effects of high temperature on a mix of carbohydrates and fat include synthesis of the toxic and carcinogenic compound acrylamide. This was recently found in a variety of processed foods, including breakfast cereals, cakes and biscuits. Changes have been introduced in Europe to reduce the problem.

CHANGES OCCURRING AFTER COOKING

In the home, food is usually consumed immediately after cooking, but this may well not be the case in commercial and industrial catering. Studies of catering in schools, hospitals and restaurants in

Table 16.1 Summary of nutrient losses during preparation and cooking of food

Food	Process involved	Loss caused by	Examples of nutrient lost
Animal			
Chopped or ground meat, fish	Freeze–thaw	Thaw drip	Protein, B vitamins – especially niacin
Meat joints	Microwave cooking, grilling, roasting	Cooking drip	Fat, fat-soluble vitamins
All	Braising or stewing	Leaching	Water-soluble vitamins
All	Lengthy heating or high temperature as in baking or roasting	Oxidation or breakdown of nutrients	Thiamin, essential amino acids and fatty acids
Plant			
Fruit, vegetables	Bruising, long storage	Spoilage	Vitamin C
	Cutting, chopping	Damage to cellular structure	
All	Cooking, washing, soaking in water	Leaching	Loss of water-soluble vitamins – vitamin C, thiamin, folic acid, pyridoxine
All	Lengthy heating or high temperature as in baking or roasting	Oxidation or breakdown of nutrients	Vitamin C, riboflavin, essential fatty acids and amino acids
All	Discarded cooking water	Leaching	Loss of water-soluble vitamins – vitamin C, thiamin, riboflavin, zinc

many countries have shown that cooked food was kept warm for 0–7.5 hours before it was consumed. In the UK a study of the 'Meals-on-Wheels' service showed that food was kept warm for 50 minutes to 3.5 hours and that the internal temperature of the food varied from 38 to 47°C.

Provided that food is stored above 65°C microorganisms are unable to grow; below this temperature there is the possibility of microbial growth. If food is stored at safe temperatures above 65°C, however, there will be fairly rapid destruction of heat-sensitive nutrients, particularly vitamins. The study of the Meals-on-Wheels service showed that 31–54 per cent of vitamin C was lost between the end of cooking and the first meal served. More recently, developments have seen the introduction of the cook-chill process to such meal services for the elderly. Here food is prepared, cooked, chilled for up to 3 days and then reheated prior to service. It is possible that the heat-labile vitamins are greatly depleted from such food. In general, vitamin C is the vitamin most rapidly destroyed when food is kept hot, thiamin is less rapidly destroyed and only small amounts of riboflavin and niacin are lost. The antioxidant flavonoids are well preserved during cooking.

MOIST HEAT METHODS

Moist heat methods of cooking employ relatively low temperatures and destruction of nutrients by heat is therefore not great. Cooking times at such low temperatures tend to be long, however, and this results in extensive loss of water-soluble nutrients into the liquid used for cooking. Vitamin C is the nutrient which is most easily destroyed in cooking and hence loss of this vitamin may be taken as an index of the severity of the cooking process. If little vitamin C is lost it may be taken that the cooking process is a mild one and that there will have been little loss of other nutrients. The losses of vitamin C that occur when vegetables are boiled are shown in Table 16.2 and the data demonstrate that the loss can be severe.

It needs to be emphasized that nutrient losses in cooking quoted in the literature should be treated with caution. The figures quoted for a given food may show considerable variation and this is because nutrient losses depend to a large extent on the way in which the cooking is carried out and also on the physical state of the food. For example, the quality of the fresh food, the treatment that the food receives before it is cooked, the time of cooking, the amount of liquid used, the extent to which air is excluded and the time for which the food is kept hot before it is consumed all affect the extent to which nutrients are lost. Figures quoted for nutrient loss during cooking must therefore be considered in conjunction with the conditions of the experiment. Unless this is done, data in the literature appear to be contradictory.

In moist heat cooking, nutrients may be lost in a variety of ways. The most important is the leaching of water-soluble nutrients, primarily vitamins and mineral elements, into the cooking water. Nutrients are also lost by the action of heat in the presence of air. Vitamin C, for example, is very sensitive to such oxidative loss. The action of oxidizing enzymes also causes loss of nutrients and again vitamin C is easily lost, being rapidly destroyed by such oxidases in the presence of oxygen in the cooking water. As enzymes are destroyed by heat – ascorbic acid oxidase is rapidly destroyed at 100°C – loss of nutrients by enzymes is

Table 16.2 Vitamin C content of raw and boiled vegetables

| Vegetable | Vitamin C (mg/100 g) | | |
	Raw	Boiled	Per cent loss of vitamin C
Brussels sprouts	115	60	48
Cabbage	49	20	59
Carrots	6	2	67
Fresh peas	24	16	33
Old potatoes	11	6	45
Runner beans	18	10	44

Table 16.3 Relation between cooking time and retention of vitamin C

| Cooking time (minutes) | Per cent retention of vitamin C during boiling | | | |
	Brussels sprouts	Cabbage	Carrots	Potatoes
20	49	40	35	55
30	36	70–78	22	53–56
60	–	53–58	–	40–50
90	–	13	–	17

greatly reduced if food (particularly vegetables) is put into boiling water rather than being put into cold water which is then heated.

Boiling

Boiling is a common method of moist heat cooking; it utilizes the fact that because water has a high specific heat capacity it is an efficient heat reservoir and therefore is a convenient medium in which to transfer heat to food. Its ready availability is another important factor. One disadvantage of water as a medium for heat transfer is that, because of its good solvent action, food cooked in it may lose a considerable proportion of its soluble matter. Vegetables, for example, are commonly cooked by boiling and this results in an inevitable loss of some mineral elements and vitamins, the loss of the latter being the more important from a nutritional point of view. Although little or no carotene is lost when vegetables are boiled, considerable amounts of thiamin and ascorbic acid are destroyed, as both these vitamins are water-soluble and easily destroyed by heat. In general, about one-third of the thiamin and two-thirds of the ascorbic acid are lost, although, as discussed below, the amount lost varies considerably with changing conditions.

Although some loss of water-soluble nutrients by leaching is inevitable during boiling, the extent of this loss is governed to some extent by the amount of water used. The loss of both mineral elements and water-soluble vitamins increases as the amount of water used increases. For example, in a series of experiments it was found that cabbage, which lost 60 per cent ascorbic acid when cooked in a small volume of water, lost 70 per cent when cooked in a larger amount. Losses of thiamin, which

are important when boiling cereal foods, follow a similar pattern and, for example, it was found that rice which lost about 30 per cent thiamin when cooked in a small volume of water, lost 50 per cent when cooked in a larger amount.

The time for which foods are boiled also affects nutrient loss. There is, for example, a drastic loss of ascorbic acid when prolonged cooking times are used, as can be seen from Table 16.3 which shows how ascorbic acid loss increases with cooking time for a number of vegetables. Another factor affecting nutrient loss is the treatment that the food receives before it is boiled. For example, the greater the surface area of a food the greater is the loss of water-soluble nutrients into the cooking water. Crushing, chopping, slicing and shredding of food not only increase the surface area but also release enzymes that cause further loss. In one study, over one-third of vitamin C was destroyed during initial shredding and washing of spring cabbage prior to cooking.

Table 16.4 shows the effect that the size of food has upon the loss of nutrients that occurs during the boiling of vegetables, such as carrots, Swedes and sprouts. Peeling vegetables before cooking also increases loss of nutrients and it has been found that whereas whole, unpeeled potatoes lost about one-third ascorbic acid when boiled, peeled potatoes lost an additional 10 per cent.

Table 16.4 Effect of size on per cent nutrient loss occurring in boiled vegetables

Nutrient	Large pieces	Small pieces
Vitamin C	22–23	32–50
Sugars	10–21	19–35
Mineral salts	8–16	17–30
Proteins	2–8	14–22

Steaming and pressure cooking

Steaming involves using the steam produced from boiling water. As the contact between the food and water is less than in boiling there is smaller loss of soluble matter but, as a longer time of cooking is required, the amount of ascorbic acid which is decomposed by heat is increased.

The rate of cooking in steaming may be increased by the use of steam under pressure, this being the principle of the pressure-cooker. As increase of pressure raises the temperature at which water boils, the cooking temperature is greater than 100°C, for example, when a pressure-cooker is used at its highest working pressure of 1.05 kg/cm² the boiling point is 120°C. It is found that the amount of ascorbic acid lost because of the increased temperature is more than compensated for by the amount conserved as a result of the shorter cooking time, though the difference is small. The relatively short cooking times involved in pressure cooking are illustrated by the fact that, using the highest pressure setting, potatoes cook in about 5 minutes and a beef casserole in 20 minutes.

Stewing

Stewing involves cooking food in hot water, the temperature of which is kept below its boiling point. The changes that occur in stewing are, therefore, similar in character to those that occur during boiling, although they occur at a slower rate. Stewing, as a slow method of cooking, results in considerable loss of soluble matter. For example, when stewing fish, one-third of the mineral salts and extractives may be lost as well as water-soluble vitamins. Stewed fish, therefore, lacks flavour and has less nutritional value than when it is raw. However, in a stew, the liquor in which the food has been cooked is usually eaten or used for making a sauce or soup, thus the passage of nutrients into the cooking water involves no loss of nutritional value and the liquor retains the flavour lost from the stewed food.

One of the advantages of stewing is that, because of the low temperature used, protein is only lightly coagulated and is, therefore, in its most digestible form. Another advantage is that it exerts a tenderizing effect on protein food as insoluble, tough collagen is converted into soluble gelatin by prolonged

Table 16.5 Loss of vitamins when fruits are stewed

Vitamin	Percentage loss
Folate	80
Thiamin	75
Biotin	33
Pantothenic acid	25
Riboflavin	25
Vitamin B_6	20
Vitamin C	25
Niacin	0

Based on figures for stewed apples in *The Composition of Foods*.

contact with hot water. Stewing is, therefore, a particularly suitable method for cooking tough meat.

Many fruits, such as strawberries and melons, are best eaten raw but others, such as rhubarb and damsons, are undoubtedly improved by cooking. Fruit may be cooked by stewing in water to which sugar has been added. Dried fruits are soaked before cooking to allow maximum absorption of water by osmosis, and less sugar is added to the cooking water because, during soaking, sugar diffuses out of the fruit. During stewing, cellulose is softened, protein is lightly coagulated and soluble matter is lost to the cooking liquor. At the same time, where stewing is done in syrup, sugar is absorbed by the fruit. Because of the low temperature used and the presence of fruit acids, which maintain pH below 7, destruction of thiamin (which is present only in small amounts) and ascorbic acid is small, though, owing to their solubility, they gradually diffuse into the surrounding liquor. The loss of vitamins that occurs during the stewing of fruit is shown in Table 16.5.

DRY HEAT METHODS

Dry heat methods of cooking are characterized by the use of higher temperatures than in moist heat methods, and the use of air as the intermediate medium conveying heat from the heat source to the surface of the food. When food is placed in a hot oven, about 80 per cent of heat reaching its surface is conveyed by convection and about 20 per cent by radiation. Heat is conveyed from the surface of the food to the interior by conduction, this being a

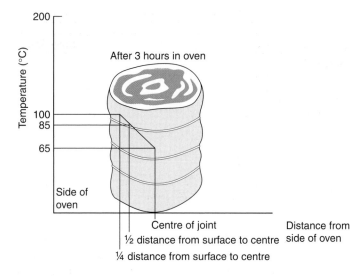

After 3 hours in oven

Side of oven

Centre of joint
½ distance from surface to centre
¼ distance from surface to centre

Distance from side of oven

Figure 16.1 *The temperature gradient through meat being cooked in an oven*

relatively slow process because of the poor thermal conductivity of food.

The rate of heat transfer in dry heat cooking can be illustrated by considering the roasting of a joint of beef. If the meat is to be cooked so that it is 'rare' the centre of the meat should reach a temperature of about 63°C, while if it is to be 'well done' the temperature should be in the range 80–88°C. If a joint of meat weighing 4 kg is placed in a hot oven, heat is conducted from the surface towards the centre of the joint. The temperature gradient through the meat after 3 hours' cooking is shown in Fig. 16.1. This figure illustrates that heat is conducted through the meat slowly and that after 3 hours' cooking the meat is in a 'rare' state. If the meat is removed from the oven after 3 hours, heat continues to be transferred from the hot outer surface towards the cooler interior, so that cooking continues for some time after the meat is removed from the heat source.

The higher temperatures used in dry heat compared with moist heat cooking means that loss of nutrients which are sensitive to heat is correspondingly greater. Apart from mineral salts, which are stable to heat, all nutrients are affected to some extent by dry heating. Fats are stable to moderate heating and, although they darken, little breakdown occurs unless they are heated to high temperatures when they start to decompose with the formation of acrolein, which has an unpleasant acrid odour (see Frying). Carbohydrates are affected by dry heat: starch is converted into pyrodextrins which

Table 16.6 Percentage loss of B vitamins when meat and fish are cooked using dry heat

Vitamin	Meat	Fish	
	Roasted and grilled	Baked	Grilled
Folate	–	20	–
Pantothenic acid	20	20	20
Pyridoxine	20	10	20
Niacin	20	20	20
Riboflavin	20	20	20
Thiamin	20	30	20

are brown in colour and which contribute colour to toast and breadcrust; sucrose is converted into dark-coloured caramel in a complex multistage reaction that involves its initial breakdown into monosaccharides and its final polymerization into coloured substances.

Dry heat cooking destroys those vitamins that are unstable to heat, notably ascorbic acid, which, as we have already noted, is destroyed at quite low temperatures.

Table 16.6 shows the average percentage losses of B vitamins which occurs when meat and fish are cooked using dry heat. It is apparent from this table that 20 per cent of B vitamins are destroyed.

Proteins, as we saw in Chapter 10, are extremely sensitive to heat but their nutritive value is not significantly affected unless they are heated to a fairly high temperature, such as occurs in roasting. Loss of nutritive value depends not only on the cooking temperature, but also on the time of cooking and the presence of other nutrients, particularly carbohydrates.

Amino acids are only destroyed at high temperatures such as are employed in roasting, and even then the loss of protein is small and confined to the surface of the food. A much greater loss of nutritive value results from a change in protein structure which affects the linkages between amino acids in such a way that they become resistant to enzymic hydrolysis. Amino acids affected in this way – notably aspartic acid, glutamic acid and lysine – cannot be released by enzymes during digestion and are therefore unavailable to the body.

Non-enzymic browning

As already mentioned, when protein and carbohydrate exist together in the same food an additional loss of nutritive value may occur due to non-enzymic browning (also called the Maillard reaction). Reaction occurs between amino groups projecting from a protein chain or peptide or amino acid and the carbonyl group of a reducing substance such as glucose. The details of the reaction are not completely understood, but it involves a number of steps, the first of which is an addition reaction between the amino and carbonyl groups, and the last is a polymerization to form a brown substance. Several amino acids undergo this reaction, notably lysine and methionine. The reaction results in the formation of substances that cannot be hydrolysed by enzymes, and the proteins affected are thus unavailable to the body.

Non-enzymic browning occurs particularly at high temperatures and at pH values of 7 and above; a certain amount of moisture is also necessary. The reduction in nutritive value of protein as a result of non-enzymic browning has been studied intensively in terms of the loss of lysine during cooking. For example, it has been found that bread loses 10–15 per cent during toasting. Some lysine is also lost during the roasting of meat, though in home cooking the loss has been found to be small.

In addition to causing some loss in the nutritive value of proteins during dry heat cooking, non-enzymic browning is also responsible for producing some desirable changes in the flavour, colour and aroma of food during roasting, baking and toasting. For example, it improves the quality of bread during baking and toasting, and of nuts and coffee beans during roasting. It is also partly responsible for the flavour of such diverse products as meat extract, biscuits and breakfast cereals.

Frying

Frying is a convenient method of cooking where a high temperature and rapid cooking are desired. Fat is the medium used in frying to provide the necessary high temperature. It is chosen because of its high boiling point, and because it can be heated almost to its boiling point without much decomposition occurring. There are two methods of frying, the most important being deep frying.

Deep frying, as the name suggests, is done in a deep pan, the food being lowered into the fat when it is very hot, normally between 175 and 200°C. As soon as the food comes into contact with the hot fat there is a violent bubbling as the water on the surface of the food is vaporized. When potato chips are immersed in oil at 190°C, the steam produced forms a layer around the chips in the form of a 'stationary layer' which greatly reduces the rate of heat transfer from the oil to the potato surface. However, once heat has passed through this barrier, it is conducted rapidly from the surface of the food to its interior, because of the high temperature of the oil. Cooking proceeds so rapidly that loss of mineral salts and nitrogenous substances is reduced to a minimum. Cooking is complete when the outside of the food is crisp and usually golden-brown in colour.

The second method of frying is shallow frying, which is done in a shallow pan, the bottom of which is covered with fat. The main role of the fat is to prevent the food from adhering to the pan, the cooking being done mainly by direct conducted heat. In this method of cooking, heat is applied only to one surface of the food at a time, so that uneven cooking may result unless the food is turned regularly.

Fats used for frying must be pure because impurities are likely to decompose at the high temperatures employed, producing unpleasant flavours and odours. Vegetable oils, providing that they have been carefully refined, may be used for frying and such oils can often be heated to higher temperatures than the more conventional fats without decomposition occurring. When using a fat or oil for deep frying, the temperature of the fat should be checked with a thermometer and it should not be allowed to rise above the value recommended. This is because if the temperature used is too high the smoke point of the fat may be reached, at which temperature blue smoke appears indicating incipient decomposition. If the temperature is raised above the smoke point the rate of decomposition increases rapidly. The smoke point for oils and fats is in the range 135–245°C, coconut oil being at the lower end of this range and pure groundnut oil at the top.

Causes of fat deterioration during frying:

1 *Too high a temperature.* If the frying temperature is high, steam generated during frying causes some hydrolysis of fat and glycerol and free fatty acids are formed; the latter may undergo dehydration with the formation of acrolein. This is a simple unsaturated aldehyde having an unpleasant acrid odour. It is probably present in small quantities in the smoke from the fat:

$$CH_2OHCHOHCH_2OH \rightarrow CH_2{=}CHCHO$$
$$+ 2H_2O$$

  Glycerol   Acrolein

2 *Access of air.* At high temperatures oxygen in air causes rapid oxidation, and consequent deterioration of oils used for cooking. Such deterioration is accelerated by light. Provided, however, that pans used for deep frying have lids, the hot cooking oil is covered at its surface by a layer of steam released from the food being fried and this prevents access of oxygen to the surface of the oil.

3 *Contamination caused by food residues.* When food is cooked by deep frying, particles of food become detached and should be removed from the oil before it is used again for frying. If such food residues are not removed repeated reheating will cause them to become charred and cause deterioration and darkening of the oil.

4 *Loss of natural antioxidants.* Natural oils and fats contain antioxidants that help to prevent oxidative changes which produce rancidity. When food is fried, the concentration of antioxidants is reduced and, in continuous frying, the removal of food reduces the amount of cooking oil in the pan, which further reduces the amount of antioxidant present. The loss of antioxidants can be reduced by 'topping up' the cooking oil as frying proceeds and by using fresh oil regularly.

5 *Effect of traces of copper.* Copper is a pro-oxidant. Extremely small traces of copper at levels of 0.1 ppm promotes oxidation and can lead to the development of rancidity in cooking oil. It is therefore important to use pans made of a copper-free metal, for example stainless steel.

It is evident from the above that repeated use of oil leads to deterioration, and consequently that oil used for cooking should be changed frequently.

Other factors which affect the choice of fat for frying are flavour and spattering properties. Spattering is caused by the presence of water in the fat; the water vaporizes on heating and causes the fat to bubble and froth. When the bubbles burst, the fat is said to 'spatter'. Pure cooking fats do not contain water and so give smoother frying than butter and margarine. Efforts are usually made to reduce the spattering properties of margarine by the addition of lecithin, which also improves emulsification.

Nutritional changes

When food is fried in oil, some of the fat used as a heat transfer agent becomes a part of the cooked product and this clearly affects its nutritional value. For example, while the fat content of raw potatoes is negligible (0.2 g fat/100 g potatoes) the fat content of the potatoes when fried as chips increases to 7–15 g fat/100 g potatoes depending on the method used for frying. Such an increase in fat content is clearly of considerable nutritional significance, especially in view of the weight of opinion advocating a reduction in fat intake as an important health goal. Experiments to discover how the increase in fat content of food varies with the way in which frying is carried out have shown that the increase can be minimized by using a combination of steaming, dipping in hot oil and baking in an oven rather than traditional deep frying.

When food is added to very hot oil, there is rapid evaporation of water and natural juices from the surface of the food leading to rapid dehydration of the food surface. This produces the crisp texture and attractive flavour associated with fried food. Losses of nutrients which occur during frying have not been extensively investigated, but in general they appear to be similar to losses that occur during roasting. Vegetables suffer a greater loss of vitamins when fried than when they are boiled. The loss of ascorbic acid in potatoes that are fried has been investigated but the results show considerable variation according to the cooking conditions. Retention of ascorbic acid was found to be greatest when the potatoes were cooked rapidly in deep fat and lowest when they were cooked slowly in shallow fat. When meat is fried, some loss of B vitamins occurs, the results being similar to those given for roasting in Table 16.6.

Microwave cooking

In the methods of cooking considered so far, heat is applied to food from an outside heat source. In microwave cooking, heat is generated within the food and the dramatic reduction in cooking time that results is the main advantage of this method of cooking.

The essential component of a microwave oven is a magnetron which converts electrical energy into microwave energy. The magnetron receives electrical energy at very high voltage and converts it into microwaves with an extremely high frequency (2450 MHz). Such microwaves come into the same category as visible, infrared and radio waves, all of which are non-ionizing forms of radiation (unlike X-rays). Microwaves travel in straight lines and are reflected by metals. Microwaves pass into the oven, being evenly distributed with the help of a stirrer or paddles, and are reflected by the metal sides, base and roof of the oven onto the food to be cooked. Food molecules which absorb the high frequency microwaves start to oscillate at the same frequency as the microwaves, namely 2450 million cycles per second. This rapid oscillation of the food molecules releases energy as heat.

The degree to which microwaves are absorbed by substances depends upon the dielectric constant of the material. Materials with a high dielectric constant absorb microwaves to a greater extent than those with low dielectric constants. Water has a particularly high dielectric constant compared with solid materials and thus in microwave cooking it is the water in the food which mainly absorbs the microwave radiation. Hence foods with a high water content cook more rapidly than those containing less water.

Fat has a much lower dielectric constant than water and consequently fatty parts of food heat up much more slowly than those with a high water content.

It follows that foods containing a mixture of watery and fatty tissues, such as bacon, cook unevenly in a microwave oven. Sugar has a high dielectric constant, and heats more rapidly and to a higher temperature than water. This can result in hazardous hot spots in foods with uneven sugar distribution if cooked by this method. The more homogeneous a food is, the more evenly it is cooked by microwaves.

Some materials such as glass, plastic, china and earthenware have very low dielectric constants and absorb very little microwave radiation. Consequently, they are heated only to a small extent by microwaves and so make suitable containers for food which is cooked in this way. (Metal containers cannot be used because they reflect microwaves.)

Microwaves penetrate food to a depth of 3–5 cm depending on the composition of the food. Thus, when small pieces of food are exposed to microwaves the radiation completely penetrates it and heat is generated throughout the food resulting in rapid cooking. Larger pieces of food are cooked more slowly because those parts of the food that are not penetrated by microwaves are heated by conduction from the outer layers which have been penetrated by the radiation. Similarly, foods having an irregular distribution of water do not heat up uniformly as the water is heated rapidly by microwaves and surrounding regions are then heated more slowly by conduction.

Food cooked by microwave heating differs in some respects from food cooked by other methods. For example, the cooking time required when using microwaves is so short that slow chemical changes, which are important in slow cooking methods, do not have time to occur. Thus, food cooked by microwaves does not turn brown or develop crispness, but it does retain most volatile substances; consequently, the food has a different flavour from usual and this may make it less acceptable.

The fact that a simple microwave oven is unable to brown and crisp food has led to the development of combination ovens in which microwave heating is complemented by convection heating or heating with halogen lamps. Some combination ovens also provide a grill. The use of such ovens produces cooked food with similar characteristics to that produced in conventional ovens.

It is difficult to ensure even distribution of microwaves within a microwave oven and this can result in 'hot spots' within the food. To obviate this difficulty food may be cooked on a rotating turntable. Alternatively a stirrer fan situated in the roof of the oven and having rotating blades, which deflect microwaves off the metal walls of the oven, may be used.

The particular merit of microwave cooking is the short cooking time required. The time of cooking depends upon the power level (measured in watts) that is selected. For example, a medium-sized domestic microwave oven might have a maximum power output of 650 or 750 W. Full power (100 per cent) could be used for rapidly bringing liquids to boiling point and for the fast cooking of meat, fish, vegetables and fruit. Medium high power (70 per cent) could be used to cook these foods more slowly, thus improving flavour, texture and appearance. Medium power (50 per cent) could be used for slower cooking of soups and casseroles, while a low setting (10 per cent) would be used for keeping foods warm.

The time taken to cook a variety of foods in a microwave oven is shown in Table 16.7. The rapidity with which microwaves heat food makes them very useful as a means of quickly reheating pre-cooked foods. For example, a bread roll may be heated through in 20 seconds, a bowl of soup in 1–2 minutes, a fruit crumble (four servings) in 3–4 minutes and a casserole (four servings) in 12–13 minutes. Medium-high (70 per cent) power is suitable for reheating.

In canteens, restaurants and hospitals cooked food often has to be kept hot for long periods, with consequent loss of flavour and nutritional value, before it is eaten. In these circumstances the use of microwaves enables cooked food to be reheated rapidly just before it is eaten, thus eliminating the need for keeping the food hot. The use of this technique is the basis of most fast-food establishments.

It is apparent that microwave cooking is convenient for both the fast cooking and the fast reheating of food. It is also valuable for a third purpose, namely the fast defrosting of frozen food.

Frozen food is normally thawed by allowing it to stand at room temperature. However, this is a lengthy process because most frozen food has a high water content – at least 60 per cent – and because water has a high specific latent heat of fusion. This means that to convert ice at 0°C to water at 0°C requires a large amount of energy supplied as heat. Microwaves, however, penetrate, heat and thaw frozen food very rapidly so making rapid thawing practical. For example, small food items such as small cakes or slices of bread may be thawed in a matter of seconds using full power (100 per cent). Larger items such as poultry may be thawed on low power (30 per cent) and the time in the microwave should be followed by a standing time to allow the food to come to an even temperature throughout by normal conduction of heat. A turkey requires a defrosting time of 5–7 minutes per 450 g, plus a standing time of 1–2 hours.

Microwave cooking can be used to heat pre-cooked frozen food very rapidly and this is an important advantage of this technique.

Nutritional changes

In theory, nutrient losses should be less in microwave cooking than with other methods because it involves

Table 16.7 The time taken to cook foods in a microwave oven (power rating 650 W)

Food	Type	Example	Power level (%)	Time (min) per 450 g
Vegetables	Fresh	Potatoes, boiled	100	10–12
	Fresh	Cabbage, boiled	100	8–10
	Frozen	Cabbage, boiled	100	10–11
Meat	Fresh	Lamb, leg	70	9–12
	Fresh	Sausages	100	9–10
Poultry	Fresh	Chicken, whole	100	5–7
		Chicken, whole	70	9–10
	Frozen	Chicken, whole	100	15–18
Fish	Fresh	Plaice, whole	100	4–5
	Frozen	Plaice, whole	100	11–12

Table 16.8 Comparison of vitamin C content in mg/100 g of fresh vegetables when cooked by microwave or boiling

Vegetable	Microwave	Boiled
Asparagus	20	18
Broccoli	117	73
Cabbage	43	25
Cauliflower	85	48
Runner beans	6	5
Spinach	24	15
Turnips	26	14

a shorter cooking time, a lower temperature at the surface of the food and the use of little or no added water. In practice, the changes or losses of nutrients that occur in microwave cooking are comparable to those occurring in other methods. Research on animal proteins and minerals suggests that microwaves have little effect on those nutrients.

The loss of water-soluble vitamins, particularly vitamin C, in microwave cooking has been extensively investigated. Early experiments showed little difference in the loss of vitamin C in fruit and vegetables when cooked by microwave and by conventional means. However, more recent research, some results of which are summarized in Table 16.8, shows that the vitamin C content of vegetables cooked by microwave is higher than when they are boiled. It is considered that this is because of shorter cooking times and the use of little added water rather than any effect of microwave heating.

RAISING AGENTS

The baking of a dough or batter used in making bread, cakes or buns involves the use of an aerator which causes the mixture to rise during baking to give a product of even texture and, in the case of bread and sponge cakes, of large volume and open cellular structure.

Sometimes enough air may be incorporated by mechanical mixing to produce sufficient aeration during baking. Usually, however, carbon dioxide is used as an additional aerating agent. In bread making, carbon dioxide is normally produced by fermentation as described earlier, but in making other types of baked confectionery and Irish soda bread carbon dioxide is produced by a chemical raising agent or baking powder.

The simplest raising agent is sodium bicarbonate (strictly called sodium hydrogen carbonate) or 'baking soda' which produces carbon dioxide when it is heated:

$$2NaHCO_3 \xrightarrow{\text{heat}} Na_2CO_3 + H_2O + CO_2$$

It will be seen from the equation that the sodium bicarbonate is converted into sodium carbonate. If sodium carbonate is present in appreciable quantities it imparts an alkaline taste and a yellow colour to the product. This unfortunate result is sometimes noticeable in home-made scones in which too much baking soda has been used. For this reason, sodium bicarbonate is only used in making products such as gingerbread and chocolate cake, which have a strong flavour and colour of their own.

A baking powder is a mixture of substances which, when mixed with water and heated, produces carbon dioxide. For most purposes, a baking powder is a more suitable aerator than baking soda. It consists of three ingredients: sodium bicarbonate as the source of carbon dioxide, an acid or acid salt to liberate the gas from the bicarbonate, and some form of starch, often cornflour or ground rice, as an inert filler to absorb moisture. A typical baking powder might contain 20 per cent sodium bicarbonate, 40 per cent acidic material and 40 per cent filler.

The action of a baking powder is most simply illustrated by the reaction of a solution of hydrochloric acid with sodium bicarbonate. On mixing, carbon dioxide is given off in the cold without any unpleasant tasting residue being left behind:

$$NaHCO_3 + HCl \rightarrow NaCl + H_2O + CO_2$$

In practice, this mixture is not used, because reaction is so rapid that much gas would be lost before baking started. Also, the use of an acid in solution is inconvenient and the amount of acid needed would have to be most carefully controlled so that no free acid remained in the product after baking.

If hydrochloric acid is replaced by tartaric acid the evolution of gas, which occurs when water is added to the baking powder, is rather slower. On reaction with sodium bicarbonate, tartaric acid is converted into the harmless salt, sodium tartrate. In modern baking powders the acid is replaced by the acid salt, potassium hydrogen tartrate, better known as cream of tartar. This salt is less soluble in cold water than the acid, so that when the baking powder is mixed with water very little reaction occurs; when the mixture is warmed, however, a copious stream of gas is produced:

$$\begin{array}{l} \text{CHOHCOOH} \\ | \\ \text{CHOHCOOK} \end{array} + NaHCO_3 \xrightarrow{\text{heat}}$$

Cream of tartar

$$\begin{array}{l} \text{CHOHCOONa} \\ | \\ \text{CHOHCOOK} \end{array} + CO_2 + H_2O$$

Sodium potassium tartrate

A baking powder containing cream of tartar keeps better than one containing tartaric acid, because exposure to moisture has less effect. Also, it is more convenient to use because carbon dioxide is not evolved in large quantities until the dough reaches the oven. Since both the acid and the acid salt cost approximately the same, cream of tartar is normally preferred.

Several other acid salts may be used in place of cream of tartar. Calcium hydrogen phosphate, $CaH_4(PO_4)_2$, often called acid calcium phosphate (ACP), has the virtue of cheapness but, like tartaric acid, it reacts slowly with sodium bicarbonate in the cold when moisture is present; hence baking powders containing it have poor keeping qualities. Disodium dihydrogen pyrophosphate, $Na_2H_2P_2O_7$, usually referred to as acid sodium pyrophosphate (ASP), is preferred because of its superior keeping qualities. It is the acid salt of pyrophosphoric acid, $H_4P_2O_7$. Sometimes the two salts are used together. Sodium aluminium sulphate may also be used to replace cream of tartar.

Glucono-delta-lactone (GDL) is also used as the acid component in baking powder, particularly when making chemically leavened bread. It slowly hydrolyses in water or in a dough at room temperature producing gluconic acid and the rate of hydrolysis, and hence the rate of production of carbon dioxide, is markedly increased at higher temperatures.

The effectiveness of an acidic component of baking powder is measured in terms of its 'neutralizing value' or 'strength', and is defined as the parts of sodium bicarbonate neutralized by 100 parts of the acidic component. On this basis the strength of acidic substances used is as follows: ACP 80; ASP 74; cream of tartar 45; and GDL 45.

Instead of adding a calculated amount of baking powder to flour it is sometimes more convenient to use a self-raising flour. This is flour to which sodium bicarbonate and an acid substance are added in such proportions that on reaction the correct amount of carbon dioxide is produced to aerate the flour. One of the advantages of self-raising flour is that because the baking powder and flour are present in the correct proportions, there is no danger of too much or too little aeration, and unpleasant tastes are avoided.

The acid substances added to self-raising flour are the same as those used in baking powders. Both acid calcium phosphate and acid sodium pyrophosphate are used to a large extent, both singly and together. The large excess of flour present absorbs any moisture and so prevents the deterioration of the acid calcium phosphate.

The use of baking powder or self-raising flour causes some loss of nutritive value, notably of thiamin, during baking. Thiamin is stable at low pH values but at pH values of 6 or above it is rapidly destroyed by heat. Baked goods involving the use of self-raising flour or baking powder usually have a pH of about 6.8–7.3, and at this pH thiamin is rapidly destroyed during baking. Losses of thiamin may be very high in such baked goods, and during the baking of cakes, for example, all the thiamin may be destroyed.

Key points

- Cooking is used to increase the variety of flavours and textures of foods, to generate blends which cannot be found in raw foods, and to make some inedible things edible
- The effects of cooking depend on temperatures, and rate of transfer of heat and of water – either into or out of the food
- Specific effects of cooking include killing bacteria, inactivating enzymes, accelerated oxidation or 'browning'

Chapter summary

Cooking methods can be divided into those which use water (e.g. stewing), which limit the temperature to 100°C, or steaming which maintains the high water content at higher temperatures, and those which do not use water (e.g. baking, frying) which generate much greater temperatures. Microwave cooking is unique in employing an internal, and instantaneous heat source which cooks so rapidly that there is no time for the chemical reactions normally associated with cooking.

FURTHER READING

FOOD STANDARDS AGENCY/INSTITUTE OF FOOD RESEARCH (2002). *McCance and Widdowson's 'The Composition of Foods'*, 6th edn. Cambridge: Royal Society of Chemistry, and Food Standards Agency. (Contains a wealth of data about raw and cooked food.)

HOLLAND, B. *et al.* (1991). *McCance and Widdowson's 'The Composition of Foods'*, 5th edn. Cambridge: Royal Society of Chemistry, and Food Standards Agency. (Contains a wealth of data about raw and cooked food.)

MCGEE, H. (1986). *On Food and Cooking.* London: Allen & Unwin. (An interesting and unusual book on the physics and chemistry of cooking.)

MCGEE, H. (1992). *The Curious Cook.* London: HarperCollins. (A general survey of kitchen facts and fallacies.)

17

Diet and health

There is no such thing as a perfect or complete food, which means that there is no single food that provides sufficient of all of the essential nutrients to keep us healthy or which we would be happy to eat on its own to the exclusion of all other foods. It follows that we need to eat a variety of foods to satisfy and nourish us; also, because different foods have widely differing nutritional contents we need to select the foods we eat in such a way that they provide us with a satisfactory or healthy diet as well as providing interest to the senses. The information given in other parts of this book will not be of great practical value unless it can be applied so as to establish the nature of satisfactory patterns of eating. A discussion of diet therefore forms a practical and logical conclusion to the principles of nutrition discussed earlier.

THE NATURE OF DIET

The nature of our diet is crucial to our well-being. As explained in Chapter 3, until recently the aim was to have a diet that was 'balanced', that is, one that provided a mixture of foods which included sufficient of all the essential nutrients for the prevention of deficiency diseases. This could be achieved by eating plenty of animal-derived foods, such as meat, fish, cheese, butter, eggs and milk which have a high nutrient content, particularly of protein and fat, together with vegetables and fruit as a source of minerals and vitamins. This rather naive approach neglected the issues of quantification or the balance of these nutrient-rich foods within an appropriate energy provision. The high-carbohydrate staple foods (potatoes, pasta, rice, bread, etc.) tended to be ignored and high fat provision tended to result.

However, as under-nutrition and deficiency diseases recede in both western and developing countries, obesity and the related 'diseases of affluence' such as coronary heart disease (CHD) and cancer have become commonplace. As explained in Chapter 3, such modern diseases are widely believed to be associated with diet. It is now considered that a more healthy diet can be achieved, not by a better balancing of nutrients, but by a careful selection of foods that will promote health. Thus, animal foods should be eaten in moderation so as to reduce intake of fat, particularly saturated fat, while cereal foods, particularly unrefined cereal foods such as wholemeal bread, should be eaten plentifully so as to provide sufficient intake of non-starch polysaccharide (NSP) and low-fat energy.

The pursuit of 'healthy diets' is promoted in many countries by governmental and other official bodies who issue guidelines on healthy eating. In the UK, understanding of the term 'healthy diet' has been promoted in a number of official reports (see Further reading). It is important to recognize the extent to which 'healthy eating' or 'healthy diet' has been interpreted as a slimming diet by the media and public. As intended by nutritionists and health planners, healthy eating will reduce the burden from a large number of diet-related diseases over time-spans measured in generations. The same pattern of healthy eating will help to reduce weight gain and obesity over the same period. But different methods are needed if weight loss is required by obese people, even if the same 'healthy diet' is appropriate as a starting point and for long-term health after weight loss.

Energy density

The energy density of foods expressed as kcal/100 g or kJ/100 g is quoted in the 'nutritional information' required for food labelling. The enormous differences in energy densities of common foods depend partly on whether the main source of energy is fat (9 kcal/g), protein (4 kcal/g), carbohydrate (3.75 kcal/g) or alcohol (7 kcal/g). However, the biggest factor is the amount of water present as this contributes to the weight of the food but contributes nothing to the energy value. Energy density is an important factor in determining energy intake. People end up eating more energy with energy-dense foods. For most nutritional purposes, water content is irrelevant and foods are better characterized in terms of nutrient density.

Nutrient density

In considering diet it is useful to be able to compare nutrient values of different foods. The simplest way of doing this is to consider the relative amounts of a particular nutrient expressed per 100 g of food. This has already been done many times in this book. Another way is to describe the amount of nutrient present in relation to a unit of energy, that is the nutrient density of the food. An example will make this clearer.

Cheddar cheese has an energy value of 1682 kJ/100 g and a protein content of 26 g/100 g. Milk has an energy value of 272 kJ/100 g and a protein content of 3.2 g/100 g. The protein density of these foods is the amount of protein they contain per 1000 kJ.

The protein density of Cheddar cheese is

$$26 \times \left(\frac{1000}{1682}\right) = 15.5 \text{ g/1000 kJ}$$

The protein density of milk is

$$3.2 \times \left(\frac{1000}{272}\right) = 11.8 \text{ g/1000 kJ}$$

Such a comparison makes it very clear that the protein density of Cheddar cheese is much greater than that of milk.

Nutrient densities can be calculated for any food for all the nutrients that it contains. Some foods, such as processed foods, tend to have very low nutrient densities. This may be because nutrients are removed during the refining process, as happens in the production of flour of low extraction rate. During the milling process the outer layers of the wheat grain, which are relatively rich in thiamin, calcium and iron, are discarded, so that flour of low extraction rate is relatively high in starch (and therefore energy) and relatively low in other nutrients. It follows that as the extraction rate is lowered the nutrient density of the flour falls. The nutrient density of processed foods may also be low because fat or sugar are added during processing, thus increasing the proportion of energy-providing nutrients. For example, fruit yoghurt has a lower nutrient density than natural yoghurt because of the sugar added during the production of fruit yoghurt.

The use of the nutrient density concept is well illustrated in considering the diet of young children. Such children have a high requirement of energy and nutrients relative to their size in order to sustain a rapid growth rate. However, because they have small stomachs they cannot consume large quantities of food and so they require to eat foods with a high nutrient density. If they eat a bulky high-fibre diet with a low energy content, they will not receive sufficient nutrients to sustain growth.

Nutrient content and contribution to diet

It is very important to make a clear distinction between the nutrient content or density of a food and the nutrient contribution which that food makes to our diet. Some examples will illustrate the point. Dried peas have a high energy value and are rich in protein (over 20 per cent) and some vitamins, notably thiamin. Yet the quantity of dried peas consumed in an average diet is so small that their contribution to our nutritional needs is very low indeed. Moreover, it is misleading to consider the nutrient content of dried foods if, before being eaten, they are soaked in water. When dried peas are soaked in water and cooked, their water content increases by about 60 per cent with consequent decrease in their nutrient density. The contribution of all pulses (peas, beans and lentils) to an average diet is extremely small – less than 1 per cent of the total energy and protein and less than 2 per cent of the thiamin.

Compared with peas, the nutrient content of potatoes is small. Their energy value is only one-third that of dried peas and they contain little protein (about 2 per cent) or vitamin C (10–20 mg/100 g). Yet, because considerable quantities are eaten (on average about 1 kg/week) they contribute about five times more energy and protein to the diet than pulses. They also contribute over one-fifth of the vitamin C intake. Similarly, no-one would claim potatoes as a food rich in iron. They contain only one-twentieth as much iron as liver. Yet, because we eat so much potato and so little liver, potatoes contribute over five times as much iron to the average diet as liver.

Variety in diet

A study of food habits of different races in different parts of the world reveals the fact that although nutritional needs remain essentially the same, the ways in which those needs may be met are unlimited. Diets may vary in an infinite number of ways and yet each diet may supply adequate amounts of the essential nutrients. Many variable factors, such as standard of living, custom, local abundance of certain foods and religious taboos all influence diet.

In highly industrialized countries such as the UK, a wide variety of foods is available, whereas in less developed parts of the world the choice of foodstuffs may be more restricted. Such restricted diets, however, may be satisfactory and supply adequate amounts of all the nutrients. For example, a Central African tribe called the Masai lived traditionally on a diet often largely composed of milk, meat and blood, supplemented by concoctions made from barks of trees and certain roots which are drunk as beverages. This may seem a Spartan and even repulsive diet to our more sophisticated taste, yet it apparently kept the tribe in good health.

During the Second World War, when great efforts were being made by Britain to reduce food imports,

a simple diet which would have been adequate nutritionally and would have required a minimum of imported food, was worked out. The main articles of this diet were milk, wholemeal bread and green vegetables, with a daily meat ration which some regarded as restrictive, but for others was a bonus. Scientifically such a diet would have been quite satisfactory, but it was never adopted because it was thought that it would have been too unattractive for a modern industrialized nation.

These examples are not intended to show that diets restricted to a few foods only have some special virtue, but they do make it clear that such diets may be nutritionally satisfactory, provided that the foods selected are chosen with care.

Any diet is based on certain staple foods that form the bulk of the diet. The nature of these staple foods varies in different parts of the world. The traditional Masai diet already quoted contains three staple foods: milk, meat and blood. For the Inuit, fish and seal were staples. The wartime diet proposed for Britain in 1940 was based on three staple foods: milk, wholemeal bread and green vegetables. More generally regional diets are often defined by a high-carbohydrate staple food – either cereals, such as wheat and rice, or starchy roots and tubers, such as potatoes and cassava. These staple foods provide a considerable proportion of the total energy and nutrients of the diet. In undeveloped countries a plentiful and reliable staple food is particularly important and when supply of that food is restricted or cut off because of crop failure, famine and death can quickly result. In western countries, staple foods are less important because a much greater variety of foods is available.

Although staple foods are the basis for any diet, the complete diet contains a number of other foods which contribute both variety and the supply of essential nutrients. Although, as we have seen above, satisfactory healthy diets may be achieved using only a few foods, it is normally desirable to eat a wide variety of foods. However, variety in diet does not of itself guarantee that the diet is a healthy one, so that even in this situation food choice remains important. The concept of food groups is often useful, when considering meals as a combination of components (food groups) within which there are a range of more-or-less interchangeable specific foods. The American Food Guide Pyramid (Fig. 17.1) is probably the best known way to use food groups in health

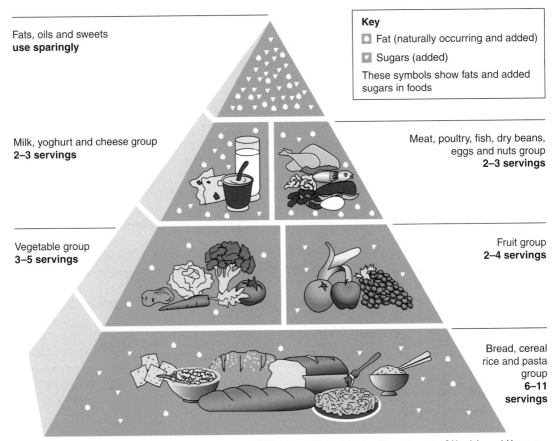

Figure 17.1 *United States Department of Agriculture (USDA) and United States Department of Health and Human Services (DHHS) food guide pyramid*

promotion. The 'Balance of Good Health' model of foods displayed on a plate table is an alternative. These models do not suit health promotion ideally, because the size of the components are based on nutritional consideration (for example, milk and dairy foods should supply a relatively small proportion of energy); however, these foods are bulky, because they contain a lot of water, so they would actually fill a relatively large part of a table or shopping trolley. The nutritional guidelines discussed later in the chapter provide information that enable sensible choices to be made in the selection of food.

ESTABLISHING DIET AND HEALTH LINKS

The idea that foods, or dietary patterns, affect health is not new. Many foods were attributed with magical, health-giving properties in ancient times. These beliefs often arose because of colours or shapes of foods, but some were based on anecdotes at least of some influence of food on health. A few examples exist of foods that have specific links to health which can be demonstrated and explained using modern scientific methods.

These links are difficult to research, because we do not eat isolated foods, but complicated mixtures of foods in 'diets'. Diet composition can be assessed after periods such as a year, a month, a week or a day, or even a meal, in terms of influence over health-related factors (such as blood pressure or cholesterol), but it makes no sense to describe individual foods in terms of nutritional health outcome. The smallest unit of nutrition is the meal. It makes sense to discuss the nutritional balance and possible health implications of a meal, but the nutrient content of foods can only be described in the terminology of food science (e.g. mg/100 g net weight).

A variety of approaches is needed to research diet and health, which form a cascade, from the cheapest and simplest to the most detailed and prolonged, as evidence creeps towards proof, or to the point where it is deemed sufficient to justify action. This was shown as a diagram in Fig. 3.2 on p. 26.

The simplest type of research, ecological surveys, use existing data collected for other reasons (so seldom perfect) about health, and about food provision (most usually as 'food disappearance' from suppliers, and taking account of wastage) in different countries. Patterns of high or low consumption can be related to high frequencies of diseases to postulate links between the disease and diet.

The second level of sophistication, the case-control study involves identifying patients with a disease, collecting dietary information (intended to reflect diet at the time the disease was developing) and collecting the same information from 'control' subjects that do not show signs of the disease. This type of research is time-consuming and becomes expensive if enough subjects are studied (usually hundreds) to be confident of the results.

Because of vagaries of the memory, better information usually comes from the next stage of epidemiological research, the prospective cohort study. Here dietary information is collected, preferably more than once, on healthy people who are then followed up with regular examinations and scrutiny of medical records. The diets of people who go on to develop a particular disease can then be compared with the diets of those that have not (yet) developed the disease in question.

All these research approaches can identify associations between diet, or food exposure, and disease. With good quality dietary data, corroborated by blood tests, links with specific nutrients can be established, but they remain at the level of association. If proof is required, then the only appropriate type of research is a randomized controlled intervention. Large numbers, sometimes tens of thousands, have their diets characterized as in the cohort studies, and are then randomly allocated to a 'treatment' (e.g. to take a vitamin pill or to follow a low-fat diet) and asked to follow that treatment for a number of years. At the same time, other subjects are asked to follow a different 'treatment' (e.g. a dummy or 'placebo' pill, or a higher-fat diet). All

the subjects are then assessed at intervals over the years to see if any diseases are more or less frequent on one or other treatment. This type of research is extremely expensive and would not be undertaken without having consistent results about associations of the 'treatments' with diseases. Even with evidence from controlled interventions, it is often reassuring to have further corroboration from laboratory studies or animal research which shed light on the mechanisms of the disease. Sometimes pharmaceutical trials (e.g. those which showed that cholesterol-lowering drugs increase survival) can provide important support for epidemiological studies (that lower cholesterol is associated with less heart disease).

The purpose of research on diet and disease is to help make decisions aimed at reducing disease in the population. If the action under consideration is expensive or has potential adverse effects, then proof from controlled intervention studies may be needed. If the action is cheap or uncontroversial, then policies may be put into place before proof is available (i.e. on the basis of association). When relying on observational research, it is vital to seek any sources of error or bias, and adjust for them. Getting the same answer from several different study designs or settings is valuable – a method known as 'triangulation'.

Evidence gathered in this way forms the basis of a number of well-established health statements (see Approved Generic Statements for Health Claims on p. 269), which can legitimately form the basis of health claims for foods. The Food Standards Agency commissioned a report from the Joint Health Claims Initiative which can be viewed on the www.jhci.co.uk site or www.food.gov.uk/multimedia/pdfs/jhci_healthreport.pdf.

THE BRITISH DIET

Food and nutrition surveillance

There is ample evidence, from international epidemiology supported by experimental evidence in humans and animals, that diet contributes to a wide variety of disease, and to protection against these diseases. If this is accepted, then a responsible society must take action to protect its citizens. Surveillance of nutrition and diet is an essential component, in order to monitor over time the patterns of diet-related diseases, nutritional status among citizens, and food choice and consumption. Nutritional surveys need to consider all these components, and may shed new light on links between diet and disease. Dietary surveys seek information about food choice, purchases, consumption and wastage, from which it is possible to build a profile of the nutrient balance to which people are exposed. Nutrition surveys often attempt to obtain information on health, nutritional status and diet in the same individuals. Dietary surveys usually attempt only to describe average dietary intake of populations or subgroups. For all such surveys there are major possible sources of error and of bias.

All food choice and consumption data require the involvement of individual subjects, either describing past eating habits from their memory (retrospective methods, e.g. 24-hour diet recall, or dietary history, or food frequency questionnaires) or describing present eating habits (prospective methods, e.g. food diary, 7-day weighed food inventory) using various methods. There is substantial misreporting, including intentional misreporting (particularly under-reporting of 20–50 per cent by people with weight problems). Ideally, food consumption data should be corroborated by independent information on food supply. The 2003 World Health Organization report (WHO, 2003) collected data to show that fat consumption is rising in most countries, whereas reported consumption (in increasingly overweight populations) is apparently falling.

In the past, nutritionists have sometimes been too eager to apply tables of average food consumption to incomplete dietary intake records, to provide improbably low nutrient consumptions. Again, corroboration is desirable, such as blood measures of nutrients or other 'biomarkers' which provide a quantitative marker of dietary exposure. Food tables can only provide average data on nutrient compositions of foods, whereas many foods vary very substantially in nutrient contents. For surveillance in population or large groups, average nutrient intakes may be reasonably accurate, but the estimates of the nutrient intakes of individuals can be misleading.

Information on the British diet comes from surveys which are carried out, and repeated regularly, diets being analysed not only in terms of nutrient content but also in terms of geographical and sociological differences. The National Food Survey provides valuable information on the way diet is changing in the country as a whole, in different regions of the country and in different classes of society. This survey of household food consumption was conducted annually from 1940 to 2000. It has now been replaced by the Expenditure and Food Survey.

Since 1986/87 comprehensive dietary and nutritional surveys of British adults and children have been undertaken. In the most recent survey, over 2000 people aged 19–64 years kept a careful record of all that they ate or drank over a 7-day period. The results of this survey have the advantage over those from the older National Food Surveys in that they include food eaten both inside and outside the home. The data contained in Tables 17.1 and 17.2 are obtained from

Table 17.1 Per cent contributions made by important food groups to the diet of British adults

Food group	Energy	Protein	Fat	Calcium	Iron
Cereal products	31	23	19	30	44
Eggs and egg dishes	2	3	4	2	3
Fat spreads	4	0	12	0	0
Fish and fish dishes	3	7	3	2	3
Fruit and nuts	2	2	2	1	3
Meat and meat products	15	36	23	6	17
Milk and dairy products	10	16	14	43	1
Potatoes and savoury snacks	9	4	10	1	7
Sugar, confectionery and preserves	6	1	3	2	2
Vegetables (excluding potatoes)	4	5	4	5	10

this source and include everything eaten except for a few very minor foods; they also exclude beverages.

A study of the results of the dietary and nutritional survey enable a number of generalizations to be made about the nature of the British diet.

The importance of cereal products is evident from Tables 17.1 and 17.2. They make a major contribution to every class of nutrient and are the most important source of energy in the diet. Bread is an important source of food energy, accounting for 13 per cent of the total intake. Although cereals are not notably rich in riboflavin or niacin, they provide a substantial proportion of our intake of those vitamins. This is because some cereal products, such as breakfast cereals, are fortified with these vitamins and because some cereal products are made with milk and eggs which provide them.

Milk and milk products are an outstanding source of calcium, and despite its low protein density, milk provides the diet with a useful amount of protein because of the relatively large amounts consumed.

Fat spreads include all the culinary fats in the British diet. But they provide only 12 per cent of the fat in the diet. The different types of spreads make the following contributions to this total: butter, 4 per cent; margarines, 1 per cent; reduced fat spreads (60–80 per cent fat), 5 per cent; and low-fat spreads, 1 per cent. As a very broad generalization, about a quarter of total fats are from spreads and oils (visible fat), a quarter from meat and meat products, a quarter from dairy products and a quarter from baked foods and confectionery.

Meat and meat products are prominent in the British diet and make major contributions to all the nutrients shown in the tables, except calcium and vitamin C. They are the major sources of protein, fat, niacin and retinol, although in the last case it needs to be appreciated that nearly all of this comes from liver.

Fish has a similar nutrient content to meat but contributes little to most peoples' diets because of the small quantities that are eaten. Fish makes a significant contribution to one micronutrient, namely vitamin D, because of the high vitamin D content of fatty fish such as herring and tuna, which provide 25 per cent of the total dietary intake of vitamin D. Like meat, fish supplies haem iron, which is important for non-meat eaters.

Vegetables are particularly valuable as a source of vitamin C and including potatoes provide over one-third the total intake. Vegetables (not including potatoes) are also the main source of carotene (shown as retinol equivalents in Table 17.2 in the diet.

Potatoes used to be the most important single source of vitamin C, but fruit and nuts now contribute almost 20 per cent with fruit juice providing a further 19 per cent. This means fruit and fruit juices provide nearly half of the total intake of vitamin C.

The tables highlight the fact that sugar, confectionery and preserves make little contribution to the diet apart from a small contribution to food energy.

Although beverages are not included in the tables, they do make a major contribution to one

Table 17.2 Per cent contributions made by important food groups to vitamins in the diets of British adults

Food group	Vitamin A (Retinol equivalents)	Thiamin	Ribo-flavin	Niacin	Folate	Vitamin C	Vitamin D
Cereal products	7	34	24	27	33	5	21
Egg and egg dishes	5	1	4	2	3	0	9
Fat spreads	10	0	0	0	0	0	17
Fish and fish dishes	1	1	2	6	2	0	25
Fruit and nuts	1	3	2	2	3	19	0
Meat and products	28	21	15	34	7	4	22
Milk and products	14	9	33	8	8	5	3
Potatoes and savoury snacks	1	13	2	5	12	15	1
Sugar, confectionery and preserves	0	1	2	1	0	0	0
Vegetables (excluding potatoes)	27	15	4	4	15	22	1

nutrient, namely vitamin C. Fruit juices contribute more vitamin C to the diet than fruit, namely 19 per cent, while soft drinks contribute a further 4 per cent.

Alcohol consumption was included in the survey and, excluding those in the sample who did not drink alcohol, men obtained 9 per cent of their energy intake from alcohol compared with 7 per cent for women.

Trends in the British diet

Over the past 50 years, Britain has experienced extensive social, economic and cultural changes. Social changes that have taken place over recent years have altered considerably the pattern of British eating habits. Formal family meals have been replaced to some extent by more informal eating styles and 'grazing'. Cooked school meals planned to give a balance of nutrients have been replaced by individual choice and cafeteria-style eating or packed meals, so that even young people have become accustomed to making their own spur-of-the-minute choices about what they will eat. Workers are increasingly likely to have a midday snack often while on the move rather than a complete meal. In the home, breakfast is often not eaten, while TV snacks in the evening may replace a family meal. All these social changes tend to reinforce personal choice and increase the likelihood that an unbalanced mixture of processed foods, which are easily and quickly prepared, will be eaten instead of more conventional meals prepared from fresh foods. When full meals are eaten, they are increasingly

ready-made. These changes have been facilitated by the increasing use of domestic freezers and microwave ovens. Increasingly, therefore, consumers have diminished influence over the nutrient composition of their meals.

Manufacturers and caterers are beginning to recognize the responsibility they have for the long-term health of consumers. This manifests in calls for training in nutrition for caterers and manufacturers for improvement in the nutrient profile of meals and in improved labelling to inform consumers about nutrition.

The nature of the changes in our diet over the past 50 years can be appreciated from Fig. 17.2. Although these changes are considerable, the British diet is still based largely on four staple foods: bread, milk, meat and potatoes. Consumption of fruit and vegetables remains low compared with other European countries. Optimists are pleased that small changes in recent years towards more fruit and less fat may relate to consistent health promotion. In countries where diets and health have improved, e.g. Finland, changes in catering and the composition of ready meals have been important, but slowly over 20–25 years.

During the past 60 years, the main changes in the British diet have been as follows:

1 *Bread.* There has been a gradual decline in bread consumption, and the fall in consumption of white bread has been only partly offset by an increase in consumption of brown bread, which occurred between 1978 and 1986, but has now ceased.

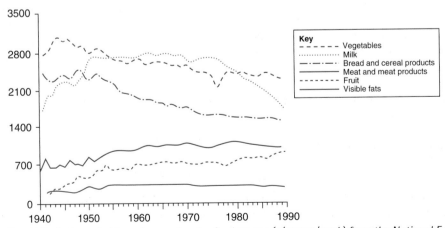

Figure 17.2 *Trends in the household purchases of major food groups (g/person/week) from the National Food Survey in the UK between 1940 and 1990*

2 *Vegetables and fruit.* When potatoes are excluded, vegetable consumption has increased only slightly over the period 1942–2000. While consumption of fresh green vegetables has fallen, consumption of frozen vegetables, especially peas, has risen since the 1960s. Consumption of fruit increased rapidly between 1945 and 1955, but thereafter has increased steadily. Although apples and pears, and bananas, followed by oranges, remain the most popular fruits, the most dramatic rise has been in consumption of fruit juice which has risen from negligible levels in 1970 to about over 300 ml per person per week. Potatoes, included in the totals for vegetables in the National Food Survey, have seen a marked fall in consumption – for fresh potatoes from 2 kg/week to around 700 g in the late 1990s. However, this has partly been replaced by an increased consumption of potato products such as chips.

3 *Milk and milk products.* Milk consumption rose between 1940 and 1950, remained at a high level until 1970 and thereafter decreased. The consumption of whole milk, however, has halved since the 1970s. Since 1984 there has been a considerable increase in the use of lower fat milks, especially semi-skimmed milk. Consumption of low-fat milks is now higher than that of whole milk. However, the fat skimmed from milk is still sold back into the human food supply, for example in cream cheeses, 'Greek style' yoghurt and baked foods. Of other milk products, the most dramatic change has been the increase in yoghurt consumption which has risen rapidly since the early 1970s. Overall, within this group, there has been a marked change towards low-fat varieties, such as low-fat milks, low-fat yoghurts and low-fat cheeses, including fromage frais.

4 *Meat.* Meat consumption has been declining in recent years, although consumption of poultry has gradually increased from 1950 until the early 1990s. Beef consumption dropped dramatically in the early 1990s due to concern about bovine spongiform encephalopathy (BSE). Meat and meat products containing less fat are in increasing demand. The fat content of carcases has been falling, because of younger age at slaughter, and improved feeding, and carcases are more carefully trimmed before sale. There is still a ready market for the fat however, and surplus fat is actually bought by the UK from more enlightened European countries to be put into 'meat pies' and sausages.

5 *Visible fats.* The overall consumption of visible fats in 1990 was not very different from what it was in 1940. After rising in the late 1940s and early 1950s, it remained steady at about 340 g/week from the mid-1950s until the 1970s, but has since declined to about 270 g/week. However, there have been considerable changes in the nature of fats eaten within this period. Butter consumption has declined since about 1970 while margarine consumption, mainly of the soft varieties, has increased since 1975, so that since 1980 margarine consumption has exceeded that of butter. However, margarine consumption has fallen from its peak in the early 1980s, having been partly replaced by low-fat and reduced-fat spreads. Consumption of vegetable oil has been increasing steadily since the late 1960s to a peak in 1996 while that of solid cooking fats, such as lard, has been decreasing since the mid-1970s.

DIETARY NEEDS OF SPECIAL GROUPS

The preceding discussion has been concerned with the average diet in the UK, as assessed by dietary surveys. While this is valuable because it allows general trends to be recognized, it does not help in evaluating the dietary needs of particular groups of people who have special needs. Such groups include pregnant and nursing women, babies and young children, elderly people and immigrants.

There are also other groups of people with special dietary needs, such as those who are ill, those who for reasons of health or fashion are slimming and those who, for reasons of conscience or preference, are vegetarians. Examples of the nutritional needs of special groups are given below.

Babies' diets

Breastfeeding

Mother's milk is the ideal food for a baby and all mothers should be encouraged to breastfeed. It is desirable that breastfeeding continues throughout the first year but especially for the first 3 months of a baby's life. There is some evidence that introducing carefully chosen additional food may benefit some infants between 3 and 6 months, but the WHO recently produced a global strategy on infant and young child feeding recommending that infants should be exclusively breastfed for the first 6 months of life. In the UK, the proportion of babies that are breast fed initially has been rising in recent years, from 66 per cent in 1995 to 69 per cent in 2000. However, 2 weeks after the birth, 52 per cent of mothers were breastfeeding and 6 weeks after the birth, 42 per cent of mothers were still breastfeeding their babies. These percentages are similar to 1995 (53 per cent breast-feeding at 2 weeks and 42 per cent at 6 weeks).

The advantages of breastfeeding are well documented. Mother's milk provides the correct balance of nutrients for the baby's needs. The infant's requirements of energy and protein (Table 17.3) over the first four months of life are provided naturally and easily by breastfeeding, and no extra food or nutrient supplements should be required as long as the mother is receiving an adequate diet. Nursing mothers are advised to take vitamin D supplements to increase their intake to the reference nutrient intake (RNI) of 10 μg per day.

Another advantage of breastfeeding is that the milk is available at the right temperature and generally in the right quantity. Also, with breastfeeding, the risk of infection is much less than in bottle feeding: the young baby is protected by antibodies and other substances in the mother's milk at a time when its own protective defences are not properly developed. Breastfeeding reduces the risk of diarrhoea from contaminated milk because the milk passes directly from mother to baby without any external contact.

Non-nutritional advantages of breastfeeding include the fostering of a close physical relationship between mother and baby and a beneficial effect on the health of the mother. Finally, it is worth mentioning that babies are less likely to become obese when breastfed than when they are bottle fed because in the latter method there is a tendency to make feeds too strong and to add energy-rich cereal foods to the milk. Recent research has identified the importance of n-3 long-chain fatty acids in breast milk, particularly docosahexanoic acid (DHA) which babies cannot adequately synthesize. They are needed for normal brain development, so their absence from most milk substitutes is a worry.

Bottle feeding

For some mothers there may be a good reason why they cannot or should not breastfeed, in which case they will bottle feed their baby using a commercial baby milk. Cow's milk has a composition very different from that of human milk and on its own is an incomplete food for babies. It also contains much more sodium than breast milk and less lactose, hence many attempts have been made to modify it so as to make it equivalent to breast milk. Although such attempts have not been completely successful many commercial products are available.

Commercial baby milks are normally in concentrated form – either dried or evaporated – and are reconstituted by the addition of water. Cow's milk is modified in a number of ways, so that it more closely resembles human milk. The main objects are to reduce the mineral and protein content and increase the lactose content. In addition, such products are usually fortified with vitamin D as neither mother's milk nor cow's milk contain sufficient for the baby's needs. In some products the animal fat of cow's milk is replaced by vegetable oils. Ordinary skimmed milk is not suitable for babies because it contains less vitamin A and has a lower energy content than cow's milk. A hazard with formula feeds is the habit of increasing the strength in a mistaken belief that this will satisfy a baby more readily.

Weaning and solid food

Although weaning, that is, the transition from milk to solid food, will take place at different ages, the WHO recommend that most babies should not be

Table 17.3 Estimated average requirements (EARs) for energy and protein for infants

Age in months	EAR for energy (kcal/day)		EAR for protein (g/day)
	Boys	Girls	
0–3	545	515	n/a
4–6	690	645	10.6
7–9	825	765	11.0
10–12	920	865	11.2

given solid food before the age of 6 months, although previous recommendations in the UK mean that babies are often weaned around 4 months, or even earlier.

There is no sound nutritional reason for introducing solid foods before 4 months and indeed there are positive dangers related to earlier weaning. For example, early addition of solids with high energy-density to feeds can produce obesity in babies and the early use of cereal foods containing wheat gluten can predispose the baby to coeliac disease (see Chapter 3) and allergies.

When solid foods are introduced, babies can be given most of the foods eaten by the rest of the family (except for strongly spiced ones), provided that they are minced or sieved. Such ordinary food is to be preferred to commercial baby foods, which are often sweetened and salted. Babies should not be given ordinary cow's milk, because of risks of gastrointestinal bleeding and they should start receiving vitamin supplements, particularly of vitamin D if there is too little exposure to sunlight to synthesize enough for the baby's needs. Cod-liver oil will supply vitamins A and D and orange juice will supply vitamin C. Alternatively, all three vitamins may be supplied as a vitamin supplement given in the form of drops. Such supplements should be continued until the age of 2 years and preferably up to 5 years.

Despite the availability of suitable vitamin supplements, the diets of some babies and young children are lacking in these vitamins, and in a very small minority this deficiency is sufficiently serious to produce rickets and scurvy. It should be emphasized, however, that the number of children suffering from vitamin deficiency diseases in the UK is extremely small. With increasing understanding of the dietary needs of the young, better dissemination of such knowledge to mothers and better availability of vitamin supplements and fortified foods, rickets, which, at the beginning of the twentieth century was a common disease among children, is now rare among most children in the UK. Unfortunately, it is not uncommon among the children of some ethnic groups, in particularly vegetarians who are covered against sunlight.

Apart from vitamins, the main nutrient likely to be lacking in an infant's diet is iron. At birth babies have a reserve supply of iron which lasts for several months and this, together with the relatively small amount of iron received from human or cow's milk, supplies their needs for some 4–5 months. After this time, however, they need to be given foods containing iron – fish, minced meat, cereals and eggs all being suitable. Although severe iron deficiency resulting in anaemia is not common in most UK children, it is frequently found among children from countries, such as the West Indies, in which the traditional infants' diet is lacking in iron. Cow's milk can induce bleeding into the bowel resulting in anaemia.

Diet of the elderly

Elderly people may suffer from an inadequate diet for a variety of reasons, including loneliness, poverty, reduced enjoyment of food due to loss of teeth, taste and smell, mental and physical lethargy, immobility, or illness with depression and inability to chew and digest food properly. Many elderly people have altered nutrient requirements through diabetes and other diseases. For these and other reasons elderly people more often suffer from malnutrition than the rest of the population. As the proportion of elderly people in the UK is increasing, the task of ensuring that they receive an adequate diet is of growing importance. Many elderly people depend on others for virtually all their food and nutrient provision, through institutional or other provided catering (e.g. 'Meals on Wheels').

Although dietary reference values (DRVs) deal to some extent with elderly people, their nutritional needs require further investigation. It is known that energy needs decrease with age because of the reduction in physical activity and the DRVs concerning the levels of food energy intake appropriate to different age groups take this into account. The requirements of older people for vitamins and trace elements appears to be little different from the requirements of younger people. For example, the need for thiamin, riboflavin, vitamin B_6 and vitamin B_{12} are similar, so there may be problems for elderly people obtaining adequate vitamin intakes from a reduced food intake.

Several studies have been carried out on the diet of the healthy elderly. These conclude that the number of malnourished people is probably small and does not constitute a serious problem; it is believed that it is disease rather than malnutrition that is the primary problem. Among those that are malnourished, the nutrients most likely to be deficient are vitamins C and D and folate. Many old people have inadequate intakes of folate and this may be because they eat few green leafy vegetables. Obesity in elderly people, however, is a more important cause of nutritional disorder than lack of nutrients in the diet.

There are some particular hazards for older people. For example, old people who have difficulty in peeling fruit or cooking potatoes may lack sufficient vitamin C, while the housebound will have little or no chance of being in the sunshine and, consequently, may lack vitamin D. Vitamin D supplements may well be beneficial for older people, particularly in winter. Finally, old people suffer from loss of calcium from bone – a disease called osteoporosis. Although this condition cannot be prevented or remedied by diet, foods that are rich in calcium such as milk or cheese should be included in diets for the elderly.

'Slimming' diets

The nature and effects of obesity and its prevalence in the UK and other western countries where it is a major health problem have already been considered in Chapter 3. Here, we shall consider ways in which diet can be used to reduce weight.

Some people try to slim for the simple reason that it is fashionable to be slim, but it is becoming increasingly recognized that many people are too fat and that this is objectionable not only for aesthetic reasons, but for health reasons as well. People who are overweight impose a strain on the heart and other organs and they are more likely to suffer from mechanical disabilities, owing to the strain put upon joints and ligaments, than slim people. Moreover, fat people are predisposed to metabolic disorders. Statistics show that for men who are 10 per cent overweight life expectancy is reduced by 13 per cent, while for those who are 30 per cent overweight it is reduced by 42 per cent.

Most people who try to slim do so by modifying their eating habits in some way and in traditional methods of slimming energy intake is reduced by cutting down the amount of food eaten. This is because people become fat when the energy intake derived from food is greater than the total energy used by the body. The food which is surplus to the body's

energy requirements is stored as fat. In this connection it is important to appreciate that it is not only fatty foods that contribute to fat reserves; excess carbohydrate and protein also contribute.

It is evident from the above that fat reserves may be depleted by reducing the energy intake to below that used by the body. Alternatively, the energy intake can be maintained and the energy used increased by greater physical activity. Unfortunately, a great deal of exercise is needed to have much effect – about 2 hours' strenuous exercise is needed to dispose of a good meal, and since increased exercise leads to increased appetite, loss of weight achieved through exercise is likely to be counteracted by a subsequent increase in weight through extra eating and drinking.

In surveying different types of slimming diet some distinct trends can be recognized. In the 1960s and 1970s, low-carbohydrate diets and calorie-counting diets were recommended, while in the 1980s low-fat or high-fibre (i.e. high in NSP) diets were in vogue. Scientific evidence favours the low fat approach, but is often overwhelmed by marketing hype. The same diet does not suit everyone equally.

The essence of the low-carbohydrate diet is simple: if intake of carbohydrate foods is restricted there will be a considerable reduction in energy intake. It is argued that fat consumption will also be reduced. For example, if less bread is eaten then less butter will also be eaten. Thus, although the low-carbohydrate diet allows foods rich in fat and/or protein to be eaten without restriction, the hope is that reduction in bread consumption will also reduce consumption of fat associated with it.

Although the low-carbohydrate diet has in the past enjoyed great popularity, it has helped create some of the nonsense that surrounds the subject of slimming. Carbohydrates have gained a bad reputation because they are considered to be particularly 'fattening' which is quite untrue. In this blanket condemnation of carbohydrates, sugar and starch are both included. This view is in direct conflict with current nutritional opinion which attaches considerable importance to maintaining our intake of starch (and NSP) while reducing sugar consumption.

Calorie-counting diets, once so popular, are now much less used. In such diets the slimmer can eat any foods provided that a selected energy intake is not exceeded. Such diets have the advantage that they permit complete freedom of choice but the disadvantage that all food eaten must be weighed and energy values calculated. These are tedious activities and provide a strong disincentive for adopting this type of diet as a 'normal' way of eating. Calorie counting has been criticised as nutritionally naïve, that unless the calories are counted, and balanced, agonising over other important nutrients is misguided.

Low-fat diets exclude or severely limit foods that are high in fat but allow other foods to be eaten freely. Fats have more than twice the energy value of carbohydrates or proteins, so that a low-fat diet is likely to be a low-energy diet. This type of diet is currently recommended by many doctors because lowering fat intake, and particularly lowering intake of saturated fat, is considered to be healthy and may be a way of reducing the risk of CHD.

Wholefood diets are now very popular and aim at establishing a diet that has a low energy value but a high NSP content. Wholefoods rich in NSP have the advantage that they have a low energy value while, because of their capacity to 'hold' considerable amounts of water, they provide bulk, which gives a feeling of fullness. Moreover, as already mentioned, it is believed that an increased NSP intake is desirable in itself, particularly an increased intake of cereal NSP. Another advantage of such a diet is that wholefoods are eaten in place of refined convenience foods.

Dietary aids to slimming

Many commercial products are available which are intended to aid slimming. The most drastic of these are complete diets in the sense that they replace normal foods completely. 'Very low calorie diets' have been developed as complete diets intended to produce very rapid loss in weight. They provide less than 2.5 MJ/day and a typical product would provide as little as 1.3 MJ/day. They also provide enough of all the micronutrients to satisfy recommended intakes for healthy people. Such products are usually based on milk powder to which minerals and vitamins are added; they are often produced in the form of drinks that completely replace meals.

Very low calorie diets are adopted because they lead to rapid weight reduction; as much as 1.5 kg/week may be lost. They are most useful for very obese people who probably lose proportionately less body protein to fat than only moderately obese people

when energy intake is severely restricted. Such diets are considered to be reasonably safe and tolerable for many. However, these diets should only be used under medical advice, having excluded active heart disease. Dehydration with headaches and dizziness and constipation are common problems, which can be ameliorated and to some extent solved by drinking and maintaining a high NSP consumption.

One obvious disadvantage of very low calorie diets and similar artificial eating regimes is that they do nothing to change habitual eating habits or restrain appetite in the long term. Once weight loss has been achieved through such a diet, there is a strong likelihood that the slimmer will revert to previous eating habits and that the weight lost will soon be regained. Such diets can be commended for the extremely obese who require a brief form of 'dietary shock treatment' to initiate rapid weight loss. They should then transfer to a diet such as the low-fat or wholefood diets already discussed, which will allow them to form new and permanent eating habits.

Apart from very low calorie diets there are a number of products available intended to aid slimming without replacing normal meals. The main types of such products are shown in Table 17.4.

Various appetite-reducing tablets containing glucose (in attempt to reduce appetite acutely) or methyl-cellulose which when consumed is supposed to absorb water and swell in the stomach, giving a feeling of fullness. Such a product provides bulk but has no energy or nutrient value whatever. The amount of methyl cellulose contained in commercial products is so small, however, and there is no evidence that they are of any benefit. Newer, heavily marketed preparations contain ground shellfish. Results do not match the extravagant marketing claims, usually considered fraudulent.

Meal replacement products are used to replace some (but not all) normal meals as part of an energy-controlled diet. They may be in the form of biscuits or confectionery bars or a powder that is added to milk. Such products contain a variety of nutrients as well as ingredients designed to make the slimmer feel full. Carrageenan, methyl cellulose and bran are all used for this purpose, the first being an interesting substance which is extracted from red seaweeds and which acts as a thickening agent by binding water. Thus, the presence of carrageenan gives body to what would otherwise be a 'watery'

Table 17.4 The popularity and effectiveness of slimming aids

Type	Per cent of slimmers using them	Verdict
Appetite reducers	17% for methyl cellulose type, 22% for glucose type	Very few found them effective
Meal replacement	50% had tried them, meals in drink form and in tins were best liked	35% thought them helpful (calorie-counted meals)
Low energy foods	90% had tried them	Majority found them helpful
(a) Sugar substitutes	50% for pellet forms, 25% for liquid forms	80% thought them helpful
(b) Low-calorie drinks	67% had tried them	
(c) Low-fat spreads	Most had tried them	Over 66% found them helpful

From Consumers' Association Survey.

drink and psychologically this gives slimmers the feeling that they have had a satisfying meal rather than a mere drink. Such products offer a convenient but expensive approach to slimming and suffer from the disadvantage that they do not help to establish better eating habits, unless it is adopted as a lifelong meal replacement without compensation from the other meals: this is rare, mainly because commercial meal replacements are expensive and do not taste pleasant. Many are very sweet and tend to perpetuate a demand for sweet foods. A bowl of porridge is a better meal replacement.

The most popular dietary slimming aids are low-energy versions of ordinary foods. The objective is to make products that resemble the original as closely as possible but which have a much reduced energy content. This is usually achieved by replacing energy-rich substances such as fat and sugar by energy-free substances such as air, water, bran and saccharin. Such products include sugar substitutes, low-energy drinks and soups, low-energy salad dressings and fats, starch-reduced breads and rolls, low-energy crisp breads and high-fibre bars and biscuits. Some 'low fat' products are in fact high in energy density, or larger in size so do not help weight control. However, routine use of low-fat products does result in eating less and prevents or reduces weight gain.

Vegetarian diets

There are many reasons for people avoiding meat or being vegetarian. Meat is prohibited by some

religions, like Hinduism and Jainism. Some avoid meat because they believe that farmed animals suffer. Others hold political conditions about optimal use of agricultural resources. Health consciousness provides another reason – including the erroneous belief that red meat is fattening. The recent publicity over BSE and foot and mouth disease led to large-scale rejection of meat for a short time. The term 'vegetarian' is often applied loosely to all meat-avoiders, including fish eaters. Fish has a number of positive advantages and is associated with health in the Mediterranean diet. Many untutored vegetarians have diets undesirably high in fat and saturated fat (from dairy products), while others can be well balanced nutritionally.

There are three main types of 'vegetarian' regime: the ovo-lacto-vegetarian diet, which consists of foods of plant origin together with eggs and dairy products; the lacto-vegetarian diet, which is similar but excludes eggs; and the vegan diet, which excludes all foods not of plant origin. Vegetarians in the first two categories get animal protein from eggs and dairy products and can easily obtain a nutritionally adequate diet if care is taken to eat a sufficient variety and quantity of food. Vegans also can achieve a diet which is satisfactory in most respects, but unless care is taken, it is difficult for them to receive sufficient vitamin B_{12}, and possibly vitamin D, from their very restrictive diet.

The water content of fruit and vegetables is usually high and their energy densities correspondingly low. Wholemeal grains and some dairy products, on the other hand, have a high energy density and so food

Table 17.5 Essential amino acid composition of 'vegetarian' food groups[b]

Food groups	'Weaknesses'	'Strengths'
Cereals	Lysine, isoleucine	Tryptophan, methionine, cysteine[a]
Dairy foods	None	Lysine
Eggs	None	Tryptophan, lysine, methionine, cysteine[a]
Pulses or legumes	Tryptophan, methionine	Lysine, isoleucine, cysteine[a]
Other 'vegetable'	Isoleucine, methionine	Tryptophan, lysine, cysteine[a]
Seeds and nuts	Lysine	Tryptophan, methionine, cysteine[a]

[a]Cysteine is not an essential amino acid because the body can make it from methionine but its presence 'spares' methionine.
[b]Assuming a cereal staple, pulses or legumes are needed if animal products are not eaten in sufficient amounts.

energy requirements can easily be met by a vegetarian diet, provided that enough food, including a reasonable amount of cereal products, is eaten. However, it is less easy to overeat when following a vegetarian diet, and vegetarians tend to be leaner than the population in general. Nevertheless, the energy intake of adult vegetarians has been found to be similar to that of meat-eaters, but that of vegetarian children tends to be lower than average. Care must be taken when children are following vegan diets to ensure that their food is not too bulky, so that enough can be eaten to provide the energy needs and nutrient requirements for growth.

Although a carefully contrived vegan diet can be nutritionally adequate, it should be borne in mind that plant proteins are usually of lower biological value than animal proteins. They will be less efficiently used by the body than animal proteins unless a variety of plant proteins is eaten on the same day, and preferably as part of the same meal, so that the absence of an essential amino acid in the proteins of one food can be complemented by its presence in another. Table 17.5 shows the amino acid 'strengths' and 'weaknesses' of foods that figure prominently in vegetarian diets. The maximum nutritional benefit will be obtained by combining foods in such a way that the amino acid 'weaknesses' of one group are compensated for by the 'strengths' of another. For example, when food of cereal origin is eaten at the same time as a pulse (as in the case of baked beans on toast) the two proteins combined provide high-quality protein. It is important that young children are provided with sufficient high-quality protein to sustain a high rate of growth so protein in the diets of vegetarian children, and especially vegan children, should be from mixed sources.

Vegetarians tend to consume more starch and NSP than meat-eaters because of their preference for wholemeal grains, nuts and fruit. Their total sugar intake may also be higher, despite the fact that many vegetarians do not 'take sugar', because of the intrinsic sugar content of their higher fruit and vegetable intake.

Vegetarian diets provide, on average, about 35 per cent of their food energy as fat. In most vegan diets, only about 10 per cent of dietary energy is provided by saturated fat. Lacto-vegetarian diets may contain more fat because of the amount of cheese and other dairy products consumed. Vegetarian and vegan diets are normally richer in the essential fatty acid linoleic acid than the diets of non-vegetarians.

The calcium intake of lacto- and ovo-lacto-vegetarians is usually high but that of vegans may be very low. Many vegans do not eat white bread and hence do not have the benefit of the calcium carbonate which is added to all white flour in the UK. In addition, the high phytate and NSP content of wholemeal bread may hinder the absorption of what little calcium there is in the remainder of their diet. Nevertheless, adult vegans are not normally deficient in calcium. This may be because of the body's ability to increase the efficiency of calcium absorption (provided that vitamin D intake is adequate) at times when the dietary intake is low.

Iron is poorly absorbed from plant sources and so the iron content of a vegetarian diet needs to be higher than that of a non-vegetarian diet to provide the same amount of iron to the body. Unfortunately, wholemeal bread and wholegrain cereals, which are likely to figure prominently in the diet, may lower the absorption rate even further because of their phytate and NSP content. However, the higher vitamin C content of vegetarian diets promotes the absorption of non-haem iron and thus can offset the effect of phytate and NSP. Vegetarian meals can valuably be complemented by fruit juice. Tea, which impairs iron absorption, is best avoided during vegetarian meals.

Vegetarians who consume milk and dairy products usually have an adequate vitamin intake and are unlikely to suffer from vitamin deficiencies, but vegan diets may lack vitamin D and vitamin B_{12}. Natural vitamin D is found almost exclusively in animal foods, particularly dairy foods, which are not eaten by vegans. A deficiency may be avoided by eating margarine which, in the UK, must be fortified with synthetic vitamin D. Fish oils are often used in the manufacture of margarine, however, and only margarine made exclusively from vegetable oil is acceptable to vegans. Vitamin B_{12} is only found in foods of animal origin and, at one time, it was difficult for a strict vegan to avoid a deficiency. Fortunately, the vitamin is now produced commercially by growing bacteria on a vegetable growth-medium and it is used to supplement a number of foods produced for vegans.

Many studies have compared the health and life expectancy of vegetarians and vegans with the population as a whole. It is doubtful whether vegetarians, as a group, live much longer than non-vegetarians, but it has been shown that there is a favourable correlation between vegetarianism and specific diseases. It is fairly clear that many intestinal diseases such as bowel disorders, including gallstone formation, constipation, haemorrhoids and diverticular disease, are less prevalent among vegetarians than in the population in general. The incidence of diabetes also appears to be lower among vegetarians. Vegetarians also have, on average, lower blood pressures than omnivores and CHD has been shown to be less prevalent among vegetarians than the population in general. It should be borne in mind however, that the general population consumes undesirably high amounts of high-fat meat products. An ideal human diet may still include modest amounts of fish and meat.

It is extremely difficult to be sure that any observed differences are related only to diet and not to other differences in lifestyle which may affect health and life expectancy. Vegetarians tend to be highly motivated and well-informed about nutritional matters and to be aware of the dangers of other health-threatening habits such as smoking, excessive alcohol consumption and overeating. Although it is difficult to be sure whether any health benefits are obtained by following a vegetarian diet, it is clear that such diets, if properly planned and controlled, are not harmful and that those that follow them are confident of the beneficial effect on their health.

TYPES OF DIETARY INTERVENTION TO IMPROVE HEALTH

Once it is accepted that dietary change can reasonably be expected to improve health for a majority of people, without detriment to others, there are two types of interventions possible.

High-risk targeted strategy

This approach requires a screening procedure to identify people with high risk of a disease, who would benefit from diet change. Screening is often expensive, the individual counselling is labour-intensive and only effective with high compliance (difficult for individuals within family meals). The individual then needs personal follow-up and assessment for reduced risk. This approach thus has huge implications for professional time and resources. It can induce anxiety, or paradoxically promote adverse dietary behaviours in people who screen negative. It should be remembered that among people with low cholesterol, the commonest cause of death is still CHD.

Population-directed interventions

This approach promotes, or imposes, dietary changes on the whole population, or at least on targeted subgroups. Education and nutritional changes to the composition of common foods are examples. No screening is needed and no information is collected about individuals. Part of the aim of this approach is to reduce the numbers of individuals who reach a 'high-risk' status. The main obstacles to this approach are the resistance of the food industry to changes, even very gradually, which would improve health. There is no escape from the obvious fact that if diet-related health is to improve, then there has to be change in the foods provided. That was very apparent in the North Karelia projects in Finland: farmers agreed to diversify away from continued high-dairy production, and this had knock-on consequences for food retailing and catering, which were matched by altered consumer demand.

One of the active debates is whether to inform consumers of changes in food composition. Consumers are generally intelligent and respect honest information from the food industry about changing composition of foods. A good example is the response to the UK SACN Report (2003) 'Salt and Health' which urges reduced sodium consumption mainly from salt added during food processing: 80 per cent of all salt consumed is added during processing, so outside the control of concerned consumers. Cost implications are minimal, and manufacturers who declare reduced sodium content in products are being met by consumers looking for them.

In general, consumers have benefited from health education in terms of their understanding of the main nutritional messages, but need quantitative guidance to help make appropriate changes. They are not looking for, indeed will not accept, high-priced 'healthy alternative' foods, but would be pleased to see foods with undesirable compositions replaced by improved versions. The human palate changes remarkably quickly: most people now prefer the taste of the reduced-fat milk that it is widely available. That was not the case 10–20 years ago.

It is worth noting that nutrition education alone may help, but its benefit is largely restricted to educated people. Education tends to exaggerate health inequalities. Changing the food environment benefits everyone.

Guidelines for a healthier diet

Many people are interested in following a healthier diet and there has been a considerable improvement in dietary standards in recent years. Over 60 per cent of milk consumed is now skimmed or semi-skimmed, meat is leaner, butter consumption is much reduced and margarine or low-fat spreads have taken its place, consumption of white bread has fallen (but that of wholemeal bread has stayed at a very low level of 100 g per person per week in the last 8 years), fresh fruit consumption (particularly bananas) has increased and, finally, sugar intake has been much reduced.

Despite these changes, so-called 'diseases of affluence' such as CHD and cancer, which in many instances are diet-related, are major health problems in most industrialized countries. In the UK, CHD is the main cause of death for those over the age of 65. The nature of the link between these diseases of affluence and diet has been explored in Chapter 3, and the role that specific nutrients may play in their causation has been dealt with in the chapters concerned with those nutrients.

The UK Committee on Medical Aspects of Food Policy (COMA) report 'Dietary Reference Values of Food Energy and Nutrients for the UK' was published in 1991. This specifies desirable levels of intake for about 40 nutrients, and when used in conjunction with information obtained from dietary surveys, it provides a sound basis for evaluating individual diets and for deciding how best to improve the average British diet. It expanded on the 1990 WHO report on Diet and Chronic Disease which has recently been updated (2003). The population nutrient intake goals (see Table 17.6) provide guidance for national bodies wishing to establish dietary recommendations for the prevention of diet-related chronic diseases (primarily obesity, CHD, cancer, diabetes, dental disease and osteoporosis).

Although the changes in the British diet mentioned above are considerable and help to meet nutritional guidelines, there is still room for improvement. Surveys of household food consumption show that dietary intakes of fat, saturated fatty acids and non-milk extrinsic sugars are all higher, and NSP intake lower, than the Dietary Reference Values specified in the 1991 COMA report.

Table 17.7 indicates how the average British diet might have to change in order to meet the dietary reference values specified in the 1991 COMA report. The changes needed, namely a considerable increase in the consumption of bread and vegetables and a halving in the consumption of the other foods listed, would amount to a revolution in dietary habits.

It is possible that improved or worsened dietary habits can be brought about by other changes. On the positive side, sugar and preserve consumption has decreased beyond expectation since 1992. However, soft drink consumption has increased such that the percentage of energy obtained from non-milk extrinsic sugars has reduced very little in the last 8 years or so. There has been an increase in fruit consumption but not vegetable consumption, suggesting that the population may prefer this

Table 17.6 Ranges of population nutrient intake goals[g]

Dietary factor	Goal (% of total energy, unless otherwise stated)
Total fat	15–30%
Saturated fatty acids	<10%
Polyunsaturated fatty acids (PUFAs)	6–10%
n-6 PUFAs	5–8%
n-3 PUFAs	1–2%
trans-Fatty acids	<1%
Monounsaturated fatty acids (MUFAs)	By difference[a]
Total carbohydrate	55–75%[b]
Free sugars[c]	<10%
Protein	10–15%[d]
Cholesterol	<300 mg/day
Sodium chloride (sodium)[e]	<5 g per day (<2 g/day)
Fruits and vegetables	≥400 g/day
Total dietary fibre	From foods[f]
Non-starch polysaccharides (NSP)	From foods[f]

[a]This is calculated as: total fat – (saturated fatty acids + polyunsaturated fatty acids + trans-fatty acids).

[b]The percentage of total energy available after taking into account that consumed as protein and fat, hence the wide range.

[c]The term 'free sugars' refers to all monosaccharides and disaccharides added to foods by the manufacturer, cook or consumer, plus sugars naturally present in honey, syrups and fruit juices.

[d]The suggested range should be seen in the light of the Joint WHO/FAO/UNU Expert Consultation on Protein and Amino Acid Requirements in Human Nutrition, held in Geneva from 9–16 April 2002.

[e]Salt should be iodized appropriately. The need to adjust salt iodization, depending on observed sodium intake and surveillance of iodine status of the population, should be recognized.

[f]See page 98, under Non-starch polysaccharides.

[g]Reproduced with permission from WHO Technical Report 916, Diet, Nutrition and the Prevention of Chronic Disease, WHO, Geneva 2003 (http://www.who.int/dietphysicalactivity/publications/trs916/download/en/).

method of increasing fruit and vegetable consumption (and thus vitamin C and NSP) rather than by a doubling of vegetable intake, as suggested in the 1994 COMA report (Department of Health, 1994). New ground was broken by two reports from Scotland. The 1993 Scottish Diet Report (www.scotland.gov.uk/library5/health/msdt-05.asp), calculated out all the interacting nutritional complexities of a national diet and health plan, to provide quantitative food-based targets. The 1996 Scottish Diet Action Plan (Scottish Office, 1996) evaluated the measures necessary along the complete pathway from food production, through processing, retailing and catering, and supported by education and media activity to its consumption, in order to achieve nutritional targets for improved health. The evidence from the North Karelia Study, in Finland, was seminal in the adoption of this document as policy by three successive governments.

Reduction in saturated fat and salt, with increases in fruit and vegetables and fish consumption in Finland have been associated with a 60–70 per cent reduction in heart disease, stroke and cancers. It is not possible to identify one key element in these changes, and the improvement took place over 20–25 years. Engaging many different sectors and complementary interventions with strong central coordination and better general education were the key elements.

Moderate alcohol consumption is not judged to be harmful, indeed 10–20 g of alcohol daily (1–2 units) is associated with relative freedom from heart disease, but it is recommended that consumption be limited, because large amounts increase blood pressure and are associated with more liver disease, cancers and accidental injuries. Recent advice is that alcohol consumption should not exceed 3–4 units a day for men and no more than 2–3 units for women to a maximum of 21 units per week for men and

Table 17.7 Some changes required in the British diet (1991) in order to meet Committee on Medical Aspects of Food Policy (COMA) dietary reference value (DRV) guidelines

Food	Average household food consumption 1992 (g per person per day)	Average household food consumption 2000 (g per person per day)	Desirable intake to meet COMA DRV (g per person per day)	Comments
Bread	108	103	161	Increase from 3 slices to 4.5 slices per day with at least one slice of wholemeal
Buns, cakes and biscuits	32	33	21	Reduce from 3–4/day to 1–2/day
Fish and fish products	20	20	27	Maintain one portion/week of white fish. Increase oil-rich fish from half to one portion per week
Fruit	133	160	184	Increase from 1–2 to 3 portions per day
Potatoes	129	101	180	Increase from average of 2 to 3 medium potatoes per day
Sugar and preserves	29	20	27	Reduction from equivalent of 6 teaspoons to 5 teaspoons a day (achieved by 2000)
Vegetables (excluding potatoes)	185	183	241	Increase from 2–3 to 4 portions each day

Adapted from Department of Health. *Nutritional Aspects of Cardiovascular Disease. Report on Health and Social Subjects No 46.* HMSO, London, 1994. Crown copyright material is reproduced with the permission of the Controller of HMSO and the Queen's Printer for Scotland.

14 units per week for women. This is equivalent to nearly 32 g alcohol per day for a man with average energy intake or, in everyday terms, about one and a half pints of beer or three to four measures of spirits or two large glasses of table wine per day. Alcohol consumption has been rising in recent years, and at present average intakes for consumers (about 80 per cent of men and 70 per cent of women) is 8 and 6 per cent of dietary energy intake for men and women, respectively. However it is estimated that about 36 per cent of men and 22 per cent of women drink amounts of alcohol that may put their health at risk in the long term. More worryingly, alcohol intake in young people is much higher than in previous generations, with unknown potential for future adverse health.

Key points

- An influence of diet composition on health and disease processes has been known since biblical times (Daniel 2, 1)
- Modern evidence-based policies require detailed information on the population – from representative samples (hard to get) – on their health and disease status, or risk factors (harder to get) and - detailed information about quantitative exposure to foods, nutrients and other food components
- Established links between diet and health is difficult because of the long time-scale of diet-related disease development, and the pervasive problems over truthful reporting or recording of food composition

---

Chapter summary

Despite these limitations, observations from a huge range of studies, in different settings, allows high confidence and agreement amongst informed experts that optimal ranges for diet composition can be broadly described. The dietary guidelines for health published by independent scientific committees in many countries are now very similar, since the same diet and profiles (e.g. high in fruits and vegetables, low in saturated fat and salt) offer benefits for preventing many diseases (e.g. diabetes, heart diseases, stroke, cancers). Although designed for population targets, these dietary guidelines are useful benchmarks for individual eating habits.

FURTHER READING

DEPARTMENT OF THE ENVIRONMENT (2003). *Family Food in 2001/2002. A National Statistics. A National Statistics Publication by Defra.* London: The Stationery Office.

DEPARTMENT OF THE ENVIRONMENT (2004). *Family Food. A report on the 2002/2003 Expenditure and Food Survey. A National Statistics Publication by Defra.* London: The Stationery Office.

(also available at http://statistics.defra.gov.uk/esg/ publications/efs/2003/familyfood.pdf).

DEPARTMENT OF THE ENVIRONMENT (2001). *National Food Survey 2000. Annual Report on Food Expenditure, Consumption and Nutrient Intakes.* London: The Stationery Office.

DEPARTMENT OF HEALTH (1994). *Nutritional Aspects of Cardiovascular Disease. Report on Health and Social Subjects No. 46.* London: HMSO.

FINCH S, DOYLE W, LOWE C et al. (1998). *National Diet and Nutrition Survey: People Aged 65 Years and Over. Vol. 1: Report of the Diet And Nutrition Survey.* London: HMSO.

GARROW JS, JAMES WPT, RALPH A (2000). *Human Nutrition and Dietetics,* 10th edn. Edinburgh: Churchill Livingstone.

GIBNEY M, VORSTER H, KOK FJ (eds) (2002). *Introduction to Human Nutrition, The Nutrition Society Textbook Series*. Oxford: Blackwell Publishing.

HENDERSON L, GREGORY J, IRVING K (2003). *The National Diet and Nutrition Survey: Adults Aged 19 to 64 Years, Energy, Protein, Carbohydrate, Fat And Alcohol Intake*, Vol. 2. London: The Stationary Office.

INSEL P, TURNER RE, ROSS D (2001). *Nutrition*. Sudbury: Jones and Bartlett Publishers.

JOINT HEALTH CLAIMS INITIATIVE (2003). *Final Technical Report*. JHCI Ref JHCI/76/03. www.food.gov.uk/multimedia/pdfs/jhci_healthreport.pdf

MANN J & TRUSSWELL S (2002). *Essentials of Human Nutrition*, 2nd edn. Oxford: Oxford University Press.

SCIENTIFIC ADVISORY COMMITTEE ON NUTRITION (SACN) (2003). *Salt and Health*. London: HMSO.

SCOTTISH OFFICE (1996). *Scotland's Health A Challenge To Us All – Eating For Health: A Diet Action Plan for Scotland. Scottish Office Department of Health*. Edinburgh: HMSO.

THE CAROLINE WALKER TRUST (1995). *Eating Well for Older People. Practical and Nutritional Guidelines for Food In Residential And Nursing Homes And For Community Meals*. Abbots Langley: The Caroline Walker Trust.

WORLD HEALTH ORGANIZATION (2003). *The World Health Report 2003 – shaping the future*. Geneva: WHO.

APPROVED GENERIC STATEMENTS FOR HEALTH CLAIMS

These should only be used after reference to the JHCI website [www.jhci.co.uk].

1 Decreasing dietary saturates (saturated fat) can help lower blood cholesterol
2 People with a healthy heart tend to eat more wholegrain foods as part of a healthy lifestyle
3 The inclusion of at least 25 g soya protein per day as part of a diet low in saturated fat can help reduce blood cholesterol

18

Food spoilage and preservation

FOOD SPOILAGE

Much of our food is perishable within days or weeks and, in the natural course of events, it becomes inedible fairly quickly. Food spoilage occurs mainly as a result of chemical reactions involved in the processes of ageing and decay, through the action of microorganisms, or through a combination of both. A knowledge of why and how food spoilage occurs enables steps to be taken to prevent or minimize it. This, in essence, is the subject matter of this chapter.

Food that is not fresh is not necessarily harmful, but it is usually less attractive to the consumer than fresher food. It may also be less nutritious and normally commands a lower price. Flavour can change within even minutes or hours of harvesting (e.g. tomatoes, strawberries and fish). Most unprocessed foods deteriorate fairly rapidly if kept at normal temperatures, but some dry foods, such as cereal grains, will remain wholesome for long periods. Processed foods originate from a desire to make use of seasonal surpluses by prolonging the period for which they remain wholesome, so that they can be used throughout the year. Butter, cheese, bacon and dried fruit are examples of early processed foods.

In addition to chemical spoilage and attack by microorganisms, drying, staling, contamination with dirt or chemicals and damage by animals or insect pests all play their parts in food spoilage. In many cases, spoilage of this type can be avoided if care is taken in the transport and storage of food. Even though we now know a great deal about how food spoilage takes place, vast losses still occur and it has been estimated that between 10 and 20 per cent more food would be made available if such wastage could be completely prevented.

Chemical spoilage

Almost all our food is produced by living organisms, whether they be animals or plants, and it is mainly composed, as we have seen, of organic compounds. In the living plant or animal, these compounds are involved in a variety of complex and carefully controlled chemical reactions which, in the main, depend upon the presence of enzymes. When a plant is harvested or an animal is slaughtered, many of these reactions cease. The enzymes present, however, will still be active and are able to continue catalysing reactions which can adversely affect the quality of the food.

When fruit is picked growth stops, but it is still alive and may undergo changes in metabolism as a result of stress, altered light exposure, and temperature, to change its composition. Ripening is often able to continue. Once ripe, however, it will deteriorate rapidly, owing to the combined actions of enzymes and microorganisms, unless precautions are taken.

Vegetables, like fruit, remain alive after harvesting and they are prone to deterioration in the same way through the actions of enzymes and microorganisms and through loss of water. The ways in which fruit and vegetables deteriorate when stored are described in Chapter 15.

Meat is dead as soon as an animal is killed and changes occur in meat after an animal has been slaughtered. The initial changes are beneficial for culinary use. Freshly slaughtered meat is liable to be tough and lacking in flavour. It is not usually eaten until certain posthumous changes have occurred which make it more tender and flavoursome. This process of 'hanging' or 'conditioning', as it is known, is discussed in Chapter 11 (see p. 154).

If meat is kept for too long at room temperature it becomes 'soggy' and unwholesome, partly owing to the breakdown of its proteins by proteolytic enzymes. Putrefaction will eventually set in since it is always contaminated with some bacteria, for example with production of slime and foul odours caused by *Pseudomonas* bacilli the meat will be offensive and inedible. For reasons that are not entirely clear, the distinctive flavour of mild putrefaction is held to be desirable when venison, hare, pheasant and other game is eaten. Because of this, these delicacies are hung for much longer than other meats.

In addition to spoilage caused by protein breakdown, meat may also suffer through oxidation of fats which are always present. Unsaturated fats are more likely to become rancid through oxidation and for this reason poultry, pork, lamb and veal cannot be kept as long as beef because they have a higher proportion of unsaturated fats. Oxidized fats are one of the main causes of 'off' flavours in cooked meats.

What has been said above about spoilage of meat applies also to fish but with greater force. The reason is that fish are cold-blooded creatures and their enzymes are designed to be able to operate efficiently at lower temperatures than those found in land-based animals. They continue to operate at freezing point and this is why fish 'goes off' more quickly than meat, even if it is kept in a refrigerator. If fish is kept at room temperature, then processes are accelerated. Fish is less likely to be contaminated by harmful bacteria because cold-blooded animals do not normally have pathogenic bacteria responsible for food poisoning in their intestines.

Microbial food spoilage

Microbes, or microorganisms, are extremely small living things. They range in size from certain algae just large enough to be seen by the naked eye (about 100 μm) to viruses which are too small (about 0.1 μm) to be seen by a normal microscope. They can, however, be seen by using an electron microscope.

Microorganisms need water and nutrients before they can multiply. They cannot multiply on clean dry surfaces. Some of them, called aerobes, also need oxygen from the air; others called anaerobes can do without it.

Microorganisms like much the same type of food as we do and moist food kept in a warm place is likely to be attacked by microorganisms which will feed on it and grow on its surface. Most microorganisms do not multiply at low temperatures and are killed by high temperatures.

In addition to causing food spoilage some microorganisms, or the toxins they produce, are harmful to human beings, and if food contaminated by them is eaten food poisoning may result (see Chapter 19).

Food that has been attacked by microorganisms may look offensive or have a peculiar smell. In many instances, however, it is not possible to tell by looking at a sample of food, or by tasting it, whether it has been attacked. In fact, food may be heavily infected and still appear to be wholesome and such foods are more likely to cause food poisoning than those that have obviously deteriorated. It must be emphasized, however, that the presence of microorganisms is not always harmful. Indeed, many of the most highly prized food flavours are a consequence of microbial activity. For example, blue cheeses such as Roquefort, Stilton and Gorgonzola owe their characteristic flavours to the presence of the mould *Penicillium roqueforti*.

Microorganisms attack food because they require energy and raw materials to support their metabolic processes and explosively rapid growth. In other words, like us, they need food – only more so. Microorganisms break down the complex molecules of the foods on which they are growing and convert them into smaller absorbable molecules. If microbes are allowed to grow unhindered their presence on food often (but not always) becomes apparent to the eye and, especially in the case of meat and fish, to the nose.

Microbial growth usually ceases when food has become really foul because the microorganisms themselves can no longer tolerate the conditions they have created. Organic acids are among the substances produced during microbial breakdown of food and these accumulate and eventually suppress further microbial growth. Given time, another species of microorganism may appear which is able to tolerate the more acidic conditions and attack on the food will then continue.

Vegetables and fruit have dry, relatively non-porous skins and their cell juices are mildly acidic. They are thus more likely to suffer from the growth of moulds and yeasts than from attack by bacteria. Yeast and mould spores are always present in the air, but intact fruit and vegetables are not at great risk. However, if they are over-ripe or damaged, so that cell fluids leak onto the surface, mould or yeast growth is highly likely. If other conditions are favourable the food will deteriorate quickly. It is well known that 'one rotten apple in a barrel' can have a devastating effect. The reason is, of course, that the rotting specimen generates many millions of voracious microbes which quickly attack adjacent wholesome apples.

Fruit and vegetables will remain in good condition for the maximum possible time if they are clean, kept cool and handled with care.

Meat spoilage is mainly caused by bacteria and moulds, although meat is not immune from attack by yeasts. Healthy carcass meat should be free from bacteria. In practice, the surface is usually contaminated by bacteria from the hide and intestines when the animal is slaughtered and when the carcass is cut up. Poultry is particularly prone to bacterial contamination and the skin and interior surfaces usually harbour great numbers of bacteria.

When microbes grow on the surface of meat, they break down the protein molecules and grow to form a film of bacterial slime. Carbon dioxide, hydrogen and ammonia are formed and the surface layer of meat becomes greyish-brown in colour owing to conversion of myoglobin to metmyoglobin. As putrefaction continues, hydrogen sulphide, mercaptans and amines, all of which are foul-smelling, are formed and collectively demonstrate the inedible state of the meat.

It is very difficult to ensure that meat is completely free from bacteria and it almost always has some surface contamination. The bad effects of this can be minimized by storing meat at a low temperature (below 5°C) to prevent bacterial growth. Before cooking it should always be wiped with a clean damp cloth to remove bacterial slime.

The microorganisms principally responsible for food spoilage are moulds, bacteria and yeasts.

Moulds

Moulds are a form of fungi. Unlike yeasts and bacteria, they are multicellular organisms. They grow as fine threads or filaments which extend in length and eventually form a complex branched network or mat called a mycelium. At this stage mould growth on foods is easily visible as a 'fluff'. Moulds also produce spores, or seeds, and these can be carried considerable distances by air currents and in this way infect other foods. Mould spores are almost always present in the atmosphere and large numbers may be literally 'floating around' in food premises.

Most moulds require oxygen for development and this is why they are usually found only on the surface of foods. Meat, cheese and sweet foods are especially likely to be attacked by moulds. In alkaline or very acid foods (pH below 2), mould growth is usually inhibited, although some moulds will grow even under these conditions. Moulds grow best at a pH of 4–6 and a temperature of about 30°C; as the temperature decreases so does the rate of growth, although slow growth can continue at the temperature of a domestic refrigerator. Mould growth does not occur above normal body temperature, but it is very difficult to kill moulds and their spores by heat treatment. To ensure complete destruction of all moulds and their spores, sterilization under pressure is necessary (i.e. at above 100°C). Alternatively, the food may be heated to 70–80°C on two or more successive days so that any spores germinating between the heat treatments will be destroyed.

Poisonous mycotoxins are produced by some moulds and these can be harmful if eaten (see p. 293).

Bacteria

Bacteria are simple single-cell organisms. They are minute living particles, either spherical (cocci), rod-shaped (bacilli) or spiral (spirella). It is difficult to get any idea of the size of bacteria but 10^{13} of them (i.e. about 2000 times the population of the world) would weigh only about a gram. Bacteria and their spores are widely distributed. They are present in the soil, in the air and in and on human and animal bodies. Uncooked food of all descriptions will almost certainly be contaminated with bacteria. In fact, they occur so universally that it is exceedingly difficult to get away from them.

Bacteria grow by absorbing simple substances from their environment and when they reach a certain size, the parent organism splits to form two new ones. In favourable circumstances this fission may occur every 20 minutes or so and in 12 hours one bacterium can provide a colony of some 10^{10} bacteria.

When bacteria multiply in or on food, their presence becomes obvious when they are present to the extent of 10^6–10^7 per gram of foodstuff. Bacteria grow most readily in neutral conditions and growth is usually inhibited by acids. Some bacteria, however, will tolerate fairly low pH; for example, *Lactobacillus*, which causes souring of milk with the production of lactic acid, and *Acetobacter*, which convert ethyl alcohol to acetic acid, flourish in acid conditions. Aerobic bacteria will only grow in the presence of oxygen, whereas anaerobes will only grow in its absence.

Bacteria grow best within a given temperature range and in their vegetative stage (i.e. when they are actually growing). All of them can be killed by exposure to a temperature near to 100°C and at this temperature they are destroyed instantly. Bacteria, like moulds, can form spores. The heat resistance of bacterial spores varies from species to species and with the pH of the surrounding medium. This is considered in more detail on p. 283.

The commonest food spoilage organisms are mesophilic bacteria which originate in warm-blooded animals, but are also found in soil, water and sewage. Mesophilic bacteria grow best at about normal body temperature between 30 and 40°C and do not grow below 5°C. Psychrophilic bacteria, which have their origin in air, soil and water, grow best at a somewhat lower temperature – about 20°C – although some are quite happy at considerably lower temperatures. Such psychrophilic bacteria can grow quite easily at the temperature of a domestic refrigerator. A small group of bacteria can grow at temperatures up to 60°C and these are known as thermophilic bacteria. The spores of thermophilic bacteria can be very heat resistant.

Bacteria are not necessarily harmful to man and the species *Escherichia coli* exists in vast numbers in the human gut. However certain types, particularly verocytotoxin-producing *E. coli* (VTEC) (e.g. *E. coli* 0157-H7 serotype) are capable of causing severe bloody diarrhoea (haemorrhagic colitis) and further symptoms which can prove fatal to weakened individuals (e.g. elderly or infants). Some bacteria present in the gut are positively beneficial because they synthesize some absorbable B group vitamins and vitamin K from the contents of the large intestine. Bacteria which do no harm to man are, nevertheless, capable of spoiling food.

Some foods are specifically produced by introducing bacteria. For example, the large range of fermented milks and yoghurts available are made by introducing *Lactobacillus bulgaricus* and *Streptococcus thermophilus* to ferment the lactose in milk. This improves the keeping properties of the product and makes it easier to digest by large numbers of people who would otherwise be unable to tolerate the amount of lactose in milk.

Yeasts

Yeasts are microscopic, unicellular fungi but, unlike moulds, they reproduce themselves by budding (i.e. by the formation of a small off-shoot or bud which becomes detached from the parent yeast cell when it reaches a certain size and assumes an independent existence). Yeasts can also form spores but these are far less heat-resistant than mould spores and bacterial spores. Yeasts occur in the soil and on the surface of fruits; the presence of yeasts on the skin of grapes is the reason why grape juice ferments to become wine. Yeasts can grow in quite varied conditions but the majority prefer acid foods (pH 4–4.5) with a reasonable moisture content. Most yeasts grow best in the presence of oxygen between 25 and 30°C. Some yeasts can grow at 0°C and below. Yeasts and yeast spores are easily killed by heating to 100°C.

Yeasts are used for making bread (and other fermented goods), beer and vinegar. They cause spoilage of many foods including fruit, fruit juices, jam, wines and meat. Although they may spoil food, yeasts are not pathogenic (i.e. they do not cause diseases such as food poisoning).

FOOD PRESERVATION

Microorganisms are present in the air, in dust, soil, sewage and on the hands and other parts of the body. They are so widely distributed that their presence in or on food is inevitable unless special steps are taken to kill them. If food is to be kept in good condition for any length of time it is essential that the growth of microorganisms be prevented. This can be done either by killing them and then storing the food in conditions where further infection is impossible or by creating an environment which slows down or stops their growth.

The ability to preserve food in good condition for long periods is an undoubted boon. The amount of food wasted is reduced and the incidence of food poisoning is minimized. A wider range of foods is available including foods 'out of season' and foods from overseas that could not be transported and stocked in former times. The widespread use of preservatives, refrigerators, 'deep-freeze' equipment and canned and dehydrated food has made it easy for the consumer or caterer to have available a wide range of wholesome food at all times of the year.

As well as suppressing the growth of microorganisms, an effective method of food preservation must retain, as far as possible, the original characteristics of the food and impair its nutritive value as little as possible.

Chemical preservatives

Chemicals have been used in the preservation of foods for many centuries; sodium chloride, sodium and potassium nitrate, sugars, vinegar, alcohol, wood smoke and various spices have come to be regarded as traditional preservatives.

An example of the preservative action of concentrated sugar solutions has already been encountered in Chapter 9 in connection with jams and other sugar preserves. Condensed sweetened milk, which contains large amounts of sugar, is another excellent example of this principle. It can be kept for several weeks after opening the can without growth of microorganisms occurring. Microorganisms cannot tolerate high concentrations of alcohol and this is why fortified wines, such as sherry and port wine, keep better than unfortified wines. Similarly, vinegar discourages the growth of many microorganisms and it performs this function in 'pickled' foods.

Preservation by salting and smoking

Meat and fish have been preserved by salting (or curing) since ancient times. The method is still used, often in combination with drying or smoking, in even the most primitive societies where salt is available. In medieval Britain, weaker animals were killed off in the autumn because insufficient feeding stuff was available to keep them alive through the winter. Whole bullocks were salted and little or no fresh meat was available during the winter months.

Meat and fish are now preserved by refrigeration and the importance of curing as a method of preservation has diminished. In western societies, nevertheless, heavily salted bacon and ham, salami-style sausage and corned beef all still feature in our diet and to some extent serve to maintain excessive salt addition to a wide range of other foods (bread, cereals, etc.), which otherwise would taste bland. 'Lighter' cures are used today so that bacon, for example, is not as salty or as dry as in the past. In consequence, it is more prone to bacterial spoilage and has to be treated almost as carefully as fresh pork.

Dry salting, in which meat or fish was buried in granular salt containing some sodium nitrate/nitrite, is now rare. In wet curing processes a concentrated salt solution, or brine, is used. Sodium nitrate is traditionally added to the brine and some of it is reduced to sodium nitrite during the curing process. It is actually the nitrite which acts as the preservative and now sodium nitrite itself is often used in place of sodium nitrate.

Cured meat (mainly pork) is usually made today by injecting the meat with a concentrated salt solution containing about 5 per cent sodium nitrate/nitrite and, for 'sweetcure' bacon, a little sugar. The meat is then immersed in a similar solution for a few days. Prepacked sliced bacon sometimes starts out as sliced raw pork and the curing solution is included in the pack. Curing takes place (or is supposed to take place) within the pack. Inevitably, the product is somewhat wetter than traditionally cured bacon and it is not to everyone's taste.

Curing changes the colour of uncooked meat as a result of partial conversion of the protein myoglobin to the redder nitrosomyoglobin by nitrites present in the curing liquor. When bacon or ham is cooked (or 'corned beef' is further preserved by canning) the colour deepens owing to formation of a more complex nitrosoprotein. The presence of nitrites in food may be harmful owing to the risk of nitrosamine formation (see p. 277).

Although nitrite ions (NO_2^-) are the main antimicrobial agents in cured meats, the other salts present also help because they dissolve in the meat fluids to form a concentrated solution in which microbes cannot flourish. The dissolved salts 'capture' some of the water molecules so making them unavailable to microorganisms. The apparent water content (as far as the microorganism is concerned) is lower than the actual water content. The amount available is expressed as the water activity, a_w, of a sample of food. Water itself has an a_w value of 1.00 and a saturated salt solution an a_w value of 0.75. The water activity of some foods is given in Table 18.1.

Bacteria flourish best on food with a high a_w value, provided of course, that other conditions are also favourable. Many bacteria will not grow below an a_w value of 0.95 and an a_w value of 0.91 is the lowest water activity level tolerable by normal bacteria. Yeasts and moulds can tolerate much lower a_w values than bacteria. The minimum a_w figures tolerable by normal yeasts and moulds are 0.88 and 0.80, respectively.

Smoking is another ancient technique of chemical food preservation. Originally, smoke from an open fire was probably used but smoking was later carried out by hanging meat or fish (usually heavily salted) above smouldering wood chips in smoke houses. Traditionally smoked food has an outer layer consisting of condensed tars, phenols and aldehydes, which have a powerful antimicrobial effect as well as a characteristic taste. The preservative effect is more or less limited to the surface of the food, but spoilage of the interior is delayed because the outer layer acts as a bactericidal skin. Smoking is now used mainly to give flavour and colour to meat and fish and its preservative effect is of secondary importance.

Smoke contains many organic compounds and over 200 components have been identified. Among them are polycyclic hydrocarbons which are known to be carcinogenic. It is possible, therefore, that eating large amounts of traditionally smoked food over a long period could be harmful. As a precautionary measure smoke substitutes are now often used in place of real smoke. The smoke substitutes (known, somewhat improbably, as 'liquid smoke') are made by condensing the volatile substances present in smoke and separating the water-soluble components from the non-soluble carcinogenic polycyclic hydrocarbons.

Genuinely smoked foods have a brown smoky appearance as well as a smokey taste, although the colour of well-smoked food is lighter than many consumers expect. 'Counterfeit' smoked food is often dyed to give the impression of thorough smoking. Kippers, for example, may be dyed with the permitted colour Brown FK (E154) – literally Brown For Kippers! Given the choice, most people would prefer their food undyed.

Use of permitted preservatives

Historically, many toxic substances have been used as food preservatives. Borates, fluorides and various phenols have all been used, but over the course of time it became apparent that their efficiency in killing microorganisms was coupled with considerable toxicity to man. However, this did not deter unscrupulous individuals from using them, often in injurious amounts. Preservatives were often used to mitigate the effect of unhygienic practices in the production and distribution of food. Milk, for example, remains fresh for comparatively long periods if first treated with formalin and this practice was once prevalent. Formalin is an aqueous solution of formaldehyde; it is extremely toxic and is widely used for preserving zoological specimens. The addition of any preservative to milk is now forbidden.

In the UK the use of chemicals to preserve food is strictly controlled by the The Miscellaneous Food Additives Regulations (1995). In these regulations the word preservative means 'any substance which prolongs the shelf-life of a food by protecting it against deterioration caused by micro-organisms'. The regulations list the conditionally permitted preservatives

Table 18.1 Water content and water activity (a_w) of some foodstuffs

	Water content (%)	Typical a_w value
Uncooked meat	55–60	0.98
Bread	38–40	0.95
Cheese (Cheddar)	35–40	0.97
Jam	33–35	0.88
Cured meat	30–35	0.83
Honey	20–23	0.75
Dried fruit	18–20	0.76
Flour	14–16	0.75

antioxidants, and the foods in which they may be used and specifies the maximum permissible amount of preservative which may be present.

Most of the traditional preservatives such as salt, sugar and vinegar are not included in this list and hence, from a legal point of view, are not regarded as preservatives at all.

Permitted preservatives and examples of the foods in which they may be used are listed in Table 18.2. Each permitted preservative is identified by a serial number which may be used in place of the full name on food labels. The serial numbers are in the 200s and if the preservative is approved for use throughout the European Union the number is preceded by an E. Although there are 35 permitted preservatives many of them are actually alternative forms of a smaller number of 'parent' compounds.

Sorbic acid and its salts (E200–E203) are inhibitors of mould and yeast growth. The acid is used in soft drinks and yoghurt and the salts mainly in pastry-type products. Sorbic acid is a non-toxic unsaturated acid and it is probably dealt with by the body in the same way as naturally occurring unsaturated fatty acids.

$$CH_3—CH=CH—CH=CH—COOH$$
Sorbic acid

Benzoic acid, C_6H_5COOH, is the parent compound of another group of widely used permitted

Table 18.2 Permitted preservatives

Number	Name	Examples of use
E200	Sorbic acid	Low fat spreads, fruit yoghurt, processed cheese
E202	Potassium sorbate	Fruit-flavoured soft drinks
E203	Calcium sorbate	Soft drinks
E210	Benzoic acid	Fruit-flavoured soft drinks
E211	Sodium benzoate	Soft drinks
E212	Potassium benzoate	
E213	Calcium benzoate	
E214	Ethyl p-hydroxybenzoate	
E215	Sodium ethyl p-hydroxybenzoate	
E216	Propyl p-hydroxybenzoate	
E217	Sodium propyl p-hydroxybenzoate	
E218	Methyl p-hydroxybenzoate	
E219	Sodium methyl p-hydroxybenzoate	
E220	Sulphur dioxide	Dried fruit, dehydrated vegetables,
E221	Sodium sulphite	fruit juices and syrups, sausages
E222	Sodium hydrogen sulphite	fruit-based dairy products, cider,
E223	Sodium metabisulphite	Fruit flavoured soft drinks
E224	Potassium metabisulphite	
E226	Calcium sulphite	
E227	Calcium hydrogen sulphite	
E230	Diphenyl	Surface treatment of citrus fruits
E231	2-Hydroxydiphenyl	
E232	Sodium 2-phenylphenate	
E234	Nisin	Cheese, clotted cream
E249	Potassium nitrite	Bacon, ham, cured meats,
E250	Sodium nitrite	corned beef and some cheeses
E251	Potassium nitrate	
E252	Sodium nitrate	
E280	Propionic acid	Bread and flour, confectionery,
E281	Sodium propionate	Christmas pudding
E282	Calcium propionate	
E283	Potassium propionate	

preservatives comprising the acid itself, its salts and esters and the salts and esters of *p*-hydroxybenzoic acid (E210–E219).

Benzoic acid   Methyl 4-hydroxybenzoate

Benzoic acid is present naturally in some foods. In the body it combines with the amino acid glycine and is excreted as hippuric acid.

$$C_6H_5COOH + H_2NCH_2COOH \rightarrow$$
Benzoic acid   Glycine

$$C_6H_5CONHCH_2COOH$$
Hippuric acid

The derivatives of benzoic acid are metabolized in the same way.

Sulphur dioxide and sulphites (E220–E227) are among the most widely used preservatives. Sulphur dioxide itself, SO_2, is a gas which has been used since antiquity to prevent the growth of unwanted organisms in wine. The free gas is now rarely used as a food preservative because its salts – sulphites, hydrogen sulphites and metabisulphites – are more convenient and equally effective. Unfortunately, sulphur dioxide and sulphites have a disagreeable taste and an after-taste that can be detected at very low concentrations by some people. When sulphites are used in foods which are to be boiled or cooked in some other way, however, most of the sulphur dioxide is driven off and so after-taste does not present a problem. Another disadvantage of sulphites is the fact that they rapidly destroy thiamin. Peeled potatoes kept in a sulphite solution (to prevent browning) lose a considerable part of their thiamin content.

Diphenyl and its derivatives (E230–E232) and thiabendazole (E233) are used to prevent moulds and other imperfections developing on the peel of citrus fruits and bananas.

Diphenyl   *o*-hydroxydiphenyl

Nisin (E234) is the only antibiotic which may be used as a food preservative. It is produced by certain strains of the organism *Streptococcus lactis* and it occurs naturally in milk and Cheshire and Cheddar cheeses. Its presence makes these cheeses relatively immune to spoilage by gas-forming bacteria. These bacteria, which are mainly *Clostridia*, cause blow-holes and sometimes cracks to appear in cheeses. Nisin is effective against a very limited range of organisms. It is not effective against gram-negative organisms, moulds or yeasts but only against certain species of gram-positive organisms. For this reason it is not suitable as a general-purpose food preservative but is attractive as a 'mopping-up' preservative for heat-processed foods, such as canned foods, as heat-resistant spores are found only among the gram-positive bacteria.

There are no medical uses for nisin and there is no danger that if bacteria develop a resistance to it they will also be resistant to other antibiotics. Nisin is a polypeptide and when eaten it is digested and absorbed without ill-effect in the same way as other polypeptides.

Nisin is also used as a preservative for cheese and clotted cream. As it is harmless to man no maximum permitted quantity is specified. This would, in any case, be difficult to establish because of the variable amounts which may be present through natural causes. The quantity of nisin required to prevent clostridial spoilage is about 2–3 ppm. Nisin prevents the development of bacterial spores; it does not kill them.

The use of *sodium and potassium nitrite/nitrate* (E249–E252) for curing meat has already been discussed (see p. 274). They are also used in some cheeses.

Nitrites inhibit the growth of *Clostridium botulinum* bacteria which are responsible for the deadly form of food poisoning known as botulism. Without the use of nitrite many canned meats, especially large cans where heat processing on its own would be less effective in killing the extremely heat resistant *C. botulinum* spores, would be less safe to eat.

Unfortunately, nitrites in food may be partly converted to nitrosamines through reaction with amino compounds. Nitrosamines have been shown to cause cancer when fed to animals but the amounts used in these feeding experiments were much greater than those likely to be consumed when cured meats are eaten. Nevertheless, as a precautionary measure, the addition of nitrates or nitrites to food made for babies or young children is now prohibited.

The use of nitrites and nitrates in foods as preservatives is a subject of much debate and research. It highlights the dilemma of whether or not the use of such additives is justified. On balance, considering their contribution in reducing health hazards by destroying C. botulinum, it would appear that their continued use is justified until any ill-effects of the presence of minute amounts of nitrosamines in the body are known. In reviewing the use of nitrites and nitrates in food it has been recommended that the amount of nitrite permitted in a given food should be reduced to the minimum needed to prevent the growth of C. botulinum in that food. There is no clear evidence that nitrates and nitrites in the average British diet are dangerous, but uncertainties remain.

Even if the use of nitrates and nitrites as preservatives were no longer to be permitted we should still consume small quantities. Nitrates are widely used as agricultural fertilizers and find their way into our water supplies and vegetables. It has been estimated that the average person in the UK eats about 60 mg of nitrate per day and gets about another 10 mg from water. Vegetables are the main source in the diet, accounting for about 75 per cent of the total intake. They contain inhibitors to the formation of nitrosamines, however, and so their nitrate content may not be a problem. Beer brewed with water in which nitrate levels are high may be the major source of nitrate in the diet of 'heavy' beer drinkers.

Propionic acid, CH_3CH_2COOH, and its salts (E280–E283) are used in bread and other baked flour products as mould suppressants. Some bakers (perhaps bread manufacturers would be a more accurate term) use acetic acid, CH_3COOH, in the form of vinegar as an anti-mould agent rather than the more effective propionic acid. Vinegar is a 'traditional' preservative – not a permitted preservative – and hence it is not associated on the label with one of the E numbers which consumers unjustly regard with suspicion.

Antioxidants

The preservatives discussed above prevent or reduce attack by microorganisms, but they do not prevent deterioration of food through oxidation. Fatty foods and foods such as cakes and biscuits, which contain fat, are particularly prone to this type of spoilage and become rancid or 'tallowy' on keeping. The rancidity is caused by oxidation of the unsaturated fatty acid radicals in the triglycerides of which fat is composed. Fat-soluble vitamins are also destroyed by oxidation.

Antioxidants, which occur naturally in fats, tend to prevent the oxidative changes that produce rancidity. Chief among these is vitamin E, which is found widely distributed in vegetable oil-bearing tissues and to a lesser extent in animal tissues. These natural antioxidants, however, are usually not present in sufficient amounts to prevent completely oxidative changes which occur when food is stored and so antioxidants which are, in effect, preservatives with a special function, may be added.

Table 18.3 gives details of the antioxidants permitted in Britain and examples of the foods in which they may be used. The E numbers for antioxidants are in the 300s.

Dehydration

Microorganisms require water in order to grow and reproduce; preservation by dehydration makes use of this fact. The water content of the food is reduced to below a certain critical value (which varies from food to food) and growth of microorganisms becomes impossible.

Dehydration is a time-honoured method of preserving food. Sun-drying of fish and meat was practised as long ago as 2000 BC; dried vegetables have been sold for about a century and dried soups for much longer. A cake of 'portable soup', believed to have formed part of Captain Cook's provisions for his voyage round the world in 1772, is still in existence. It resembles a cake of glue and chemical analysis has shown that it has changed little in composition with the passage of years.

Dried fruits have been produced for many years by drying in the sun, but such unsophisticated techniques are not suitable for the dehydration of most other types of food. In modern practice, many types of equipment are used for dehydrating food. Drying is usually accomplished by passing air of carefully regulated temperature and humidity over or

Table 18.3 Permitted antioxidants

Number	Name	Examples of use
E300	L-ascorbic acid	Fruit drinks; also used to improve flour and bread dough
E301	Sodium L-ascorbate	
E302	Calcium L-ascorbate	
E304	L-ascorbyl palmitate	Chicken stock cubes
E306	Tocopherol-rich extract	Vegetable oils
E307	Synthetic α-tocopherol	Cereal-based baby foods
E308	Synthetic γ-tocopherol	
E309	Synthetic δ-tocopherol	
E310	Propyl gallate	Stock cubes, chewing gum
E311	Octyl gallate	
E312	Dodecyl gallate	
E315	Erythorbic acid	
E316	Sodium erythorbic acid	
E320	Butylated hydroxy anisole (BHA)	Stock cubes, cheese spread
E321	Butylated hydroxy toluene (BHT)	Chewing gum
E322	Lecithins	Low-fat spreads; as an emulsifier in chocolate

through the food in tray dryers, tunnel type dryers, rotating drum dryers or on a fluidized bed. Heated vacuum dryers are also used; the temperature necessary for dehydration under reduced pressure is much lower than that which would be required at ordinary pressures. In vacuum-drying, the atmosphere above the food contains a much lower concentration of oxygen than in the normal methods of drying and this reduces the extent to which oxidative changes occur. In spray-drying, a fine dispersion of preconcentrated food (e.g. milk) is sprayed into heated air in a large drying chamber and rapid drying takes place because of the large surface area of the droplets.

A modern development of vacuum-drying is freeze-drying in which frozen food is dried under high vacuum. It may seem surprising that frozen food can be dried at all but it is common knowledge that frozen puddles gradually 'dry out' in winter time and that washing will dry slowly on a clothes line even though it is frozen stiff. This is an example of sublimation – the ice becomes converted to water vapour without passing through the liquid phase. Drying by this method is very slow at normal pressures but it is speeded up tremendously in accelerated freeze drying (AFD) by reducing the pressure at which sublimation occurs and by supplying heat to provide the latent heat of sublimation of the ice. The rate of input of heat is carefully

controlled, so that the temperature of the food does not rise above freezing point.

Freeze-drying is particularly attractive for drying heat-sensitive foods. Dehydration occurs without discoloration and sensitive nutrients such as vitamins remain unharmed. In most methods of dehydration, the food has to be sliced or minced to present the maximum possible surface area to the hot air current which carries away the moisture. Large pieces of food, such as complete steaks, can be freeze-dried, however, and this is a great advantage. As ice at the surface of the food sublimes during freeze-drying the drying front recedes into the food until all the water has been abstracted. The highly porous product contains only a few per cent of water and it can be stored for long periods in moisture-proof packs at normal temperatures. Freeze-dried food can be rapidly rehydrated, by adding cold water, and the product closely resembles the starting material.

Freeze-drying is a relatively slow process and one that requires expensive equipment; freeze-dried products are therefore more expensive than foods dried by more conventional means.

Before vegetables are dehydrated, whether by freeze-drying or other methods, they are scalded or 'blanched' by immersion in boiling water or by treatment with steam. This inactivates oxidative enzymes such as catalase, phenolase and ascorbic acid oxidase and improves the stability of the dehydrated product. With coloured vegetables, blanching also improves the colour of the product. Some loss of water-soluble vitamins occurs during water-blanching, but this can be minimized by allowing the concentration of water-soluble substances in the blanching water to build up. Losses due to solution of water-soluble substances are much less with steam-blanching than with water-blanching. Blanching also destroys a large proportion of microorganisms present. For example, the microbial count is reduced by a factor of 2000 for peas and over 40 000 for potatoes.

It is not necessary to remove all the water from food in order to prevent the multiplication of microorganisms. Bacteria will not multiply in food with a water activity a_w (see p. 275) below 0.91. The minimum a_w level tolerable by most yeasts and moulds is 0.88 and 0.80, respectively. Most dehydrated foods contain less than 25 per cent water and have a water activity below 0.6. Freeze-dried foods contain practically no moisture.

Multiplication of microorganisms should not occur in properly processed, dehydrated food, but they are not immune to other types of food spoilage. Those containing fats are prone to develop rancidity after a period, particularly if the water content is reduced to too low a figure. This is true of potatoes but for non-fatty vegetables, such as cabbage, as much water as possible should be removed, because this helps to conserve ascorbic acid. The storage life of dehydrated food is much increased, and the loss of vitamin A and ascorbic acid much decreased, in the absence of oxygen. By completely filling the container with compressed dehydrated food the amount of oxygen can be reduced to a minimum. Replacement of the air in the container with nitrogen is more preferable: most dehydrated foods can be stored for 2 years or more in sealed tins in which the air has been replaced by nitrogen.

One of the great advantages of dehydrated foods is that they occupy very little space. Dehydrated potato in powder form, for example, has a volume only 10 per cent that of ordinary potatoes.

Refrigeration and freezing

Microorganisms do not multiply nearly as rapidly at low temperatures as at normal temperatures. This is taken advantage of in the domestic refrigerator which is used for keeping foods for short periods. The temperature in such a refrigerator is usually about 5°C, which is sufficient to chill the food and reduce the activity of microorganisms, but insufficient to give a long storage life. This is because microorganisms are not killed and can still grow and reproduce but at a much slower rate. Moreover, enzyme action continues, although at a reduced rate, leading to chemical changes in the food and loss in quality.

Commercial refrigeration or chilling is applied to many foods, including meat, eggs, fruit and vegetables. When meat is chilled, the temperature is reduced to about −1°C and it can remain in good condition for up to a month.

For large-scale use, chilling can be advantageously combined with gas storage, that is, storage in an atmosphere that has been enriched in carbon dioxide. This process is called modified- or controlled-atmosphere storage (MAS and CAS). Microbes produce carbon dioxide by their own respiration as well as the respiratory activity of fresh fruits and vegetables, and addition of this gas to the atmosphere surrounding them retards their growth. In CAS, the levels of gas are carefully monitored and controlled and this is used for storage of fruit where complete deprivation of oxygen is likely to lead to anaerobic respiration and risk the production of alcoholic off-flavours. In MAS, the atmosphere changes as oxygen is used up and carbon dioxide is produced. In modified atmosphere packaging (MAP), the food is packed in an atmosphere other than air. For example the shelf-life of fresh meat is extended from 3 to 7 days at 0–2°C by packaging in an 80 per cent O_2/20 per cent CO_2 atmosphere. The oxygen helps to maintain the red colour of the meat. Higher concentrations of carbon dioxide would be even more effective, but they are not used because they cause the meat to become brown, owing to the conversion of the haemoglobin to methaemoglobin. However, they can be used for pork, poultry and cooked meats which do not need the oxygen to maintain the colour.

Although chilling to about 5°C enables food to be stored for short periods it must be frozen and stored at a low temperature if long-term storage is required. Microorganisms, which are the main spoilage agents, become inactive at about −10°C while enzymes, which cause chemical spoilage and consequent loss of quality, are largely inactivated below −18°C. Domestic freezers store food at about −18°C, but a temperature of −29°C is employed commercially to ensure high quality and a long storage life.

Most fresh foods contain at least 60 per cent water, some of which, known as bound water, is tightly attached to the constituent cells, the rest, known as available or freezable water, being mobile. On average, plant cells contain 6 per cent bound water and animal cells 12 per cent. Available water does not freeze at 0°C because of the solids dissolved in it which lower the freezing point. For example, at −5°C, 64 per cent of the water in peas is frozen, at −15°C, 86 per cent is frozen while at −30°C, 92 per cent (virtually all the available water) is frozen.

The rate at which foods are frozen is important. Good quality is only retained if freezing is quick, usually defined as meaning that the temperature at the thermal centre of the food pack should pass through the freezing zone, 0–4°C, within 30 minutes. It is within this temperature range that most of the available water is frozen and most heat (latent heat of freezing) must be removed.

The way that freezing rate affects quality can be appreciated from Fig. 18.1. Plant cells have relatively large vacuoles which contain most of the available water. During fast freezing tiny ice crystals are formed within the vacuoles and, because they have little time to grow, they do not distort the cellular structure. However, if freezing is slow, crystals start to form in the intercellular spaces outside the cell walls and as they grow they draw water from within the cells leaving the cells dehydrated and distorted. Some ice crystals may also be formed within the vacuoles. The process in animal cells – which have smaller vacuoles and which contain less water – is broadly similar.

If food is immersed in liquid nitrogen (boiling point −196°C), or if it is sprayed with liquid nitrogen, the liquid nitrogen boils as a result of rapid heat transfer from the food. Nearly instantaneous freezing occurs and the food retains its original shape and appearance. This technique, known as cryogenic freezing, or immersion freezing, is relatively expensive but it is useful for high-cost products.

Loss of nutritional value on freezing and subsequent storage is small, but some losses do occur in the preliminary preparation of fruit and vegetables and during the storage of most frozen food.

In good commercial practice, there is little delay between harvesting vegetables and freezing and, consequently, nutritional loss is insignificant. Vegetables, and some fruits such as apples, are blanched with boiling water or steam before freezing to destroy enzymes and some microorganisms. This causes some loss of water-soluble vitamins, mainly ascorbic acid and, to a lesser extent, thiamin. The actual loss will depend on the way blanching is carried out but, overall, blanching conserves ascorbic acid by reducing the final cooking time required and by inactivating ascorbic acid oxidase, thus reducing loss of ascorbic acid on storage.

After freezing, foods are usually stored at −18°C in home freezers or at −29°C commercially. At these low temperatures there is a very slow and gradual loss of quality but little loss in nutritional value. Ascorbic acid is lost only very slowly on storage. If the temperature rises above −18°C, food starts to deteriorate more rapidly. It is a legal requirement in the UK that all frozen food be kept below −18°C throughout the food distribution chain from manufacturer to purchaser.

When frozen foods are thawed there is often some loss of liquid – known as drip – which causes loss of

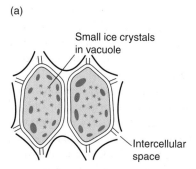

(a)

Small ice crystals in vacuole

Intercellular space

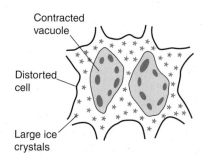

(b)

Contracted vacuole

Distorted cell

Large ice crystals

Figure 18.1 *Plant cells: (a) after quick freezing; (b) after slow freezing*

soluble nutrients from the food. The extent to which drip occurs depends on the rate at which freezing is carried out, the duration and temperature of storage and the cellular nature of food. Plant material is more liable to drip than animal food because plant cells have larger vacuoles containing more available water (Fig. 18.1) and consequently suffer greater distortion on slow freezing. Fruit, particularly soft fruit such as strawberries, may suffer extensive drip and consequent loss of vitamin C on thawing. (Thawing of vegetables may also cause some loss of vitamin C and they are best cooked without thawing.) Soft fruits also suffer partial collapse of their cell structure on thawing, which makes them mushy. When frozen meat is thawed, there may be considerable loss of soluble nutrients, including protein and B vitamins. However, loss of nutrients in drip may be avoided if the drip from meat is incorporated in gravy and the liquid (often syrup) from fruit is eaten.

In conclusion, it may be said that nutritional loss in food that has been properly frozen and stored is very small, and its nutritional value may well be superior to that of equivalent 'fresh' food which may have suffered a delay of several days between harvesting and consumption.

Preservation by heating

Canning

Canning, which is the principal method by which foods are preserved by heat treatment, developed from bottling and, in essence, both processes are the same. The principle is delightfully simple – the food is sealed in a can which is then heated to such a temperature that all harmful microorganisms and spores capable of growth during storage of the can at normal temperatures are killed. As no microorganisms can gain access to food while the can remains sealed, decomposition does not occur.

Almost any type of food may be canned and its nature largely determines which pre-canning operations are carried out. Food is first cleaned and inedible parts such as fruit stones, peel or bones are removed as far as possible. Fruit and vegetables may be subjected to a preliminary blanching before canning in order to soften them and enable a larger quantity to be pressed into the tin without damage. With vegetables, blanching also serves to displace air

and causes a certain amount of shrinkage. The food is placed in the can which is then filled to within about half an inch of the top with liquor (usually sugar syrup in the case of fruits or brine in the case of vegetables). The lid is then placed loosely in position and the can and its contents are heated to about 95°C by hot water or steam. This process, known as 'exhausting', causes the air in the headspace of the can to expand and displaces any remaining air from the fruit or vegetable tissues. Exhausting also reduces strain on the can during subsequent heat treatment. It also substantially reduces the amount of oxygen in the headspace and so minimizes internal corrosion of the can and oxidation of nutrients, particularly ascorbic acid, after sealing. The can is sealed when exhausting is complete and it is then ready for heat sterilization or 'processing' as it is called.

Most canned food is processed in batch-type cookers or retorts which are large-scale, steam-heated versions of the domestic pressure cooker. The temperature of processing is controlled by adjusting the pressure at which the equipment operates.

Continuous retorts where the cans are conveyed through the heating system and pressure is more gradually increased, permit close control over the heating process and gradual changes of pressure inside the can. These can be combined with computer controls. Different types include cooker-coolers, rotary sterilizers (which allow content of the cans to be mixed as they travel along a helix) and hydrostatic sterilizers. The continuous process is completed when the cans enter the cooling process. A great deal of work has been carried out to determine the optimum conditions for processing canned foods. Over-processing has an adverse effect on quality and it is desirable to reduce the time and temperature of processing as much as possible. Processing conditions must be severe enough, however, to ensure that all harmful microorganisms in the canned food are destroyed or inactivated. Bacterial spores are easily killed by heating in acid conditions, and the temperatures at which fruits are processed are not as high as those used for vegetables and meat.

Canned vegetables and meat are usually processed at 115°C, whereas fruits may be processed in boiling water. The size of the can and the physical nature of the food it contains are other factors that influence the amount of heat processing needed because they both affect the rate of heat penetration. If a liquid is present, heat is distributed to all parts of the can by convection currents. Conversely, with solid foods the rate of heat penetration is slower and the time of heating must be correspondingly greater. Processing times for non-solid foods can be reduced by up to two-thirds by agitating the contents of the can, as this assists heat penetration.

Ultra-high temperature (UHT)/aseptic canning By substantially increasing the temperature at which it is carried out, it is possible to reduce considerably the duration of heat processing: in theory, if very high temperatures could be used, processing times could be very short indeed. In practice, however, the rate at which heat penetrates to the centre of the food in a can imposes a limitation on such high-temperature short-time (HTST) processes and so they can only be used for processing food before canning Sterilization is carried out at about 120–140°C in special equipment designed to achieve a high rate of heat transfer. The food is then cooled somewhat before sealing into cans or the familiar flexible rectangular packages which have been previously sterilized with superheated steam. This procedure, known as aseptic canning, can be used only for liquid or semi-solid foods where a high rate of heat transfer to a thin film of the food is possible. The heating time varies from 6 seconds to about 6 minutes depending upon the type of food being canned.

An advantage of HTST processes is that since the food is cooked in thin layers there is less likelihood of some of it being over-processed to ensure that all of it is adequately processed. This, of course, is the situation with normal 'in-can' processing. Another advantage is that large cans, convenient for large-scale catering, can be used because there are no problems about heat penetration to the centre of the can.

Heat resistance of microorganisms Bacteria, moulds and yeasts are rapidly killed by the temperatures used in canning foods (see p. 271). Bacterial spores, however, can be very resistant to high temperatures. The death of bacterial spores in heat-treated food follows a logarithmic course in which equal proportions of surviving cells die in each successive unit of time. Thus, if 10 000 spores per unit volume were initially present and 9000 were killed by exposure to a particular temperature for 1 minute, 900 would be killed in the second minute, 90 in the third minute, nine in

the fourth minute and so on. One thousand times as many spores would be killed during the first minute's exposure as during the fourth.

The heat resistance of a particular microorganism can be expressed in terms of its thermal death time (TDT) at a particular temperature. The TDT, or F-value, is the time required to achieve a specific reduction in microbial numbers at a given temperature.

Conditions drastic enough to kill the spores of the organism C. *botulinum*, which are heat-resistant above pH 4.5, and particularly dangerous (see p. 291), will also kill all other harmful organisms. The heat-resistance of these spores forms a standard of comparison against which the efficiency of a heat treatment process can be judged. Such a process is referred to as a minimum safe process or, less formally, as a 'botulinum cook'. It can be calculated that a preparation of C. *botulinum* is killed by exposure to 121°C for 2.78 minutes.

A few viable microorganisms may remain in canned food but they are unobjectionable and, in normal circumstances, will not cause spoilage. Spores are unable to develop in acid foods and the processing given to fruits is designed primarily to kill moulds, yeasts and non-sporing bacteria, the presence of bacterial spores being quite acceptable. In 'non-acid' foods only highly resistant thermophiles will survive the high processing temperatures and under normal storage conditions they will be unable to develop.

Canned food cannot really be said to be sterile but it is as sterile as it need be – a condition euphemistically described as 'commercial sterility'.

Nutritive value of canned foods Some nutrient loss occurs during heat processing of canned foods and more thiamin may be lost from meat during processing than would be lost during normal cooking. Reduction in ascorbic acid content also occurs during processing, but much more disappears during the first few weeks of storage as a result of oxidation by the small amount of oxygen remaining in the headspace of the can. Losses can be as much as 80 per cent. Water-soluble nutrients may become dissolved in the canning liquid, which is usually thrown away.

Spoilage of canned foods Properly canned food remains edible for very long periods if the cans are not corroded. In 1958, a number of cans that had been sealed for many years were examined. A tin of plum-pudding prepared in 1900 was opened and the contents were found to be in excellent condition. The meat in two cans sealed in 1823 and 1849 was found to be free from bacterial spoilage but the fat was partially hydrolysed into glycerol and fatty acids. The contents of a number of cans taken to the Antarctic by Shackleton in 1908 and Scott in 1910, and brought back to this country in 1958, were found, with some exceptions, to be in good condition.

When spoilage of canned foods occurs it is commonly caused by a defect in the can. Spoilage may also arise from inadequate heat treatment which is insufficient to kill all the microorganisms present in the food. Certain heat-resistant bacterial spores produce acids when they germinate in foods and if this happens a flat sour results. No gas is produced and the spoilage is not evident until the can is opened and the unwholesome smell of the contents becomes evident. The organism particularly responsible for flat sours is *Bacillus stearothermophilus*, the spores of which are able to survive exposure to 120°C for 20 minutes. Non-acid foods, such as peas, are most likely to be affected. The organism finds its way to the food via infected equipment or ingredients such as sugar or flour, and spoilage of this type may be an indication of low standards of hygiene at the canning plant.

Another type of spoilage to which canned foods are prone is the hydrogen swell or hard swell. This is caused by heat-resistant bacteria such as *Clostridium thermosaccharolyticum* which produce hydrogen gas as they grow in the canned food. The ends of the can may bulge, as a result of increased pressure, to produce what is known as a blown can.

Improperly canned food sometimes smells offensively of bad eggs and may be very dark in colour. This is an example of sulphide spoilage (or, in more descriptive American parlance, a sulphide stinker!) and is caused by the presence in the can of *Clostridium nigrificans*. This organism produces hydrogen sulphide gas which is responsible for the foul smell. Not enough gas is produced to cause distortion of the can. Spoilage of this type is not common in the UK.

The three types of spoilage organism mentioned above are not harmful, but they make the canned food unpalatable. The fact that these organisms have survived the heat treatment process, however, indicates that the food has been inadequately heat treated and there is the possibility that more harmful organisms such as *C. botulinum* may also be present. Spoiled canned food should never be eaten.

Canned foods should be stored in dry, fairly cool conditions because storage at higher temperature will encourage the growth of any thermophiles that have survived heat processing. Cans stored in damp conditions may become rusty and, in time, penetration of the can and spoilage of the contents may occur.

Food preservation by irradiation

Food irradiation is a processing technique that exposes food to electron beams, X-rays or gamma rays. It produces a similar effect to pasteurization, cooking or other forms of heat treatment, but with less effect on look and texture.

Cobalt-60 and caesium-137 are two radioactive isotopes available as byproducts of the nuclear power industry. Both emit γ-rays with sufficient energy to kill all the microorganisms found in food, but not of such high energy that the irradiated food is itself made radioactive. Only one source of ionizing radiation is permitted for food irradiation in the UK and that is γ-rays from cobalt-60.

The unit of radiation dose is the gray (Gy). One gray is the dose of radiation received by 1 kg of matter when it absorbs 1 J of radiation energy.

γ-Rays are able to penetrate food (or any other substance, for that matter) to a considerable depth. Consequently, food can be processed in bulk or in packages made of any material and of any size without fear that the innermost parts will not be properly processed. The food is carried past the radioisotope on a conveyor and after a very brief exposure the process is complete.

Three levels of radiation treatment, known in order of severity as radurization, radicidation and radappertization, are used for extending the storage life of food.

1 *Radurization* (low doses – below 1 kGy)
   - Inhibits sprouting of vegetables such as onions and potatoes.
   - Retards ripening of fruit.
   - Kills insects in grain, rice and spices.

2 *Radicidation* (moderate doses – 1–10 kGy)
   - Kills most microorganisms and so extends storage life and reduces risk of food poisoning.

- Kills parasites in meat (e.g. larvae of *Trichina spiralis* which cause trichinosis).

3 *Radappertization* (high doses – above 10 kGy)
- Completely sterilizes food by killing all micro-organisms. Irradiation equivalent of canning: a dose of about 50 kGy is required.

As well as inhibiting sprouting and ripening, and killing pests and microorganisms, irradiation causes minor chemical changes. Some large molecules, such as those of carbohydrates or proteins, may be split and some destruction of vitamins may also occur. New compounds – called radiolytic products – may be formed, but they will be present to only a very minor extent (perhaps one or two parts per million). Nevertheless, it is possible that they might be carcinogenic or be harmful in other ways. Even such minor changes in the composition of a food can affect its flavour and texture. Irradiated meats, for example, have been said by some to have a 'goaty' flavour or, more vividly, a 'wet dog' taste. Vegetables may become soft and spongy after drastic irradiation owing to partial breakdown of their cellulose cell walls.

All the information currently available about the safety of irradiated food has been exhaustively examined by the Food Standards Agency. They state that it is a safe processing technique for herbs and spices and undertake safety inspections of the only irradiation facility in the UK. The agency also carries out regular surveys to ensure that products are correctly labeled. In the UK, food may only be irradiated under licence and only correctly labelled irradiated herbs, spices or vegetable seasonings are permitted. It can be concluded that irradiation is not an important method of food preservation in the UK.

Key points

- Food spoiling or decay can be the result of chemical contamination or microbial invasion, as well as by endogenous enzymes
- Higher temperatures and exposure to oxygen tend to accelerate food spoiling
- Preservation methods include drying, irradiating, cooking or blanching and canning, chilling or freezing, and chemical preservation with salts or organic compounds to inhibit bacterial growth

Chapter summary

Modern food manufacture and distribution, together with moves from daily to weekly shopping, have generated new demands for food preservation. To this can be added increased awareness of the risks and legal consequences, of food poisoning. Permitted chemical preservatives are regulated by European legislation.

FURTHER READING

FELLOWS PJ (2000). *Food Processing Technology: Principles and Practice*. 2nd edn. Cambridge: Woodhead Publishing Limited.

Irradiated Foods from http://www.food.gov.uk/safereating/foodadvice/irradfoodqa/?version=1

19

Toxins, food-borne infections and food hygiene

FOOD TOXINS

A surprising number of foods in their natural state contain toxic substances in small amounts which can cause symptoms if consumed in sufficient quantity. The presence of solanine in green potatoes, oxalates in rhubarb and spinach, have already been referred to. There are numerous other examples and Table 19.1 shows some of the toxins present in common foods.

Just as the body is able to deal with regular but small amounts of caffeine or ethyl alcohol, so can it deal with small amounts of the other toxins listed in Table 19.1. When one food is eaten to excess, however, even substances normally regarded as nutrients can be toxic and at least one death has occurred through retinol (vitamin A) poisoning. Admittedly, this is a rather extreme example as the person concerned, a health-food enthusiast, had drunk a gallon of carrot juice daily for 10 days. It is recorded that retinol poisoning has also been caused by eating large amounts of polar bear liver, though this is hardly likely to be a problem in the UK. There are, however, vulnerable stages of life, so eating liver of any kind must be restricted in pregnancy, because doses of retinol not toxic to a woman may harm a fetus.

The toxic substances listed in Table 19.1 usually cause little trouble and the term 'food poisoning' is normally used to refer to illness caused by eating food that has been contaminated by bacteria or, less commonly, viruses or moulds.

Bacterial gastroenteritis

Gastroenteritis with diarrhoea, often with nausea, vomiting and fevers, may occur if food containing pathogenic bacteria or toxins produced by them is eaten. This is the most common type of food poisoning and it is caused by the presence in food of harmful bacteria or poisonous substances produced by them. The general term 'food poisoning', which is used in this chapter refers, more specifically, to bacterial food poisoning. The characteristic symptoms of food poisoning – abdominal pain and diarrhoea, usually accompanied by vomiting, and sometimes fever and general malaise – which follow from 1 to 36 hours after eating such food, will be familiar to most readers from personal experience.

An outbreak of food poisoning may be caused by food that appears to be quite wholesome despite the fact that it is heavily infected by bacteria. The organisms that cause food poisoning are quite different from those involved in food spoilage, and food that is dangerously contaminated may appear to be quite normal. Food which has 'gone off' may also be infected with pathogens, but as such food is unlikely to be eaten it is not a major cause of food poisoning.

Table 19.1 Toxins present in some foods

Food	Toxin	Effects
Almonds, lima beans, kirsch, fruit stones and seeds	Cyanogens which produce cyanides	Inhibition of respiratory system with possible fatal consequences
Nutmeg, mace, black pepper, parsley, celery seed	Myristicin	Headaches, cramps, nausea, hallucination
Green or sprouting potatoes	Solanine and chaconine	Stomach upsets, nervous effects
Rhubarb (especially leaves)	Oxalic acid	Interference with calcium absorption
Alcoholic drinks	Ethanol (ethyl alcohol)	Personality changes, vomiting, unconsciousness, subsequent 'hangover'
Cabbage and other brassicas	Goitrogens	Interference with iodine absorption by thyroid gland
Most raw beans (especially soya)	Protease inhibitors	Interference with protein digestion and absorption
Bread and other cereal products	Phytates	Complexes with iron and calcium and may interfere with their absorption
Raw red beans	Haemaglutinins	Cause red blood cells to clump together
Fungi of Amanita variety (mistaken for mushrooms)	Amanitin	Inactivates metabolic enzymes causing severe illness with possible fatal results
Some algae on shellfish	Alkaloid related to strychnine	Severe and sometimes fatal illness Paralytic or amnesic illness
Fish especially puffer fish and scombroid fish (e.g. tuna, mackerel and bonito) if not fresh	Toxins from algal commensals; various toxins derived from food eaten by fish	Severe digestive upset
Mustard	Sanguinarine	Fluid retention (dropsy)
Parsnips, celery, parsley	Psoralens	Genetic mutations
Tea, coffee, cola drinks	Caffeine	Diuretic and stimulant
Some cheeses, yeast extract, red wines	Tyramine	Increased blood pressure, migraine; Interferes with some antidepressant drugs

Harmful bacteria, or pathogens as they are called, find their way into food in a number of ways. Meat and meat products may be infected at source (i.e. they may come from animals which are themselves hosts to pathogenic bacteria). Most food-borne gastroenteritis, however, occurs as a result of unhygienic behaviour by humans coupled with inappropriate food-handling practices and this means it is preventable. The human body is itself a source of potential food poisoning organisms, which are transferred easily from mouth, nose and bowel to food. Pathogens can be 'carried' and passed on to others by individuals who are themselves not ill. Such carriers may have recently suffered previous infection and still be harbouring the organisms in their body. In some instances, carriers of gut pathogens act as 'hosts' over a period of many years, having themselves acquired an immunity to the organism concerned. They are unaware of their role as reservoirs of infection and that is a particular problem with salmonellae such as *Salmonella typhi*, which causes typhoid fever. Animals may also harbour organisms pathogenic to humans and pass them on to human beings via food with which they come into contact. Rats, mice, cockroaches and domestic pets can all be instrumental in transmitting food poisoning in this way.

We know from experience of other illnesses that contact with disease-causing microbes does not always lead to infection and this is equally true of food poisoning. Acidic conditions in the stomach and the body's natural defensive mechanisms are often able to deal with food that is not too heavily infected and so it is sometimes possible to eat food contaminated with pathogenic organisms without becoming ill. This is more likely to happen if the body has previously encountered the pathogen involved and so has been able to acquire some resistance to it. A great deal depends upon the virulence of the particular microorganism. Ingestion of a small number of some pathogens may be sufficient to cause illness, whereas a much larger number might be required to produce the same effect if a different pathogen were involved. Unfortunately, even quite small numbers of microbes can quickly grow into dangerous hordes when infected food is inappropriately stored. In almost all instances of bacterial food poisoning, the food concerned has been mishandled in such a way that bacterial growth has been encouraged.

High-risk foods

Some foods are categorized as high-risk foods because they are particularly likely to become infected with pathogens and are intended to be eaten without further cooking (which kills bacteria). Any cooked food which is in contact with a raw food (or utensils and surfaces contaminated by raw food) is likely to become infected, and storage in warm conditions promotes growth. The more important high-risk foods are:

1 Cooked meat and poultry
2 Cooked meat products (e.g. pies, gravy, soups and stock)
3 Milk, cream, custards and dairy produce, artificial cream
4 Cooked rice
5 Shellfish
6 Eggs and egg products (e.g. custards, mayonnaise).

Toxic food poisoning

Some bacteria produce toxins or poisons which they release outside their cells when they are growing and multiplying in food; these toxins are known as exotoxins. Exotoxins are not living cells; they are poisonous chemicals produced by cells. The incubation period, that is, the period of time between the entry of the poison into the body and the appearance of the first symptoms, is normally short with toxic food poisoning. The toxins produce irritation of the stomach and vomiting occurs, often within 2 hours of eating the food. Abdominal pain and

diarrhoea normally follow. This is a common time-course for staphylococcal food poisoning, commonly originating from staphylococci in nasal secretions of food handlers.

Exotoxins are less easily destroyed by heating than the bacteria from which they come. Thus, if food is lightly cooked, so only heated sufficiently to kill the bacteria, the exotoxins may survive and still cause food poisoning when the food is eaten. Food-poisoning bacteria are killed in 1–2 minutes in boiling water, whereas it may take up to 30 minutes to destroy exotoxins. Food that has been contaminated and then frozen is likely to cause illness if not completely thawed before cooking.

Infective food poisoning

This type of food poisoning (or, more correctly, food infection) is caused by eating food containing live bacteria in sufficient numbers to cause illness. Infective food poisoning bacteria produce toxins within their own cells. Such toxins – called endotoxins – are not as heat-resistant as the exotoxins referred to above and if infected food is heated to a temperature high enough to destroy the bacteria, the endotoxins are also destroyed. Food poisoning may occur if infected food is not heated to a high enough temperature during cooking or if infected food (e.g. cooked meat) is eaten without further cooking. When this happens, the live organisms containing their endotoxins enter the gut and as they die the endotoxins are released and cause illness. The incubation period for infective food poisoning is normally longer than that for toxic food poisoning because it takes time for the endotoxins to be released. The symptoms of fever, headache, diarrhoea and vomiting do not usually appear for about 12 hours. Eight important types of bacteria which cause food poisoning are listed in Table 19.2.

Salmonella Gastroenteritis caused by the *Salmonella* group of bacteria is called salmonellosis. There are many different strains of *Salmonella*, some of which take their names from the places where they were first observed. Examples are *Salmonella typhimurium*, *Salmonella enteritidis*, *Salmonella newport*, *Salmonella dublin* and *Salmonella eastbourne*. The bacteria can survive outside the body for long periods and on warm, moist food multiply rapidly. Food must be

Table 19.2 Bacterial food poisoning

Bacteria responsible	Source and foods commonly affected	Illness incubation period	Duration
Infective food poisoning			
Salmonellae, especially Salmonella typhimurium *and* Salmonella enteritidis	*Raw or inadequately cooked meat, milk, eggs, poultry. 'Carried' by pets and rodents*	6–72 hours but usually 12–30 hours	1–8 days
Listeria monocytogenes	*Pre-cooked chilled foods. Untreated dairy products*		See text
Escherichia coli	*Excreta and polluted water. Raw or inadequately cooked meat and poultry*	10–72 hours but usually 12–24 hours	1–5 days
Campylobacter jejuni	*Raw or inadequately cooked foods of animal origin, raw or inadequately heat-treated milk*	3–5 days	2–3 days
Toxic food poisoning			
Staphylococcus aureus	*Human nose, mouth, skin. Boils and cuts. Raw milk and cheeses made from raw milk*	2–6 hours	6–48 hours
Bacillus cereus	*Rice, cornflour, vegetables, dairy products*	1–6 hours (vomiting type) 8–16 hours (diarrhoeal type)	24 hours
Clostridium perfringens	*Animal and human excreta. Soil, dust. Raw or inadequately cooked meat and poultry. Gravy, stews, large joints of meat*	8–22 hours but usually 12–18 hours	12–48 hours
Clostridium botulinum	*Soil, meat, fish and vegetables. Inadequately processed canned food*	6 hours–8 days but usually 12–36 hours	Death within 7 days or slow recovery

grossly infected with a large number of live bacteria (normally over 10 0000/g) before illness occurs.

Multiplication of salmonellae can be prevented by keeping food below 5°C. Meat that has been cooked and is not to be eaten at once should be cooled quickly, so that the temperature zone in which salmonellae multiply rapidly is passed through as quickly as possible.

The foods most often infected are meat (particularly processed meats, such as pies and brawn), eggs and egg products, custard cakes, trifles and artificial cream. Poultry and other animals often act as carriers of salmonellae and eggs are a common source of infection. They may be infected with *S. enteritidis* in the chicken's oviduct before they are laid or they may be infected after laying through contamination by poultry excreta. Foods containing raw eggs

(e.g. mayonnaise or cake icing) or inadequately cooked eggs (e.g. lightly boiled or scrambled eggs, meringues and omelettes) may cause salmonellosis. For this reason, no unpasteurized liquid or frozen whole egg may be used in the preparation of food in the UK. Dried egg may also be infected with salmonellae (spray-drying does not kill it) and so it should be used as soon as it is reconstituted and must be well cooked. Food poisoning caused by *S. enteritidis* is the most common type of salmonellosis in the UK.

Rats and mice may be carriers of *S. typhimurium* and are a common source of infection, especially where it is possible for their excreta to come into contact with food. Domestic animals may also excrete salmonellae without exhibiting symptoms of food poisoning. This is one good reason for excluding dogs from food shops.

Raw meat is often infected by salmonellae and meat products, particularly if they are made from meat 'trimmings' and scraps from the outside of meat carcasses, may be heavily contaminated. Fish and poultry are also often contaminated with salmonellae and there is a particular danger of food poisoning when frozen poultry is only partly thawed before cooking, especially if undercooked. Salmonellae are easily killed and provided that cooking is thorough so that the temperature at the centre of the food is high enough (i.e. at least 65°C) all such bacteria will be destroyed.

Clostridium perfringens This bacterium, which causes toxic food poisoning, is the second most common cause of food poisoning in the UK. It is found in soil, in human and animal intestines and excreta, and on raw meat and poultry. Most people harbour the bacteria in large numbers without becoming ill. It is possible that the bacteria reproduce themselves more rapidly on warm food, and produce more poisonous toxin, than they do in the intestine. The spores of *Clostridium perfringens* are very heat resistant and remain active after boiling or slow roasting. They are able to grow readily in cooked meat that is cooled slowly or kept in a warm place. *Clostridium perfringens* can reproduce every 10 minutes at its optimum temperature of 43–47°C. It can continue to grow at temperatures of up to 50°C and, as it is an anaerobe, it grows in the absence of oxygen. These are just the conditions likely to be found at the centre of a large joint of meat cooling slowly. When infected food is eaten, the enterotoxin is released in the gut and causes food poisoning.

Gastroenteritis from *C. perfringens* may occur in large-scale catering establishments where meat is cooked some time before it is required, allowed to cool, and then reheated before serving. Large pieces of meat used in catering establishments are often tightly tied into rolls before cooking. As a result, contamination at the outer surfaces may be transferred to the interior of the piece of meat where the temperature during cooking is insufficient to kill the spores.

Clostridium perfringens does not grow below 10°C and if cooked meat cannot be eaten at once it should be quickly cooled and held below this temperature. Similarly, meat and meat dishes which have to be reheated before consumption should be heated and not warmed. The Food Hygiene (General) Regulations (1970), which lays down minimum standards of hygiene for food premises in the UK, requires that high-risk foods in catering premises be kept below 10°C or above 63°C other than in the course of preparation or when exposed for sale.

Staphylococcus aureus Food poisoning produced by this organism is caused by toxins produced by the bacteria growing in food before it is eaten. The bacteria are found in abundance in whitlows, infected burns and wounds and are commonly carried in nasal secretions, released by sneezing or transmitted by nose wiping. When the bacteria find their way onto food, via the hands of an infected person, rapid growth usually occurs with production of a toxin. If the food is eaten the toxin is rapidly absorbed and this almost always causes illness. The bacteria can be killed fairly easily by heating but the toxin is more heat resistant and is only completely destroyed by boiling for at least 30 minutes. Staphylococcal food poisoning is usually caused by eating cream-filled cakes, custard cakes or by cooked meats which have been contaminated by a food handler. Staphylococci are able to grow in higher concentrations of salt than other food-poisoning bacteria and they are often responsible for food poisoning outbreaks involving salty foods, especially meats such as ham and bacon.

Listeria monocytogenes This organism may cause the disease listeriosis if food contaminated by it is eaten. It is found in a wide range of foodstuffs and raw chickens are commonly infected with it: it may also be present in untreated milk (and dairy products made from raw milk), vegetables and seafood.

Listeria bacteria can multiply at temperatures below those found in many domestic refrigerators and commercial chilled food cabinets. They may stay dormant for several days at these temperatures and then multiply rapidly. Some pre-cooked chilled meals and chilled prepacked salads have been found to be dangerously contaminated by the organism. Cook–chill foods should not be stored for more than 5 days at 4°C and they should be eaten within 12 hours if their temperature reaches 5°C. Listeria bacteria are also fairly heat-resistant and may sometimes be present in pasteurized milk. The bacteria may survive in food which has been cooked or reheated in a microwave oven because of uneven heating in such ovens. High-risk food cooked in a microwave oven should be allowed to 'stand' for the recommended time before eating, to allow heat to diffuse from hotter areas to any cold spots.

Listeria bacteria produce a toxic enzyme which may cause serious illness if it enters the blood system. Listeriosis is especially dangerous to pregnant women and it may lead to abortion or the premature birth of a baby, itself infected with the disease. Other vulnerable classes of people may also be seriously affected by listeriosis and the very young or elderly, and those whose immune systems have been impaired by illness, are especially at risk. Despite the availability of antibiotics, the mortality rate for such classes of individuals is high.

Fortunately, listeriosis occurs relatively infrequently in the UK, but because of the danger to vulnerable groups and its relatively high fatality rate, it must be regarded as a serious food-borne illness.

Campylobacter jejuni This organism is a very common and particularly unpleasant cause of infective food poisoning; it is now the commonest cause of infective intestinal disease in the UK, with about 40 000 cases reported annually. It may be possible to develop a degree of immunity to *Campylobacter* infection and this probably explains why the disease mainly affects children and young adults. The illness it causes is often quite violent and debilitating, but deaths rarely occur. *Campylobacter* may be present in a wide range of food, particularly poultry, unpasteurized milk and untreated water. It is found in up to 50 per cent of intensively farmed chickens. It can also get into food through contamination by other infected food. *Campylobacter* can survive and multiply in the intestines and so it is possible to become ill after eating food that is not heavily infected. Attempts to reduce campylobacter infections by addressing contamination of chicken farms are hampered by the global trade in chicken meat.

Clostridium botulinum Illness through poisoning by *Clostridium botulinum* – known as botulism – is extremely serious but infections with living *C. botulinum* bacteria are very rare. The bacteria produce a toxin which is the most virulent poison known, 1 g of which would be sufficient to kill as many as 10 million people if it could be uniformly distributed. The mortality rate from botulism is about 65 per cent but, fortunately, the disease rarely occurs in the UK. *Clostridium botulinum* is found in the soil and on vegetables which have been in contact with contaminated soil. It is also found in the intestines of fish and pigs and certain other animals. Like *Clostridium perfringens*, it is a spore-forming anaerobe.

Bacillus cereus This organism produces an exotoxin when it grows on food and if contaminated food is eaten illness usually follows within 12 hours. *Bacillus cereus* requires air for growth but when conditions for growth are unfavourable it is able to form tough spores. The spores are often found in cereals, especially rice, and they are able to survive in the dry cereal for long periods. Consumption of 'take-away' fried rice contaminated by *B. cereus* is a frequent cause of food poisoning. If *B. cereus* spores are present in the uncooked rice they are able to survive the boiling process, which is often carried out in bulk before the rice is fried. Rapid growth, accompanied by exotoxin formation, occurs when the mass of warm and wet boiled rice cools slowly before being fried in smaller portions for sale. One of the exotoxins produced by *B. cereus* is not destroyed by exposure to 126°C for 90 minutes and once it is present in food, reheating is unlikely to destroy it.

In order to prevent food poisoning from *B. cereus*, cooked food should be cooled rapidly and stored in a refrigerator. If the food is reheated this should be done as quickly as possible, immediately before the food is eaten.

Food poisoning caused by *B. cereus*, especially if infected fried rice has been eaten, may have a very short incubation period followed by nausea and vomiting which can be severe and last for up to a day. Another less common type starts about 8–16 hours after contaminated food has been eaten and the main symptoms are abdominal pain and diarrhoea which may last for a day or so.

Escherichia coli This organism is a common and normally harmless inhabitant of our intestines and of the intestines of all animals. There are many subtypes or strains, however, a small number of which are pathogenic and produce illness with a range of severity. The intestinal disorder known, among other colourful names, as traveller's diarrhoea, is often caused by the presence of unfamiliar strains of *Escherichia coli* living on food eaten or in drinking water. Food poisoning by *E. coli* is usually caused by eating inadequately cooked meat or poultry or where cooked meat is contaminated by *E. coli* from raw meat.

One particular strain of *E. coli* referred to as *E. coli* 157 has attracted publicity, and indeed stimulated radical changes in the food regulatory systems intermittently. *Escherichia coli* 157 is a relatively unusual strain which appears to have emerged as a result of mutations among the *E. coli* living in the bowels of cattle in the 1990s. It has caused outbreaks of severe food poisoning with systematic collapse of organ function and death in a number of cases – usually the elderly and infirm, but also some young people. Its route of infection has been traced to meat products (pies) contaminated by contact with raw meat in butchers' shops, including secondary contact of the pies with surfaces, knives or butchers' hands after they had been in contact with raw meat. Meat products are often eaten cold or warmed, without killing the *E. coli*. This route of infection is totally preventable if the handling of raw meat is kept completely separate from cooked products, with separate surfaces and tools, and hand washing. Contamination in the home, after purchase is still possible, and the same principles should apply, but the public has a right to expect proper handling of meat and meat products in retail and catering agencies, and this is now carefully regulated with severe penalties for infringement. In some countries, cooked meats (charcuterie) have been traditionally sold through completely separate shops to raw meat. This would seem ideal, and perhaps this custom did not arise by chance. Bowel contents can be kept away from meat after slaughter but even the best maintained abattoirs allow some contamination of raw meat with *E. coli* (e.g. from traces of faeces on the hides of animals). Therefore, all raw meat should be treated as if infected with *E. coli*. *E. coli* 157 will usually be there if it is present in the herd, although it is unsuspected because it causes no illness to cattle.

Other outbreaks of *E. coli* 157 infection have occurred directly from consumption of cattle and sheep faeces by children, for example when playing or camping in fields where recent animal inhabitants have carried the organism. The route of infection always involves a pathway from 'faeces to face', 'poo to plate' or 'turd to tongue', which has not been broken by heating or washing.

Questions are asked as to why farmers do not seem to suffer from *E. coli* food poisoning despite regular and heavy contact with the organisms. It is possible that they have developed resistance, or that they harbour other strains whose presence in the bowel can mollify the effects of pathogenic over *E. coli* 157.

Other types of food poisoning

Food poisoning can be caused by viruses and moulds as well as by bacteria.

Food-borne viruses

Viruses are extremely tiny particles (about 100–10 000 times smaller than the average bacterium) which span the boundary between animate and inanimate things. Virus particles are too small to be seen using optical microscopes, but they can be seen by using an electron microscope. They have none of the usual characteristics of living things and, in some respects, may be regarded as large organic molecules, mainly of genetic material (DNA or RNA) and some proteins. Outside a living cell, viruses are dormant but they can reproduce themselves inside living cells, and if they are taken into the body in or on food, they may invade the body's cells and multiply rapidly inside them. When this happens, severe gastro-enteritis or liver disease may be caused.

Some pathogenic viruses are actually infection of normally harmless bacteria and affect humans by altering the behaviour and products of the bacteria. The first outbreak of gastro-enteritis to be identified as a food-borne viral infection occurred in the USA, in 1968, at Norwalk, Ohio, and this led to the discovery of what is now known as the Norwalk virus. Detection of food-borne viruses is difficult and their importance as a cause of gastroenteritis may be seriously underestimated. Some authorities consider that outbreaks of viral food infection may outnumber those of bacterial food infection, but the latter can be far more easily identified and categorized.

Unlike bacteria, viruses cannot grow in food and they require a living host in which to multiply. A very small number of virus particles – perhaps as few as 10 – may be enough to cause illness. As a result, most people who eat food contaminated with viruses which can cause illness do in fact become ill, whereas heavy contamination is usually required before illness through bacterial food infection occurs. The very small numbers of virus particles required to cause illness multiply rapidly inside the body and the vomit and excreta of infected persons may contain millions of virus particles per gram. A minute quantity of infected food, if eaten by a food handler whose standards of personal hygiene are low, may infect many people. When viral food infection occurs, it is usually followed by rapid person-to-person spread and, in this respect, it differs from bacterial food infection.

Viruses are resistant to many food-processing and food-preservation techniques. They are not affected by chilling, freezing, ultraviolet light or acidic conditions. They are, however, destroyed or inactivated by heating and do not normally survive the temperatures involved in normal cooking processes. Consequently, viral food infection only occurs when uncooked food, or food which has been cooked and subsequently infected, is eaten.

The main type of viral food infection is gastroenteritis caused by a 'small round structured virus' (SRSV) or a Norwalk virus. The illness occurs about a day or so after infection and often involves uncontrollable vomiting. The illness typically lasts for a few days and the vomiting is accompanied by abdominal pain and diarrhoea. During this period the infection may be spread by handling food or by person-to-person contact.

The hepatitis A virus is commonly transmitted by contaminated food. This causes liver inflammation, the principal symptom of which – jaundice – may take several weeks to appear. During this symptomless period carriers of the disease may be extremely infective; in the pre-jaundiced phase, patients' viruses in faeces and urine and can be passed to others on any food (e.g. salads) or by contaminated drinking water.

Viral food infection can occur through eating raw or partly cooked shellfish, commonly oysters, mussels or cockles grown and harvested in sewage-contaminated coastal waters. Whether it is caused by shellfish or other food, however, the initial contaminant is human excreta.

Other viruses, including the poliomyelitis virus, can be transmitted by infected food. As with all food-borne viral infections, the food itself is not affected but simply acts as a vehicle for carrying the virus from one infected person to another.

Poisoning by mycotoxins

Poisonous mycotoxins are produced by some moulds, and serious illness may result if the affected foods are eaten. The mould *Aspergillus flavus*, which can grow on groundnuts (i.e. peanuts) and cereals in humid conditions, produces harmful aflatoxins some of which may be carcinogenic. We all know that moulds grow readily on some foods, including cheese and bread. Such moulds are not usually harmful, but their presence may indicate that the food is old, or that it has been stored in inappropriate conditions. It is possible, however, that the moulds may contain dangerous mycotoxins and the mouldy areas should be discarded or, to be absolutely safe, the food concerned should not be eaten.

FOOD HYGIENE

High standards of hygiene minimize food spoilage and help to ensure that when food is eaten it is as wholesome and as free from pathogenic bacteria, harmful viruses and moulds as possible.

Many factors may affect the quality and wholesomeness of food. Among them are:

1 The way in which it is grown or, in the case of animals, reared and fed
2 The design and cleanliness of farm buildings, slaughterhouses and factories in which it is processed
3 The premises, equipment and conditions in which it is stored
4 The care taken by food handlers to avoid contamination from other foods
5 The personal hygiene of food handlers.

It is not possible to deal fully with all these matters here, but the last two points listed are of concern to all food handlers and, indeed, to all those who have an interest in food.

The basic aims of good food hygiene practice can be summarized as follows:

- *Avoid contamination* of food by bacteria, viruses and moulds.
- *Prevent multiplication* of bacteria and moulds which nevertheless gain access to food before and after cooking.

- *Cook food thoroughly* to destroy any bacteria, viruses and moulds, and to inactivate any heat-sensitive toxins.

These three principles of good hygienic practice are amplified below.

Avoid contamination

- Keep raw and cooked foods separate. The same working surfaces and equipment should not be used for both raw and ready-to-eat foods. Surfaces and equipment used for raw foods (including vegetables) should be thoroughly cleaned afterwards.
- Keep animals and unauthorized persons out of food areas and make sure that birds and insects do not have access.
- Dispose of waste food promptly.
- Do not use washbasins for food preparation or food-preparation sinks for washing hands.
- Maintain high standards of personal hygiene. Thorough hand-washing is essential especially after handling raw meat or using a toilet. Clean towels, disposable towels or hot-air driers should be used for hand-drying to prevent reinfection of clean hands by dirty towels.
- Clean protective clothing (including head covering and face masks) should be worn in food areas and should be removed when leaving those areas.
- Hands should be kept away from bacteria-rich areas of the body including the mouth and nose.

This is one reason why smoking by food-handlers is prohibited by law. Soiled handkerchiefs and uncovered wounds are other potent sources of infection.

Prevent multiplication of microorganisms

- Keep foods cold or hot. Avoid the temperature zone 5–65°C in which bacteria flourish. Food should be in this temperature danger zone for as little time as possible. Bacteria can multiply quickly in warm food, and at about 40°C the number of bacteria may double every 20 minutes. At this rate, 10 bacteria can multiply to over 150 000 000 000 in 12 hours if enough food is available. Some bacteria are more resistant to heat than others but, in general, almost all pathogenic bacteria are killed in 30 minutes at temperatures

above 36°C in wet conditions. Dry heat is much less effective.

Cook food thoroughly

- Cooking times and temperatures must be sufficient to ensure that all bacteria and their toxins are destroyed. If bacteria present in food (or their spores) are not killed when the food is cooked they may multiply when it is cooling through the danger zone, or if it is kept in this temperature zone before being served.
- Meat and poultry should be completely defrosted before cooking. If this is not done some bacteria or bacterial spores may survive the cooking process.

The incidence of food poisoning

There has been a growth in the incidence of food poisoning in recent years and the number of reported cases in the UK now exceeds one million per annum and 500 people died of food poisoning in the year 2000. In other countries, the reported cases are much less frequent. There are wide variations in case ascertainment and in reporting of symptoms to, and by, doctors. The number of reported cases of symptoms of 'infections intestinal disease' (in the region of 10 million per annum in the UK) far exceeds the number of cases that are genuinely caused by intestinal pathogens, and for every one case caused by pathogens in foods, there are four or five caused by pathogens transmitted in some other way. The commonest pathogen is *Campylobacter*, with about 40 000 cases reported annually (http://www.parliament.uk/post/pn193.pdf). Food poisoning may be regarded as a preventable disease that is not being prevented, and the following are some of the reasons why so many incidents still occur.

1 *An increase in communal feeding.* Large-scale catering, whether in hospitals, schools, canteens or restaurants, provides the opportunity for a single item of infected food to produce many cases of food poisoning.
2 *Varied menus and rapid food service.* In order to have a wide menu and be able to produce dishes quickly, food may be precooked and kept warm until it is required or it may be reheated rapidly,

and perhaps inadequately, in a microwave oven or under an infrared grill when it is ordered.

3 *Increased use of convenience foods.* Although factory processes are carefully controlled and carried out under hygienic conditions, one source of infection can lead to the contamination of thousands of prepacked items. In addition, the use of convenience foods, especially meat products which are eaten cold or without being thoroughly reheated, increases the risk of food poisoning. Reheating in a microwave oven is not always sufficient to destroy food-poisoning organisms because some parts of the food may be less thoroughly heated than others.

4 *Increase in factory farming.* The intensive rearing of poultry and animals increases the possibility of large-scale infection of such food supplies, especially by *Salmonella*.

5 *Rapid increase in consumption of take-away meals.* Such food may be kept warm for long periods or briefly reheated in the home, thus allowing rapid bacterial growth. For example, 'take-away' rice may be contaminated with *Bacillus cereus*.

6 *Changing patterns of shopping and food storage in the home.* A weekly, rather than a daily, shopping routine means that food has to be stored for greater periods of time. Incorrect storage conditions may encourage the growth of bacteria. Increasing use of freezers means that meat, especially poultry, needs to be thawed before it is cooked. Incomplete thawing followed by normal cooking may not kill all bacteria, especially in the centre of the food.

7 *Increased use of packed meals.* The incidence of food poisoning is much higher in summer than in winter largely because of inadequate refrigeration. The increasing tendency to have a packed meal, often including cooked meat in sandwiches, in the middle of the day increases the risk of food poisoning in summer.

8 *Use of staff untrained in hygiene in catering establishments.* Large-scale handling of food by staff not trained or conscious of hygiene requirements is a major source of infection. In such circumstances cross-contamination, that is the transfer of bacteria from a contaminated source to an uncontaminated source, can easily occur and spread the risk of infection.

The high, and rising incidence of food poisoning in the 1980s and 1990s was a major reason for establishing the Food Standards Agency in the UK and Food Safety Authority in Europe. The Food Standards Agency is independent of influence from government or industry. It oversees the Meat Hygiene Service and has set targets for continued reductions in incidences of food poisoning.

Key points

- 'Food poisoning' which usually means acute infective gastro-enteritis, is common although fortunately only very rarely serious to health
- Many foods are normally contaminated by small numbers of harmless faecal bacteria. Pathological bacteria and viruses which produce toxins emerge sporadically
- Food may carry bacteria on the surface, be invaded by multiplying bacteria or be contaminated by toxins produced by bacteria

---

Chapter summary

Very simple rules for food hygiene, to prevent food poisoning, have been developed for the UK following a fatal outbreak of *E. coli* 157 infection which arose from unhygienic practice in a butcher's shop. Essentially, these entail ensuring, or advising, thorough cooking of potentially contaminated foods (e.g. all meat which could be exposed to the external environment or intestinal contents) and keeping entirely separate raw foods and the utensils used with them from cooked foods (which can often perfect culture media and which may not be cooked again). Risks of food poisoning can be reduced by raw and cooked foods sealed and separated in refrigerators, and ensuring the correct temperature for cooking and storage.

FURTHER READING

Websites

http://www.parliament.uk/post/pn193.pdf

Food poisoning statistics: http://www.food.gov.uk/news/pressreleases/2002/feb/46640

Pennington Report 1996: Report on the circumstances leading to the 1996 outbreak of infection with *E. coli* in Central Scotland, the implications for food safety and the lessons to be learned. www.scotland.gov.uk/library/documents-w4/pgr-00.htm

www.opsi.gov.uk/si/si1995/Uksi_19951763_en_1.htm#end

Food contaminants – adulterants and additives

Many people are concerned about the presence of 'chemical additives' in their food and worry about the possible ill-effects of eating them. 'E numbers' (which signify the presence of an additive in a food) have become notorious as unnatural components of foods, and catalogues of ill-defined effects have been attributed to them. Yet, as explained in the preceding chapters, food itself is composed of chemicals and so, for that matter, are our bodies. What is usually meant by 'chemicals' in connection with food are those substances which do not normally form a part of the food in its natural or traditional state. Their presence may arise as a result of accidental contamination, or they may be deliberately added to improve processing or keeping qualities or to supplement the nutrients already present. The adulteration of food by crude methods, such as the addition of alum to flour or water to milk, though once common, does not occur today to any extent. Many people, however, take the view that the adulterants of former times have been replaced by additives in the twentieth century. For some people, a risk of bacterial food poisoning – even a high risk – is bearable because bacteria are 'natural', but they consider all chemicals as 'unnatural' and any theoretical risk from them is unacceptable. This is a philosophical and religious issue which cannot be resolved by a study of food science or of nutrition.

FOOD CONTAMINANTS

Food can become contaminated in a multitude of ways but there are some sources of contamination which are of outstanding importance today, and it is with these that we shall be concerned here.

Agricultural contamination

Many crops are treated with insecticides to prevent infestation by insects, fungicides to prevent growth of fungi and weedkillers or growth regulators to kill weeds selectively. The treatment of growing crops with chemicals is by no means new. Insecticides containing sulphur, the arsenical spray Paris Green and Bordeaux Mixture, which contains copper, were first used over 100 years ago. Insecticides, herbicides (weedkillers), fungicides and other chemicals used to promote plant health are referred to generically as pesticides.

If chemicals were not used by farmers the amount of food available would fall considerably and its cost increase dramatically. The nineteenth-century Irish potato famine, which was caused by potato blight, is a striking example of the misery that can be caused by crop failure. Potato blight is now largely controlled by fungicidal spraying and the Colorado beetle, a modern menace which could wreak equal havoc on the potato crop, is controlled by the use of insecticides. Pesticides and fungicides are invaluable aids to efficient food production, not only when crops are growing, but also after harvesting when they are being stored.

Modern agricultural chemicals are for the most part complex organic compounds and they are becoming increasingly complex. Many of them have the capacity to be toxic to animals and human beings if eaten in sufficient amounts, but they are usually applied to the plants before the part which is eaten has appeared, or at least a sufficient length of time before harvesting to ensure that the amount remaining on the crop is so small that when it is eaten it will be wholesome. Some agricultural chemicals are applied to the soil before the crop has been planted, or soon afterwards, to ensure a healthy, disease-free and pest-free environment for the young plant.

As soon as a pesticide is applied to a field or a crop the action of light, air, microorganisms and the metabolism of the plant itself begin to break it down. In many cases, no traces can be detected on the crop when it is harvested, even though sensitive methods of analysis, able to detect and measure as little as one part of pesticide in 20 000 000 parts of plant material, are used. A permitted maximum residue level (MRL) has been set for each pesticide and the permitted amounts are extremely low – never more than a few parts per million and often even less. Toxicologists have been able to specify an acceptable daily intake (ADI), which is the quantity of a pesticide that could be taken daily for an entire lifetime without appreciable risk. In practice, the ADI is set at a very low level with a safety factor of at least 100 (i.e. the ADI is at least 100 times less than the 'no-effect' level). The amounts of pesticide actually eaten normally fall far short of this figure. For example, the MRL for the fungicide tecnazene (which is used to suppress sprouting and development of fungal diseases in potatoes) is limited to 0.05 mg/kg and daily consumption of 200 g of potatoes by a 60 kg man would only amount to about 1.5 per cent of the ADI.

The number of pesticides in use has increased dramatically in recent years. Whereas in 1926 there were only a dozen or so pesticides in common use, there are now several hundreds. All new pesticides are carefully evaluated for safety and efficiency before their use is approved. The Pesticides Safety Directorate (PSD) is an executive agency of the Department for Environment, Food and Rural Affairs

(DEFRA) and this regulates agricultural, horticultural and garden pesticides in the UK. European Community directives are incorporated into recent statutory instruments such as The Pesticides (Maximum Residue Levels in Crops, Food and Feeding Stuffs) (England and Wales) Regulations (1999) and similar regulations in Scotland and Northern Ireland, and The Water Supply (Water Quality) Regulations (2000).

Antibiotics

As well as treating soil and crops with chemicals, farmers treat animals with chemicals in the form of antibiotics. Antibiotics are used to cure animal diseases such as mastitis, enteritis, pneumonia and infected wounds and feet. By using antibiotics many animal infections which formerly were a source of great trouble to farmers can now be easily controlled. Farmers are also tempted to dose pigs and poultry with antibiotics when there is nothing apparently wrong with them. It is supposed that by doing so the animals will be given blanket protection against disease or will be better able to resist stress and hence will grow faster or give higher yields of eggs. Antibiotics are also used to stimulate growth but under European law the use of antibiotic growth-promoting feed additives will be phased out by 2006. This is because of concerns about the potential spread of antibiotic resistance.

The use of antibiotics for treating infected animals meets with general approval. Indeed, the use of antibiotics in veterinary practice has been a great boon for farmers and, even more so, to the animals themselves. The use of antibiotics as animal food supplements is a different matter, however, and this practice is widely opposed.

Indiscriminate use of antibiotics by farmers is not approved by veterinary workers and it is generally accepted that antibiotics should only be used to treat specific infections. The reason for this is that microorganisms which are continually exposed to low concentrations of an antibiotic may become antibiotic-resistant; when this occurs, the antibiotic is valueless when it is required to treat an illness caused by the organism concerned. An organism that has acquired resistance to an antibiotic can, in some circumstances, transmit this resistance, merely by contact, to a previously sensitive organism. This is known as infective drug resistance. In practice, farmers can seldom afford to call a veterinary surgeon to make a diagnosis and they have to take responsibility for some antibiotic use.

When organisms become resistant to antibiotics, it is more difficult for veterinary surgeons to deal with infected animals. Also, because there is an inevitable interchange of organisms between animals and man, similar difficulties may arise in treating infected humans. It would be most unfortunate if, as a result of veterinary use, the typhoid organism *Salmonella typhi* became resistant to the antibiotic chloramphenicol (Chloromycetin) as this is by far the most effective drug available for treating typhoid fever in humans. There are, however, no indications at present that this is likely to occur. Chloramphenicol is extensively used for treating animals but its effectiveness for the treatment of typhoid fever in humans has not diminished.

A further objection to the widespread use of antibiotics by farmers is the danger that an individual who is allergic to a particular antibiotic may be made ill if they drink milk in which the antibiotic is present. To prevent this happening, farmers are required to withhold milk from treated cows until residues of antibiotic have reached insignificant levels. Usually no traces can be detected after 48 hours but in some cases up to 14 days may elapse before the milk is acceptable. Less than 1 per cent of samples of bulk milk tested are found to contain antibiotics but, even so, the danger of an allergic reaction still exists.

Lead

Fruit and vegetables grown near large towns or busy roads may have been seriously contaminated with lead deposited from the exhaust fumes of motor vehicles in the past. However, leaded petrol is now virtually unobtainable and 'unleaded' petrol is now used by most cars. Lead which has been absorbed from contaminated soil by the growing plant, however, cannot be removed and as it is a cumulative poison long-term consumption could be harmful.

Radioactive contamination

Most elements are mixtures of extremely similar isotopes differing only in the numbers of neutrons in the atoms. Some of these isotopes are unstable, and correct spontaneously to a stable parent atom. In doing so, they emit radioactivity and atomic particles, and they are known as radioisotopes. Naturally occurring radioisotopes are fortunately present in only minute amounts. Contamination of food with industrial radioisotopes, which enter the atmosphere as a result of accidents in nuclear power stations or nuclear fuel reprocessing plants and from the testing of nuclear weapons, is another serious modern problem. Although radioisotopes are unstable, some can remain active and emit radiation for a very long period. The radiation and atomic particles emitted are extremely harmful to living cells. Radioisotopes which enter the atmosphere become widely distributed and may finally reach the ground many thousands of miles away. When radioisotopes fall on soil and vegetation, they may be absorbed by plants. If these are eaten by man or animals and the nutrients absorbed, the radioisotopes may become incorporated into the body tissues with harmful consequences. A recent example was in 1986 when a major nuclear accident occurred at Chernobyl nuclear power plant in the former Soviet Union. The surrounding area was contaminated with the radioisotopes and the incidence of cancer rose in the area. There were concerns about the fallout of the radioisotopes in the UK and at the time of writing there are still restrictions on the use of lamb bred in certain areas of Scotland.

The treatment of food with ionizing radiation for preservation purposes (see p. 284) does not produce radioisotopes if it is properly carried out, and it does not make food radioactive.

Contamination from packaging materials

There has been some concern in recent years about the possible contamination of foodstuffs by migration of chemicals from the materials in which they are packed. Plastics are increasingly used as packaging materials, and while the polymers themselves are non-toxic, compounds which may have been added to them to improve their properties may not be equally innocuous. Catalysts such as organic peroxides or complex metal salts may have been used to initiate polymerization and these remain in the polymerized product. Plasticizers are incorporated in many plastic materials to increase their flexibility. They are usually viscous organic liquids such as the esters of phthalic, phosphoric or ricinoleic acids. Plastics may be adversely affected by atmospheric oxidation, especially when they are in the form of thin sheets which present a large surface to the air, and antioxidants are used to mitigate this. Unfortunately, however, the antioxidants used are not those approved for use in foods. Stabilizers, which may be organo-tin salts or calcium salts of fatty acids, may be used in some plastic materials and pigments, antistatic agents, bactericides and fungicides may also be present. When plastics are used as packaging materials for food, any of these substances may find their way into the food. Only very small amounts will be present in the food, but even these minimal amounts may prove to be toxic if ingested over a period. Studies have shown that there fat-soluble compounds may accumulate in brain and in visceral pathways.

Paper-based packaging materials are widely used for foodstuffs and even these may be a source of contamination if, as often happens, the paper or board has been treated to increase its strength when wet. Such wet-strength paper is made by impregnating paper or pulp with urea–formaldehyde or melamine–formaldehyde resin, and it is possible for formaldehyde to migrate from the treated paper to the foodstuff. The presence in foods of up to 5 ppm of formaldehyde arising from any resin used in the manufacture of wet-strength papers or of plastic food containers or utensils is permitted.

The regulation of packaging material is under review and a plethora of regulations is being updated following various European Commission (EC) directives. For example, The Plastic Materials and Articles in Contact with Food (Amendment) (Scotland) Regulations (2003), and the recently issued Materials and Articles Intended to Come into Contact with Foodstuffs (Amendment) (Scotland) Regulations.

FOOD ADDITIVES

Additives are natural or synthetic substances which are added to foods to serve particular purposes. The legal definition of an additive (The Food Labelling Regulations, 1996) is:

> any substance not normally consumed as a food in itself and not normally used as a characteristic ingredient of food, whether or not it has nutritive value, the intentional addition of which to a food for a technological purpose in the manufacture, processing, preparation, treatment, packaging, transport or storage of such food results, or may be reasonably expected to result, in it or its by-products becoming directly or indirectly a component of such.

Most processed and manufactured foods contain additives, and in the UK the use of additives in the following categories is controlled by law.

1 Colours
2 Sweeteners
3 Miscellaneous additives – this includes preservatives, antioxidants, emulsifiers and stabilizers as well as additives such as flavour enhancers, gelling agents, humectants.

In each category only substances known as permitted additives may be used in food. Any substance that does not fall into one of the controlled categories may be added to food subject to the general limitation imposed by law that it must not 'render the food injurious to health'.

Most permitted additives have been given a serial number. Where usage is also controlled by the European Union (EU) the serial number is prefixed by an 'E'.

Some permitted additives are naturally occurring substances. Pectin (E440i), for example, which is used as a gelling agent, is obtained from apples. Other permitted additives are manufactured 'copies' of naturally occurring substances. An example is L-ascorbic acid (E300) which is manufactured on a large scale for use as a food additive, and is identical in every respect to naturally occurring vitamin C. In addition to the natural or nature-identical compounds, there are a substantial number of permitted additives that do not occur naturally and are purely synthetic in character. This does not mean that they are harmful, but it is mainly to this type of additive that people object. Tartrazine (E102), which is used as a food colour (see p. 301) is an example of this type of additive.

Preservatives

Preservatives prevent microbial spoilage of food, as described in Chapter 18. There are around 38 permitted preservatives and all except one of them (nisin) may also be used throughout the EU. A list of permitted preservatives is given in Table 18.2 (see p. 276). Their serial numbers are in the 200s.

Antioxidants

Antioxidants prevent fats and oils from going rancid and their use is described in Chapter 18. There are 15 antioxidants permitted as food additives, including ascorbic acid and vitamin E. A list of permitted antioxidants is given in Table 18.3 (see p. 279). Their serial numbers are in the 300s.

Emulsifiers, stabilizers, thickeners and gelling agents

Emulsifiers are used to make stable emulsions or creamy suspensions from oils and fats and water (see p. 58). They are also used in baked food to slow down the rate of staling. Stabilizers are used to improve the stability of emulsions and prevent the separation of their components. There are 60 permitted emulsifiers and stabilizers. They include: edible gums, such as locust bean gum (carob gum), tragacanth and acacia (gum arabic); alginic acid and alginates; cellulose derivatives; monoglycerides and diglycerides of fatty acids such as glyceryl monostearate; pectins and various sorbitan derivatives. The large number of permitted emulsifiers and stabilizers reflects their widespread use in a large variety of different types of manufactured foods where 'creaminess' or 'spreadability' are required. Salad cream, ice cream, instant desserts, cheese, fish and meat spreads, margarine and low-fat spreads all contain emulsifiers or stabilizers, or both.

Most of the permitted emulsifiers and stabilizers have serial numbers in the 400s.

Food colours

Dyes and pigments used in food are known collectively as food colours or, more tersely, simply as colours. They are added to food to make it more attractive to the purchaser or consumer or to replace natural colour lost during food processing. Canned strawberries, for example, would be greyish-brown if colours were not added, and canned peas a brownish-green.

The addition of colours to foods is controlled by law in most countries; in the UK only 43 permitted colours may be used. Their serial numbers range from 100 to 180: about two-thirds of them may be used throughout the EU.

Many permitted colours are of natural origin and they include cochineal, carotenes (and the closely related xanthophylls) and anthocyanins, which colour ripe fruit. Other permitted colours are inorganic substances such as the white pigment titanium dioxide and finely divided aluminium, silver and gold, which are used in cake decoration.

The list of permitted colours includes some synthetic dyes. Thousands of such substances are known but most of them are too toxic to be used in foods and some are known to be carcinogenic. Colouring matter must not be added to meat, fish, poultry, fruit, cream, milk, honey, vegetables, wine, coffee, tea and condensed or dried milk. No colours may be added to foods intended for babies and infants except riboflavin (and its phosphate), lactoflavin and β-carotene, all of which occur naturally in other foods.

Sweetening agents

Sweetening agents, or sweeteners as they are generally known, fall into two categories. Intense sweeteners are many times sweeter than sucrose and they are therefore used in very low concentrations. Bulk sweeteners are about as sweet as sucrose and hence are used in roughly equal amounts. The relative sweetness of naturally occurring sugars and artificial sweeteners is considered in Chapter 8 (see p. 92).

There are six permitted intense sweeteners:

1 *E950* acesulfame potassium, used in canned foods, soft drinks and table-top sweeteners
2 *E951* aspartame, used in soft drinks, yoghurts, dessert and drink mixes and sweetening tablets
3 *E954* saccharin (and its sodium and calcium salts), used in soft drinks, cider, sweetening tablets
4 *E957* thaumatin, used in sweetening tablets and yoghurt
5 *E959* neohesperidine dihydrochalcone (NHDC), used in soft drinks and pharmaceutical preparations such as vitamin pills
6 *E952* cyclamic acid.

Aspartame (which is sold under the trade name Nutrasweet) is a dipeptide made from the amino acids L-aspartic acid and L-phenylalanine. It is broken down in the body to its constituent amino acids. People who suffer from the genetic disease phenylketonuria (PKU) are unable to metabolize phenylalanine and some doubts have been expressed about whether aspartame can safely be consumed by them. The government committee responsible for overseeing the use of chemicals in food has concluded, however, that aspartame can safely be used by those suffering from PKU.

The bulk sweeteners (sometimes known as nutritive sweeteners) are mostly hydrogenated sugars: hydrogenated glucose syrup, isomalt (E953) and mannitol (E421) are used in sugar-free confectionery; sorbitol (E420) is used in sugar-free confectionery xylitol, used in sugar-free chewing gum and lactitol (E966), derived from whey (a byproduct of cheese manufacture), is used in reduced-sugar jellies and jams.

Bulk sweeteners were originally developed for marketing to people with diabetes. However, nutritional guidelines for diabetes now recognize that total avoidance of sugar is unnecessary and there is no caloric saving from bulk sweeteners. They help protect teeth when used instead of sugar-containing products.

Other food additives

There are many other uses for additives and over 120 miscellaneous additives have been approved for use in foods in Britain. They are principally used as processing aids and the main types are listed in Table 20.1. Only substances which have been approved may be used for the purposes listed in this table.

Table 20.1 Additives used as processing aids

Acids and bases	Glazing agents
Anti-caking agents	Humectants
Anti-foaming agents	Liquid freezants
Buffers	Mineral oils
Bulking agents	Packaging gases
Firming agents	Propellants
Flavour modifiers	Release agents
Flour bleaching agents	Sequestrants
Flour improvers	Solvents

Flavour modifiers

A flavour modifier is a substance which is capable of enhancing, reducing or otherwise modifying the taste or odour, or both, of a food. Flavour modifiers or enhancers, are themselves practically tasteless but they intensify the flavour of soups, meat and other savoury foods.

Salt

Sodium chloride has been used since earliest recorded history to preserve foods, specifically allowing meat and fish to be eaten long after the animal's death. The necessary high concentration of salt was found to be unpalatable, but the palate can adapt remarkably to accept high-salt taste over time. It was found that if a great deal of salt was added to accompanying foods (e.g. bread, potatoes, vegetables) then the taste of highly salted meat or fish was no longer unbearable.

Nowadays, it is not necessary to salt meat or fish (refrigeration or freezing is the solution), but we have been left with manufacturing and cooking methods which still add 1 per cent salt – or even more – to common foods such as bread and breakfast cereals, and catering services which still add salt routinely to cooking. The result is that people's palates are still attuned to having 1 per cent salt in everything. It is possible to adapt the palate to a diet without salt; this takes about 2 weeks and food tastes bland while the palate is adapting.

The importance of salt in food is that it contributes, over a lifetime, to increasing blood pressure, and then to heart disease and strokes. High blood pressure is usually not symptomatic, but causes or contributes to 170 000 deaths each year in England alone. In 2003, the Scientific Advisory Committee on Nutrition completed a detailed review of evidence, concluding that salt intake should be reduced from the current 9 g/day average, to an upper limit of 6 g/day. There is no biological reason to eat even half of this amount, but the target of 6 g/day will take the food industry several years to achieve.

The most widely used flavour enhancer apart from sodium chloride is monosodium glutamate (E621), or MSG as it is commonly known. It is the sodium salt of glutamic acid, an amino acid which is a common component of proteins (see p. 135). It occurs in soy sauce, which is made by fermenting or hydrolysing soya beans and it has long been used in this form as a flavour enhancer in Chinese food. MSG itself is made on a large scale by allowing a specific bacterium to grow in a solution containing ammonium ions.

Most dehydrated soups and stock cubes contain MSG and it is also present in many other 'meaty' prepared foods. Some people react unfavourably to MSG and suffer from what has come to be known as the 'Chinese restaurant syndrome' if they eat food containing it. This manifests itself in a variety of ways including palpitations, chest or neck pain and dizziness. The cause is not known and the ill-effects soon disappear. Monosodium glutamate is not thought to be harmful but, as a precautionary measure, it is not now added to food manufactured for babies and infants.

Sodium 5*-ribonucleotide (E635) is another powerful permitted flavour enhancer. Ribonucleotides are compounds formed from the sugar ribose, phosphoric acid and an organic base such as guanine. They occur in all animal tissues and are present in yeast extracts and contribute substantially to their characteristic meaty taste. As soon as an animal is killed, however, enzymes called phosphatases begin to break down the ribonucleotides and by the time the food reaches the table a great deal of the flavour-enhancing properties of the ribonucleotides may be lost. By adding ribonucleotides to foods of animal origin such loss of flavour may be made good.

Ribonucleotide flavour enhancers are used in soups, meat and fish pastes, all types of canned meat products, sausages, meat pies and other processed food products of which the main ingredient is meat or fish. As their flavour enhancing power is very great – ten times that of MSG – only very small quantities (as little as 20 ppm) are required.

Polyphosphates

A range of phosphoric acids and their sodium, potassium and calcium salts are used as food additives. Twenty-six such substances, from the simple acid orthophosphoric acid, H_3PO_4, to complex polyphosphates are permitted for use in food.

Phosphates, particularly polyphosphates, are added to flesh foods such as meat, fish and poultry in order to permit increased retention of water and greater solubility of proteins and, it is claimed, to improve texture.

Chicken and other poultry can be made to absorb water with the aid of polyphosphates. If this is done it must be declared on a label and if the amount of added water exceeds 5 per cent that also must be stated. Water added to poultry without using polyphosphates, however, need not be declared even though some frozen poultry may contain as much as 8 per cent.

Flavouring agents

Flavour is one of the most important attributes of food and is detected by the senses of taste and smell. Taste itself is made up of the four primary tastes – sweet, sour, salt and bitter – which are detected by taste buds situated in the mouth (mainly on the tongue, palate and cheeks). Smell is detected by extremely sensitive cells situated at the top of the nasal cavity.

Flavouring agents have been used from earliest times to increase the attractiveness of food. Originally, flavourings were the dried, and sometimes powdered, forms of spices, herbs, berries, roots and stems of plants. For example, spices such as pepper, cloves and ginger were prized for their ability to add interest and palatability to a monotonous diet. Condiments and spices were invaluable not only for their flavour, but also because they were able to disguise the tainted flavour of meat which was past its best.

As the demand for flavouring agents increased, methods of extracting the active principles were devised. The most important types of natural flavouring agent are essential oils, which are extracted from plant tissues. These oils (which are chemically quite different from the oils and fats discussed in Chapter 6) are volatile (easily vaporized) and have a flavouring power many times that of the raw material from which they come. Synthetic flavours which are usually copies of the essential oils are cheaper and far more convenient to use than the corresponding natural flavours. They are usually dissolved in ethyl alcohol or another permitted solvent but powdered versions, made by spray-drying the flavouring material in a gum arabic solution, are also available. Such powders are widely used in powdered convenience foods, such as instant dessert mixes.

At present, flavouring agents, or flavourings as they are referred to by the food industry, may be used in

Table 20.2 Classification of flavouring agents

Natural	Synthetic
Herbs, spices	Acids, ethers, esters
Essential oils,	Acetals, ketals, others
extracts, distillates	Alcohols, ketones
Foods (e.g. cocoa)	Aldehyde, lactones

Table 20.3 Esters used as flavouring agents

Name	Formula	Use
Ethyl formate	$HCOOC_2H_5$	Rum, raspberry and peach essences
Ethyl acetate	$CH_3COOC_2H_5$	Apple, pear, strawberry and peach essences
Pentyl acetate	$CH_3COOC_5H_{11}$	Pear, pineapple and raspberry essences
Pentyl butyrate	$C_4H_9COOC_5H_{11}$	Banana, pineapple and peach essences
Allyl caproate	$C_5H_{11}COOC_3H_5$	Pineapple essence

foods without restriction. It is intended that they will, in time, be subject to control in the same way as the permitted additives already discussed. The problems to be overcome in doing so, however, are very great because of the large number of flavourings available and the minute concentrations in which they are often used. The blending and use of flavourings is more akin to an art than a science and hence it is more difficult to control in a scientific way.

Many thousands of flavourings are available for use by the food industry and a classification of natural and synthetic flavourings is given in Table 20.2.

Many of the simpler artificial fruit flavours are esters, which are formed when carboxylic acids react with alcohols. Ethyl acetate, for example, which is a fruity-smelling liquid, is produced when acetic acid and ethyl alcohol are heated together:

$$CH_3COOH + C_2H_5OH \rightleftharpoons CH_3COOC_2H_5 + H_2O$$
$$\text{Ethyl acetate}$$

The reaction also occurs at normal temperatures, but at a much slower rate, and esters, particularly ethyl acetate, are formed in this way during the maturing of wine and contribute to the much prized bouquet. Other esters can be easily and cheaply made in the same way by heating together the appropriate acid and alcohol, usually in the presence of a catalyst.

At one time, synthetic fruit flavours were usually made up of a single ester and consequently they were rather poor imitations. As the composition of natural flavours has become known it has become possible to blend together synthetic materials so as to imitate the natural flavour more closely. Esters are the most widely used type of flavouring and Table 20.3 shows some of those commonly used.

It is possible to analyse natural flavours by vapour-phase chromatography, which is a very sensitive technique for splitting up mixtures of volatile compounds into their components. The results of such investigations show that natural flavouring agents are usually complex mixtures of many different substances, some of which are present in extremely small amounts. Occasionally, however, the flavour of a natural flavouring agent depends very largely on the presence of a single substance which may be the main ingredient, such as eugenol in oil of cloves which constitutes 85 per cent of the oil, or a minor ingredient, such as citral in oil of lemon which constitutes only 5 per cent of the oil.

In the rare cases where a natural flavour is composed wholly or predominantly of one chemical, a synthetic substitute can be made fairly easily. Usually, however, a large number of substances must be blended together to obtain a good imitation of a natural flavour.

Added nutrients

Nutrients are added to some processed foods to improve their nutritional quality. In some cases the added nutrients replace those lost during processing. In the manufacture of dehydrated potato, for example, a great deal of the ascorbic acid (vitamin C) originally present is lost and synthetic ascorbic acid is added to replace it and to act as an antioxidant. The addition of iron, thiamin and niacin to all flour (except wholemeal) to replace losses caused by milling is another example (see p. 119).

Nutrient additives may be used not only to maintain nutritional value but also to improve it. This is known as food fortification or enrichment. Such addition of nutrients may either be a legal requirement to safeguard public health or it may be done voluntarily by the manufacturer. The enrichment of margarine with vitamins A and D so as to make its vitamin content equivalent to that of summer butter is obligatory, as is the addition of nutrients to flour. Fortification of breakfast cereals with a range of vitamins and minerals or the addition of vitamin C to soft drinks and fruit juices, on the other hand, is not legally required, but is used for marketing day-to-day foods on health grounds. In the USA, fortification of all cereal and bread products with folic acid is now mandatory and a range of health benefits have arisen since intakes are low or marginal for many people.

SAFETY OF ADDITIVES

There is widespread and understandable concern, but amounting almost to hysteria in some cases, about the presence of 'chemicals' in food. Additives, with their accompanying 'E numbers', have acquired an undeservedly poor reputation with the general public. Readers of this book will, it is hoped, be better informed and will appreciate that one of the main reasons for the presence of additives in food is to ensure that it is safe to eat and that perishable foods are available in good condition throughout the year. Some additives are completely natural compounds. Others could pose hazards if consumed in excess. Achieving safe, reliable food will always involve judging the balance between benefits and possible hazards from additives.

The object of regulations controlling the use of additives in food is to prevent abuses that might otherwise occur and the consequent dangers to health. Nevertheless, the general public views the presence of additives in food and the regulations that control their use as aspects of a vast conspiracy practised by an unscrupulous food industry without regard to possible harm. To what extent, if any, can these suspicions be justified? Is it possible that the use of food additives could make our food less safe either by concealing substandard food or from the additives themselves, or is it the case that additives make our food safer, cheaper, more varied and more attractive?

A radical view is held by some that the addition to food of chemicals of any sort, for whatever purpose,

should be banned. However, many of the traditional foods we regard as 'natural' may be far removed from their original condition as a result of treatment with chemicals which, because of long-standing usage, are not now regarded as additives. Traditional techniques for processing foods, such as cooking, smoking, pickling and curing bring about chemical and physical changes.

It is generally agreed that the use of additives in food is justified when they serve one or more of the following functions.

1 Maintenance of nutritional quality
2 Improvement of keeping quality or stability with a reduction of wastage
3 Enhancement of attractiveness in a manner which does not lead to deception
4 Provision of essential aids to processing.

Situations in which the use of food additives would not be in the interests of the consumer, and should not be permitted, include the following:

1 When faulty processing and handling techniques are disguised
2 When the consumer is deceived
3 When the result is a substantial reduction in the nutritive value of a food.

It is important that the risks of possible ill-effects from the presence of chemicals in foods should be negligible compared with the benefits which accrue, and the food additives approved for use in the UK perform useful functions without harming the vast majority of consumers. It has to be accepted, however, that some sensitive people may react adversely to some food additives. The European Community Scientific Committee for Food has estimated that 0.03–0.10 per cent (less than one in a thousand) of the population may be sensitive to a food additive. This is unfortunate, but it has to be borne in mind that the number of people who have adverse reactions to other foods – to strawberries or shellfish, for example – may exceed these figures. It has been estimated that from 0.3 to 2.0 per cent of children in the UK suffer from some kind of dietary intolerance at some stage. These figures exceed by a factor of 10–20 the numbers thought to be sensitive to food additives.

Clearly, additives should neither be condemned nor condoned as a class, but each should be considered and judged upon its merits. Some chemicals are so objectionable that their presence in food is indefensible. Formaldehyde, fluorides and similar toxic compounds which were formerly used as preservatives fall into this category, as do azo dyes known to be carcinogenic to man.

Only slightly less objectionable than the above are those substances which may conceivably cause harm when eaten. Synthetic colouring materials are somewhat suspect because, as already pointed out, some of are known to be toxic. Many thousands of synthetic dyes are known and it would appear to be easy to draw up a list of a few dozen that would be adequate for colouring food and which could be guaranteed to be safe. It is not possible, however, despite the most rigorous tests, to be sure that a compound which is apparently harmless is in fact so. The number of colours approved for use in the UK is steadily decreasing as new evidence of their toxicity becomes available. Pressure of public opinion (well-informed or not) and a 'bad press' has caused several major supermarket chains to impose bans on the presence of certain additives in their 'own brand' products. The widened global market has introduced a further complexity, since some imported foods have recently been found to contain banned additives (e.g. red dyes in Asian food). Testing procedures are difficult and expensive, so only possible for major importers.

Tartrazine (E102), a bright yellow permitted colour used extensively in soft drinks and confectionery, has acquired a reputation for provoking food intolerance and causing hyperactivity in children. The Food Advisory Committee (which gave expert scientific advice to the old Ministry of Agriculture, Fisheries and Food), however, did not consider that tartrazine posed more problems than any other colour or food ingredient, and that evidence for a causal link with hyperactivity was unconvincing.

Food colours are used in low concentrations and it has been estimated that in the UK the average daily intake is between 10 and 50 mg. The consumption of individual colours is estimated to be never greater than 10 per cent (and in most cases less than 1 per cent) of the ADI figure worked out by toxicologists.

Additives are sometimes used to give manufactured foods properties associated with the presence of traditional ingredients. Emulsifying agents used to decrease the amount of fat needed in the manufacture of cakes and bread come into this category. Although compounds of this type reduce the amount of fat required to produce familiar physical properties in cake, they do not, of course, fulfil its nutritional functions. The amount of fat lost in this way, when considered in terms of an individual, is not large, but for someone living on a barely adequate diet it may not be insignificant. Most people, however, eat too much fat and a reduction in intake would not be undesirable.

Synthetic cream and meringues are now often made from cellulose derivatives that have absolutely no nutritional value. The use of colouring matter in cakes to give an impression of richness is also open to criticism. There are numerous other examples of the use of additives which contribute nothing to the nourishment of the consumer. The more luxurious classes of foodstuffs lend themselves particularly well to such sophistication and it may be argued that these are not, in any case, eaten primarily for their nutritive value. This is a specious argument, however, and does not wholly remove the impression that the use of such substances is tantamount to a confidence trick.

One might suppose that the addition of nutrients to food would be above suspicion but this is not always so, and even here there is need for caution. The quantities of nutrients employed, however innocent they seem, should bear some relationship to the body's needs. The bad effect of an excessive intake of vitamin D, mentioned in Chapter 14, shows that it is possible to have too much of a good thing!

The risk/benefit balance

It is generally accepted that no food additive can be proved to be absolutely safe. It is impossible to prove that an additive causes no harm and in this situation it is helpful to balance possible risks against benefits conferred.

The assessment of a risk/benefit balance is well exemplified by the use of nitrites and nitrates to preserve meat products discussed in Chapter 18. The benefit of using these additives is well established; they destroy *Clostridium botulinum* bacteria and so prevent food poisoning. There is the risk, however, that nitrites in food are partly converted into nitrosamines, which are known to produce cancer in animals. At the low levels permitted in specified foods, nitrites are not known to have caused any harm to any human being. Nevertheless, the risk remains and it is a matter of judgement whether the risk is considered to be justified in the light of the known benefits.

With some types of food additive it is more difficult to assess the risks and benefits. Food colours provide a suitable example. The risk of using food colours is clear from the knowledge that some synthetic dyes are carcinogens. Conversely, the benefits arising from the use of food colours are harder to assess, although it is true that they improve the attractiveness and appearance of food. The risk in using a known carcinogen would so obviously outweigh the benefits that the use of such a substance would not be considered. Difficulties arise with substances which are not known to be carcinogenic but cannot be said with certainty not to be. The decision to permit the use of such a substance as a food additive is at best a compromise based on the risk/benefit considerations outlined above. Assessment of risk can only be made on the scientific evidence available, or obtainable, at the time. Nevertheless, evidence accumulated later during its use, and possibly by using improved scientific techniques, may show that continued use of the additive is not advisable. Great harm may have been done to consumers in the meantime, and this is why such extreme caution is necessary before the use of a food additive is permitted.

The use of synthetic colours is particularly difficult to justify. The risks, although small, are thought by many people to outweigh substantially the somewhat dubious cosmetic benefits of the additives. The number of permitted synthetic colours has decreased from 32 in 1957 to less than half this number.

Pessimistic readers may feel inclined to forgo all foods containing additives, but that would prove to be rather difficult. Fortunately, the risks, although real, are (for most people) exceedingly small and they are insignificant when measured against other hazards. Smokers, in particular, have less cause to worry about the dangers of food additives than the threat to health from smoking, which is probably many thousands of times greater. Consumption of excessive amounts of alcohol and, possibly, coffee or cola drinks is similarly not entirely free from risk.

Of more general concern (and far outweighing the dietary risks already mentioned) are the life-threatening risks associated with obesity, hypertension and coronary heart disease. All of these conditions may be diet-related (see Chapter 17) and they undoubtedly pose a far greater threat to corporate health than the presence in food of minuscule amounts of additives.

Food laws, monitoring and regulation and the control of food additives in Britain

The adulteration of food has its origins in antiquity, and in England the earliest action to prevent adulteration was taken by the guilds. For example, in the reigns of Henry II and Henry III, pepper was widely used to preserve meat and other foods but because it was expensive adulteration was common. To remedy this, the Guild of Pepperers was granted powers to sift spices so as to control quality. In the sixteenth and seventeenth centuries, adulteration of food was prevalent and practices such as the dilution of mustard with flour, the addition of leaves (e.g. scorched oak leaves) to tea, the mixing of sand, ashes and sawdust to bread doughs and the addition of water to milk became commonplace. Some forms of adulteration, such as the addition of sulphuric acid to vinegar, were even more serious and made the food poisonous.

Adulteration of food continued unabated in the eighteenth and nineteenth centuries and following increasing expressions of public concern and the publishing of the findings of a Select Parliamentary Commission, the Adulteration of Food and Drink Act was enacted in 1860. This was extensively amended and strengthened by the 1875 Sale of Food and Drugs Act which made the appointment of Public Analysts obligatory and gave inspectors the right to take samples for analysis. Over 100 years have elapsed since the passage of the 1875 Act and in this period a vast amount of legislation controlling the composition, production, distribution and sale of food has been enacted.

The statute currently in force is the Food Safety Act (1990), which consolidates previous legislation and takes into account the UK membership of the European Union. Membership imposes obligations on the UK to conform with EU Law. In recent years, many of the regulations surrounding food have been updated in order to enact EU directives.

The fundamental intention of the 1990 Food Safety Act is to ensure that food shall be in as wholesome a condition as possible when it is eaten. The Act and associated legislation prescribes legally enforceable standards of composition and treatment and makes infringement a criminal offence. It prohibits the addition to food of any substance which would make it 'injurious to health'. Ministers are also required to 'have regard to the desirability of restricting, so far as practicable, the use of substances of no nutritional value as foods or ingredients of foods'. The Food Act empowers the Food and Health Ministers to make regulations concerning foods and these, after approval by Parliament, are published as legally binding statutory instruments (SI).

Key points

- Food can be contaminated by atmosphere industrial pollutants, by agricultural chemicals or antibiotics used in farming, and by industrial chemicals during processing, distribution and storage. Some unscrupulous manufacturers introduce adulterants to enhance bulk, flavour or marketability in some way
- Some contaminants introduce unpleasant flavour, so are detectable. Most are not
- Under unusual circumstances there may be sufficient contaminants to harm health (e.g. radioactive isotopes, nitrites, allergenic antibiotics)
- A variety of non-food additives are permitted to be added to foods, after proper testing, for specific purposes – but including colouring and artificial flavours as well as preservatives

---

Chapter summary

The levels of contaminants in foods and possible adulterants are under regular surveillance by government and public health agencies. Food additives are permitted only under the regulations of the Food Standards Agency (FDA in the USA). Much public debate arises from the impossibility of proving negative relations between any/all individual food additive and any health outcome.

FURTHER READING

Websites

List of current European Union Approved additives and their E numbers (September 2002) available at: http://www.food.gov.uk/safereating/additivesbranch/enumberlist

Jukes, D. Food Law pages at http://www.foodlaw.rdg.ac.uk/index.htm

The following are available from the Stationery Office website at http://www.legislation.hmso.gov.uk/legislation/uk.htm

Statutory Instrument 1995 No. 3187 The Miscellaneous Food Additives Regulations 1995.

Statutory Instrument 1995 No. 3124 The Colours in Food Regulations 1995. London: HMSO.

Statutory Instrument 1995 No. 3123 The Sweeteners in Food Regulations 1995. London: HMSO.

Pesticides (1999). England and Wales: www.opsi.gov.uk/si/si1999/19993488.htm
Scotland: www.opsi.gov.uk/legislation/scotland/ssi20000022.htm
Northern Ireland: www.opsi.gov.uk/sr/sr2002/20020020.htm

Water Regulations (2000). www.opsi.gov.uk/si/si2000/20003184.htm

Plastic Materials (2003). www.opsi.gov.uk/legislation/scotland/ssi2003/20030009.htm
www.opsi.gov.uk/legislation/scotland/ssi2005/20050243.htm

Food Labelling (1996). www.opsi.gov.uk/si/si1996/Uksi_19961499_en_1.htm

Food Safety Act (1990). www.food.gov.uk/multimedia/pdfs/saactandyou.pdf

Index